UROLOGIC
SURGERY OF THE
DOG & CAT

ELIZABETH ARNOLD STONE,

DVM, MS

Professor
Diplomate, American College of Veterinary Surgery
Department of Companion Animals and Special Species Medicine
College of Veterinary Medicine
North Carolina State University

JEANNE A. BARSANTI, DVM, MS

Professor
Diplomate, American College of Veterinary Internal Medicine
Department of Small Animal Medicine
College of Veterinary Medicine
University of Georgia

Illustrated by
BARBARA DAVISON DEGRAVES, MA

Medical Illustrator
Biomedical Communications
College of Veterinary Medicine
North Carolina State University

UROLOGIC
SURGERY OF THE
DOG & CAT

1992
LEA & FEBIGER, PHILADELPHIA, LONDON

LEA & FEBIGER
Box 3024
200 Chester Field Parkway
Malvern, Pennsylvania 19355-9725
U.S.A.
(215) 251-2230

Executive Editor—Carroll C. Cann
Project/Manuscript Editor—Fran Klass
Production Manager—Samuel A. Rondinelli

Library of Congress Cataloging-in-Publication Data

Stone, Elizabeth A.
    Urologic surgery of the dog and cat / Elizabeth Arnold Stone,
  Jeanne A. Barsanti ; illustrated by Barbara Davison DeGraves.
        p.   cm.
    Includes index.
    ISBN 0-8121-1431-0
    1. Dogs—Surgery. 2. Cats—Surgery.
    3. Genitourinary organs—Surgery. 4. Veterinary
urology. I. Barsanti, Jeanne A. II. Title.
    SF992.U75S76 1992
    636.7'0897461—dc20   91-46620
                                                CIP

Reprints of chapters may be purchased from Lea & Febiger in
quantities of 100 or more. Contact Sally Grande in the Sales
Department.

PRINTED IN THE UNITED STATES OF AMERICA

Print number: 5 4 3 2 1

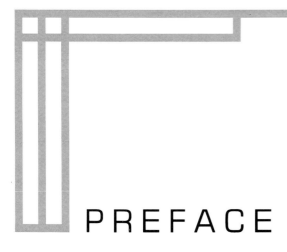

PREFACE

The purpose of this book is to provide practitioners and veterinary students with a concise source for surgical management of urologic disease. The book is not intended to be a comprehensive atlas of possible surgical procedures. We describe selected techniques that have worked for us. The chapters are cross-referenced to avoid contradiction and unnecessary repetition. Surgical choices are integrated into the total management of urologic disease because the practitioner often must choose among several possible treatments. We have strived to present the different options and to provide references for appropriate medical therapy. The indications and contraindications for each surgical procedure are discussed. This information should help practitioners decide whether to do the surgery or refer the client to a surgical specialist. Diagnosis and perioperative care are emphasized because proficiency in surgery is only one component of a successful outcome.

We are grateful to many people for their assistance with this book. Our four contributing authors provide expertise in radiologic diagnosis (Drs. Mary Mahaffey and Don Barber), anesthesia (Dr. Steve Haskins), and urologic oncology (Dr. Stephen Gilson). At North Carolina State University, Barbara Davison DeGraves transformed ideas, slides, and dissections into accurate, lifelike illustrations. Dr. N. J. E. Sharp critiqued all of the surgical chapters. Mrs. Margaret Hemingway used her editorial and word-processing skills to standardize the format. At the University of Georgia, Ms. Janet Calpin compiled the index, and Mr. Kip Carter developed illustrations. We are indebted to our surgery and medicine colleagues and residents, past and present, who have stimulated out thoughts, questioned our methods, and created new solutions. Raymond Kersey, formerly with Lea & Febiger, encouraged and advised us throughout the writing process. We appreciate the editing and production skills of Carroll Cann, Lea & Febiger Executive Editor, Samuel Rondinelli, Production Manager, Frances M. Klass, Project Editor, and Dorothy DiRienzi, Manager, Manuscript Editing.

Raleigh, North Carolina
Athens, Georgia

Elizabeth Arnold Stone, DVM, MS
Jeanne A. Barsanti, DVM, MS

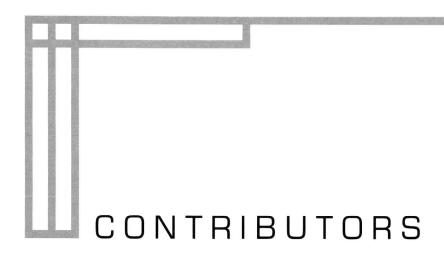

CONTRIBUTORS

MARY B. MAHAFFEY, DVM, MS

Diplomate, American College of Veterinary Radiology
Associate Professor, College of Veterinary Medicine
The University of Georgia
Athens, Georgia

DON L. BARBER, DVM, MS

Diplomate, American College of Veterinary Radiology
Professor and Head, Department of Small Animal Clinical Medicine
Virginia/Maryland Regional College of Veterinary Medicine
Virginia Polytechnic Institute and State University
Blacksburg, Virginia

STEVE C. HASKINS, DVM

Diplomate, American College of Veterinary Anesthesiology
Professor, School of Veterinary Medicine
University of California
Davis, California

STEPHEN D. GILSON, DVM

Diplomate, American College of Veterinary Surgery
Sonora Veterinary Surgery and Oncology
Phoenix, Arizona

CONTENTS

PART I

GENERAL PRINCIPLES

Section One

Urinary Tract Problems: Differential Diagnosis and Diagnostic Plan

1

Abnormal Urine Output and Voiding

DEFINITION OF TERMS

Urine output may be greater or less than normal. Greater than normal urine output is referred to as *polyuria*; urine output less than normal is *oliguria*. Total absence of urine output is *anuria*. Owners of pet dogs and cats usually detect polyuria because urination may occur in the house, the litterbox may be noted to be wetter than usual, or the animal may ask to go outdoors more frequently. Oliguria or anuria are usually not noted by owners but may be accompanied by signs that the owner can detect, such as straining to urinate or signs of uremia (e.g., vomiting, depression, anorexia).

One of the most common abnormalities of urine voiding is dysuria. *Dysuria* refers to difficult urination, characterized in animals primarily by frequently straining to pass small quantities of urine. Pain is also characteristic of dysuria in humans, but may be difficult to ascertain in dogs and cats. *Stranguria* is synonymous with dysuria. *Pollakiuria* is frequent urination. Dysuria is accompanied by pollakiuria, and, in fact, in common veterinary usage, the term dysuria implies pollakiuria; pollakiuria, however, can also result from polyuria. Because pollakiuria is nonspecific in relation to urine volume, it is a less useful term than dysuria (increased frequency with small volumes) or polyuria (increased volume; frequency may or may not be increased).

Inappropriate urination is urination at the wrong time or in the wrong place. The determination of "proper" place and time of urination is, of course, the owner's. Causes of inappropriate urination include behavioral problems, dysuria, and polyuria. *Nocturia* refers to urination during the night. Nocturia is a problem only in animals confined at night to an area inappropriate for urination. Nocturia may reflect polyuria (inability to store an increased urine volume for prolonged intervals), or dysuria (urgency). *Urinary incontinence* is another cause of inappropriate urination and refers to the involuntary passage of urine. A thorough history is nec-

essary to distinguish incontinence from dysuria, polyuria, and behavioral problems. The key is whether the animal is conscious of the act of urination during urination. Animals that have been punished for inappropriate urination may appear "guilty" after the fact, even if urine was voided involuntarily. What owners perceive as guilt is actually fear of punishment when urine is in the "wrong" place.

The purpose of this chapter is to provide a list of diagnostic possibilities for the problems of polyuria, oliguria, dysuria, and urinary incontinence. Diagnostic plans to determine the causes of these conditions are given. Subsequent chapters focus on individual diseases and their treatment.

POLYURIA

Normal Water Balance

Every animal must remain in water balance. If water input exceeds output, edema develops (Fig. 1–1). If water output exceeds input, dehydration occurs (Fig. 1–2). Voluntary water and moist food consumption is normally responsible for input. Urine formation is the major method of water output. In dogs, water may also be lost by panting, especially with exercise and increased environmental temperature. The gastrointestinal tract is another major source of water loss in dogs and cats. Normal water intake varies with environmental temperature and humidity, with exercise, and with individual preference. In dogs, normal water intake is approximately 20 to 70 ml/kg/day. In cats, normal water intake is approximately 20 to 50 ml/kg/day.[1,2] In calculating water intake, one must consider water in food, especially when the animal's diet is commercial canned foods that are at least 70% water. Cats are slower to correct dehydration by voluntary water intake than are dogs.[3] Normal urine output is slightly less than intake

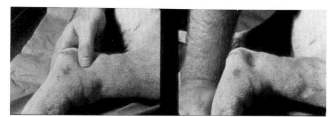

FIG. 1—1. Pitting edema in the limb of a dog.

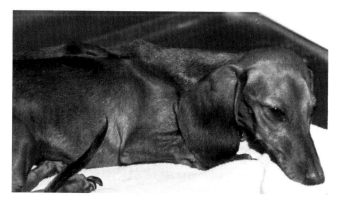

FIG. 1—2. Severe dehydration secondary to profuse vomiting.

because of nonurinary sites of water loss. Normal urine output in dogs and cats is 15 to 45 ml/kg/day.

Water balance is regulated primarily by antidiuretic hormone (ADH) acting on the collecting ducts of the kidneys.[4] The hypothalamus produces ADH and releases it via the posterior pituitary gland. The major physiologic stimuli for ADH release are hypertonicity and volume depletion. After release, ADH binds to receptors on the basolateral membrane of the collecting ducts of the kidneys. This binding initiates a series of intracellular events, leading to water reabsorption (Fig. 1–3). These intracellular events include the activation of adenylate cyclase that generates cyclic AMP, which in turn increases the permeability of luminal membranes to water. Scanning electron micrographs show the formation of water channels within collecting duct cells after ADH stimulation. The half-life of ADH is short (minutes) so the body can adjust rapidly to changes in water balance. Although ADH is required for water to enter collecting duct cells, water movement also depends on a high osmotic gradient within the renal medulla. High urea and sodium chloride concentrations, maintained by the loops of Henle, and vasa recta are responsible for this osmotic gradient.

Documentation of the Problem

Because of the necessity of being in water balance, an animal that is polyuric must be polydipsic, or it can rapidly become dehydrated. Owners are more likely to detect polydipsia than polyuria if the animal drinks from a measurable water source such as a bowl that the owner can notice requires filling more often. Owners are likely to detect polyuria in indoor pets that require litterbox or paper changing or in indoor pets that require being released or walked outside to urinate. Owners may particularly notice polyuria when the pet shares their bedroom and begins to wake them up to be let out or begins to have "accidents" when confined for long hours.

Owners are usually accurate when they present an animal for increased water intake, although they usually do not know whether the amount drunk is excessive. When owners present an animal for increased urination, a careful history is important to separate dysuria and behavioral problems from polyuria. The owner should be asked to describe exactly what the animal is doing. The normal daily routine of the pet should be ascertained. The amount of water drunk should be recorded. Whether urination is observed and whether it appears normal are important. Diet or exercise changes should be noted. Because polyuria can result from many systemic causes, a complete general history is necessary as well as a problem-specific one. The occurrence of vomiting, diarrhea, coughing, oculonasal discharge in all dogs, and estrous cycles in intact bitches should be determined.

After the animal's problem or problems have been described, a complete physical examination should be performed. All abnormalities should be noted.

To confirm that the problem is polyuria/polydipsia, water intake and urine specific gravity should be measured. Measurement of urine output is useful but is usually difficult to accomplish in a practice setting. Excessive water intake, nonconcentrated urine (specific gravity < 1.030), or both suggest that the problem exists. If water intake is excessive but urine is concentrated, there must be an extrarenal site of water loss. If water intake is normal but urine is not concentrated, the animal may be subclinically dehydrated. This is not an uncommon occurrence when animals are hospitalized for assessment. Their water consumption may initially decrease as a result of lack of familiarity with surroundings. Laboratory work should be assessed as well as body weight changes for evidence of dehydration.

Collecting Duct Cell

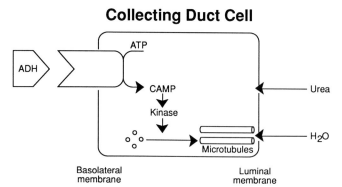

FIG. 1—3. Summary of some of the intracellular events stimulated by ADH binding to the membrane of the collecting duct.

TABLE 1-1. CAUSES OF POLYURIA/POLYDIPSIA

Primary Polyuria	Primary Polydipsia
Lack of ADH	Hyperthyroidism
Pituitary origin diabetes insipidus	Hypercalcemia
ADH inhibition	Hypokalemia
Pyometra	Hepatic failure
Bacterial pyelonephritis	"Psychogenic"
E. coli septicemia	Hypothalamic lesion
Hypoadrenaocorticism	(thirst center)
Hypokalemia	
Hypercalcemia	
Hyperadrenocorticism	
Glucocorticoid administration	
Renal inability to respond to ADH	
Nephrogenic diabetes insipidus	
Generalized renal failure	
Increased solute load	
Generalized renal failure	
Diabetes mellitus	
Increased salt intake	
Posturethral obstruction	
Hypoadrenocorticism	
Diuretics	
Decreased medullary tonicity	
Hepatic failure	
Hypokalemia	
Hyponatremia	

Differential Diagnosis

Once the problem has been defined to be polyuria/polydipsia, the question arises as to which came first. Some diseases result in polyuria, necessitating polydipsia for maintenance of water balance; some diseases cause polydipsia and, thus, polyuria; and some diseases do both (Table 1-1).

PRIMARY POLYURIA

Diseases that cause primary polyuria are more common than those that cause primary polydipsia. Diseases that cause primary polyuria involve an abnormality in the ADH-renal tubule concentrating mechanism. A complete lack of ADH (pituitary origin diabetes insipidus) results in severe polyuria with hyposthenuric urine (specific gravity < 1.008). Partial deficiencies of ADH production exist in humans, result in less severe polyuria, and are much more difficult to diagnose. Diabetes insipidus can be congenital or acquired. Acquired causes include trauma, inflammation, and neoplasia of the hypothalamus or posterior pituitary gland. Glucocorticoids have been reported to inhibit ADH release, but this effect could not be documented in dogs.[5]

In other diseases that cause polyuria, ADH is present in normal amounts, but its action at the renal tubular receptor is inhibited. Bacterial endotoxins, especially those associated with *Escherichia coli,* can compete with ADH for its binding sites on the tubular membrane. Infections that may be associated with polyuria through this mechanism include pyometra, prostatic abscessation, pyelonephritis, and septicemia. Hypercalcemia also inhibits binding of ADH to its receptor site. Glucocorticoids and increased calcium concentrations inhibit the intracellular production of cAMP that is normally stimulated by ADH. Aldosterone inhibits phosphodiesterase, the enzyme that degrades cAMP. Thus, in hypoadrenocorticism (Addison's disease), absence of aldosterone inhibits ADH action. Hyponatremia has also been associated with impaired renal concentrating ability in dogs.[6] This is another mechanism whereby hypoadrenocorticism may result in inadequate urine concentration.

The cause for polyuria may be renal inability to respond to ADH. Nephrogenic diabetes insipidus refers to renal tubular lack of ADH receptors. The kidney appears anatomically normal in this condition, which has been described in dogs as a congenital defect. The term *nephrogenic diabetes insipidus* has also been used by some to include the conditions previously listed in which ADH activity at the renal tubular receptor site is inhibited.

Generalized renal failure, in which there is a moderate decrease (>66%) in functional nephron number, is also characterized by polyuria. In generalized renal failure, a reduced number of nephrons must excrete the same quantity of solutes as when the kidney was normal. To accomplish this, each nephron must excrete more water (*obligatory polyuria*). Specific gravity gradually decreases to the isosthenuric range. This increased obligatory water loss prevents the kidney from responding adequately to sudden increases in extrarenal water losses (e.g., vomiting, diarrhea) and to decreases in water intake. Dehydration develops much more rapidly in an animal with renal failure than in one that is normal.

Similar to generalized renal failure, the kidney must excrete more water whenever it must excrete an increased solute load. An example is diabetes mellitus, in which an increased glucose load must be excreted. Another example is increased salt intake. A similar situation exists after relief of urethral obstruction. The solutes retained during obstruction must be excreted, necessitating increased water loss. Natriuresis may also partially explain the polyuria in hypoadrenocorticism.

Hepatic failure can result in polyuria through at least two postulated renal mechanisms. One is decreased hepatic production of urea. Urea is the major contributor to medullary hypertonicity. Without urea, the osmolality of the renal medulla decreases, reducing the ability of the kidney to reabsorb water. Another postulated mechanism is that increased serum concentrations of ammonia, owing to decreased hepatic conversion of ammonia to urea, is a direct renal tubular toxin.

Hypokalemia is also associated with an inability to concentrate urine well. This is thought to be caused by an inability to establish the normal osmolar gradients in the medullary interstitium, to suppression of cAMP generation, and to blunting of release of ADH from the neurohypophysis in response to hypertonicity.[7]

PRIMARY POLYDIPSIA

Causes of primary polydipsia include hyperthyroidism, hypercalcemia, hypokalemia, and hepatic failure. As discussed, hypercalcemia, hypokalemia, and hepatic failure can also cause primary polyuria. One mechanism for polydipsia in liver failure is postulated to be lack of catabolism of renin, which is a dipsogenic compound.

Some dogs and cats drink excessive water compulsively or intermittently. These animals have normal ability to concentrate urine when water is deprived. This condition has been referred to as "psychogenic" polydipsia. In humans, a similar disorder has been noted with some mental illnesses, but partial pituitary diabetes insipidus may produce findings similar to psychogenic polydipsia on diagnostic testing. Whether partial pituitary diabetes insipidus exists in dogs and cats is unknown.

Diagnostic Plan for Polyuria/Polydipsia

Once the problem is documented to be polyuria/polydipsia, the history and physical examination should be reviewed. Has the animal been receiving any drugs, such as diuretics, glucocorticoids, or anticonvulsants, which could induce polyuria? In intact bitches, when was the last estrus? On physical examination, the liver and kidneys should be palpated and size and contour noted. Endocrine alopecia, a pendulous abdomen, or both may suggest hyperadrenocorticism. Lymphadenopathy may indicate lymphosarcoma. Lymphosarcoma may result in pseudohyperparathyroidism and hypercalcemia in some dogs. The neck in old cats should be carefully palpated for thyroid enlargement. If any abnormalities are found, they should be pursued by appropriate diagnostic tests.

If there are no definitive abnormalities on physical examination, a complete urinalysis, complete blood count (CBC), and blood chemistry profile should be performed. The blood chemistry profile should include blood urea nitrogen (BUN), creatinine, liver enzymes, calcium, phosphorus, glucose, total protein, albumin, sodium, and potassium concentrations. These tests can determine whether systemic or urinary infections, renal failure, hepatic disease, hypercalcemia, diabetes mellitus, hyponatremia, or hypokalemia is present. Hypercortisolism may be suggested by a stress leukogram, elevated liver enzyme concentration, mildly elevated blood glucose concentration, and urinary tract infection without pyuria. Hypoadrenocorticism may be suggested by hyperkalemia, hyponatremia, and lack of a stress leukogram in spite of signs of a stressful illness. Hyperthyroidism can be confirmed by measurement of serum thyroid hormone concentrations.

If the cause of the polyuria and polydipsia is still unknown (all the aforementioned test results are normal), a water deprivation test should be performed. Water deprivation testing is *contraindicated* if the animal is dehydrated, azotemic, or hypercalcemic or has any major systemic disease. Laboratory work should *always* be performed before water deprivation. The test should

be carefully conducted as follows. The bladder should be emptied voluntarily or by catheterization at the beginning of the test, urine specific gravity measured, and a serum and urine sample submitted for osmolality if possible. The animal should be weighed, the time recorded, and water and food removed. The animal should be monitored for dehydration every 2 hours by reweighing and examining skin turgor and mucous membrane moisture. Urine specific gravity should be recorded and the animal allowed to empty its bladder. The test is continued until there is a 5 to 7% decrease in body weight or until the specific gravity is greater than 1.048. Serum and urine osmolalities are measured at the end of the test.

To evaluate the water deprivation test, one examines how rapidly dehydration occurred, what final specific gravity was reached, and how the pretest and post-test serum and urine osmolalities compare. Of normal dogs and cats, 95% reach a urine specific gravity of 1.048 before they lose 5% of their body weight.[8,9] It may require 2 to 3 days for them to become dehydrated. Urine osmolality rises rapidly with minimal change in serum osmolality. If the animal does not concentrate (specific gravity < 1.030) and becomes dehydrated, a marked abnormality in the ADH/renal concentrating mechanism is confirmed. If the patient concentrates to greater than 1.040 but polydipsia has been previously documented, the most likely possibility is psychogenic polydipsia. If the patient concentrates to 1.030 to 1.040, a partial ADH or renal tubular defect or primary polydipsia may be present. If the animal concentrates to 1.030 with water deprivation, water restriction to maintenance amounts is usually adequate therapy.

If the patient does not concentrate urine to greater than 1.030 with water deprivation, an ADH response test should be performed. The ADH used can be oil-based (vasopressin tannate, 0.25 units/kg to a maximum of 5 units, IM) or aqueous (dd-AVP, 10 to 20 μg, IV).[10,11] If oil-based ADH is used, the vial should be well shaken to be sure the ADH goes into suspension. Urine specific gravity should be checked at 6, 12, 24, and 48 hours. The bladder should be emptied at each check. Applying pressure to the bladder of a cat may stimulate the cat to urinate when it is placed back in the cage. The use of nonabsorbent beads in the litter pan allows collection of urine for measurement of urine specific gravity. If aqueous products are used, the urine specific gravity should be checked every hour for 6 to 8 hours. Urine osmolality should be checked at the beginning and end of the test, if available. Water consumption can also be measured. We do not generally withhold water during ADH response testing, unless the aqueous test is conducted immediately after water deprivation. There is potential danger of overhydration if an animal with pituitary diabetes insipidus were to consume large amounts of water just as ADH was administered.

A positive response to ADH is a rise in urine specific gravity to greater than 1.020 or a fivefold rise in urine osmolality.[10,12] In normal animals, response to water deprivation (endogenous ADH) is greater than response to exogenous ADH.[8,10,12,13] In general, response to

ADH in oil is greater than response to aqueous vasopressin.[10,12] In an animal with inability to respond to water deprivation, a positive response to ADH confirms pituitary diabetes insipidus. If urine specific gravity or osmolality does not rise significantly, an abnormality in renal tubular response to ADH is confirmed.

The results of water deprivation and ADH response testing are not always straightforward. Measurement of plasma ADH concentrations improves diagnostic accuracy[14] but is not yet widely available in veterinary medicine. Hypercortisolism can result in partial responses to both water deprivation and ADH administration, for example. The diseases that are often difficult to differentiate are preazotemic, chronic, generalized renal disease and atypical hypercortisolism (canine Cushing's disease without dermatologic or serum chemistry changes). In these cases, measurement of serum cortisol concentrations in conjunction with adrenocorticotropic hormone (ACTH) stimulation or dexamethasone suppression, or measurement of serum ACTH concentrations, or both should determine whether Cushing's disease exists. A creatinine clearance test can be done to determine whether renal dysfunction is the cause of the polyuria. Creatinine clearance tests are described in Chapter 5.

OLIGURIA/ANURIA

Differential Diagnosis

Oliguria is generally defined as urine production of less than 1.0 ml/kg/hour. Anuria is defined as absence of urine production. These terms include both decreased urine formation and decreased urine output from the body (Table 1–2). Decreased urine formation can be a normal response to decreased water intake or increased nonurinary losses, such as from vomiting, diarrhea, and increased exercise.

Decreased urine formation can also be caused by severe renal failure with marked reduction in glomerular filtration rate and tubular fluid flow rate. Such severe renal failure may be the result of either acute renal injury or terminal chronic renal disease. Acute renal injury can be produced by ischemia, by direct tubular toxic injury,

---

TABLE 1–2. CAUSES OF DECREASED URINE PRODUCTION

Normal urinary tract
    Decreased water intake
    Increased nonurinary losses
Inability to excrete urine
    Urethral obstruction
    Detrusor muscle dysfunction
    Bilateral ureteral obstruction
    Urinary tract rupture
Severe renal insufficiency
    Acute renal failure
    Terminal chronic renal failure

---

or both, leading to sloughing of epithelial cells and intratubular obstruction. In chronic, progressive renal diseases, inability to concentrate urine is the first clinical sign (see under "Polyuria"). Obligatory polyuria develops after loss of 66% of functional nephrons. Before this degree of loss, remaining nephrons can compensate for those lost. When 75% of nephrons are nonfunctional, above-normal elevations of BUN and serum creatinine concentrations develop, and the animal becomes more likely to develop signs of uremia. Initially, azotemia and uremia are associated with polyuria. Oliguria occurs only in the terminal phase.

Decreased urine output may also be caused by inability to eliminate urine produced. The most common example is urethral obstruction. With such an obstruction, the animal is unable to void, leading to bladder overdistention and decreased renal urine production (see Chapters 12 and 15 for further discussion). Bladder or urethral tears or ruptures also result in decreased urine output. Bilateral ureteral obstruction is another potential cause of oliguria or anuria but is uncommon.

Diagnostic Plan

The first steps are always obtaining a history and performing a physical examination. Animals are rarely presented for the problem of oliguria per se but more commonly for related problems such as dysuria or vomiting. Palpation of the bladder is essential in animals presented for decreased urine output. If the bladder is distended, an attempt should be made to pass a urinary catheter to determine whether urethral obstruction is present. If there is fluid in the abdominal cavity or in the perineal area, urinary tract rupture may be present.

The most important laboratory tests are complete urinalysis and renal function tests (BUN and serum creatinine concentrations). If the urine is concentrated (>1.035), renal failure is excluded. Urinary tract obstruction or rupture is still possible, as is compensation for extrarenal water loss. With urinary tract obstruction or rupture, azotemia would be expected if the condition has been present for more than 24 hours. If the urine is not concentrated (<1.030), the animal is azotemic, and oliguria exists, urinary tract function is abnormal. Either renal failure or urinary tract obstruction or rupture is present.

In any animal with oliguria and azotemia, a thorough search must be made for urethral obstruction or rupture and bladder rupture because these problems are surgically correctable. This search should include attempts to pass a urethral catheter and may also need to include abdominocentesis, diagnostic peritoneal lavage, survey abdominal radiographs, and contrast-enhanced radiography (see Chapters 6, 12, 15, and 21).

If urinary obstruction and rupture have been excluded and renal failure exists, differentiation of acute from chronic renal failure becomes important. Oliguria may be reversible with acute diseases but is usually a nonreversible, terminal event in chronic renal disease. Differentiation of acute from chronic renal failure may be difficult without renal biopsy. Nevertheless, certain clinical and laboratory findings are suggestive of acute or chronic disease (Table 1–3). With each individual case, it is useful to compose a table similar to Table 1-3 to list characteristics compatible with either acute or chronic disease and to determine whether a consistent pattern emerges.

With acute diseases, there is no precedent history of polyuria or azotemia. There may be exposure to a renal tubular toxin such as ethylene glycol or gentamycin, kidney size is normal to mildly symmetrically increased, and urine may contain large numbers of granular casts (indicating ongoing renal tubular injury) or oxalate crystals (ethylene glycol toxicity). Evidence may exist in the laboratory work of multisystem involvement. Acute renal injury can occur in certain infectious diseases (e.g., leptospirosis, Rocky Mountain spotted fever) as well as with trauma and heat stroke, all of which affect multiple organ systems. Ultrasonography may be useful to assist in determination of renal size and consistency.

Chronic renal failure is usually associated with progressive fibrosis, loss of nephrons, and mild interstitial mononuclear inflammation of unknown cause. This is most common with aging and in young dogs of certain breeds (e.g., Lhasa apsos, Shih Tzus). Other causes of chronic renal failure include neoplasia, urolithiasis, bacterial pyelonephritis, chronic glomerulopathies, and granulomatous infections (e.g., feline infectious peritonitis). With chronic disease of any cause, there should be a precedent history of polyuria and azotemia if the animal is well observed and if BUN concentration has been evaluated regularly. Unfortunately, because most dogs and cats with chronic renal disease compensate well and appear outwardly normal, previous laboratory work is often unavailable. Other evidence for chronic disease includes small, irregular kidney size. Irregular increases in renal size may also occur with renal neoplasia, with the presence or development of renal cysts, and with granulomatous diseases (e.g., feline infectious peritonitis). Decreased bone density occurs with advanced chronic renal disease. Clinical manifestations include increased flexibility of the mandible ("rubber jaw"), loose teeth and periodontal disease, and pathologic fractures. A nonregenerative anemia develops in advanced chronic renal failure. Urinalysis may be unremarkable other than inadequate concentrating ability, unless the chronic disease is secondary to a glomerulopathy, renal infection, or urolithiasis. With renal infection and urolithiasis, urine usually contains red blood cells, white blood cells, and bacteria. With a glomerulopathy, urine contains large amounts of protein with a normal urine sediment. Survey abdominal radiographs are useful to determine whether uroliths are present and to evaluate renal size. A rough estimate of bone density may also be made, but radiographs of the mandible would be more indicative of bone loss. Ultrasonography is useful to help determine renal size and consistency.

If the type of renal failure cannot be classified as acute or chronic, based on the aforementioned characteristics, a renal biopsy may be required. Techniques of renal biopsy are covered in Chapter 5.

If the underlying disease is acute, treatment efforts to restore urine production are warranted. If urine production cannot be restored by intravenous fluid therapy, sometimes in combination with diuretics or vasoactive drugs, supportive peritoneal dialysis or hemodialysis may be required to provide time for renal regeneration. If the underlying disease is chronic, treatment success is unlikely, unless the oliguric episode has been provoked by a reversible prerenal insult (e.g., water deprivation, severe gastroenteritis). If there is no response to intravenous fluid therapy, euthanasia is often the most humane course. Clients may suggest renal transplantation to avoid euthanasia. Renal transplantation, however, is rarely successful at the present time in dogs unless a littermate donor is available.[15–17] In any case, it should not be done as an emergency procedure.[17] Successful renal transplantation has been performed in cats using unrelated donors.[18] Dialysis should be performed if needed for stabilization. Clients should also understand that animals with renal transplants require extensive postoperative monitoring and treatment to try to prevent organ rejection.

TABLE 1–3. CHARACTERISTICS OF ACUTE AND CHRONIC RENAL FAILURE

	Acute Renal Failure	Chronic Renal Failure
History	Nephrotoxin exposure No prior PU/PD*	Prior PU/PD*
Physical examination	Normal renal size to symmetrical increase Normal bone mass	Reduced renal size or asymmetrical increase Normal to reduced bone density
Urinalysis	Normal to increased granular casts Oxalate crystals†	Normal to increased granular casts Marked proteinuria
Hemogram	Variable	Normal to nonregenerate anemia
Radiography	Normal to mild symmetrically increased renal size	Normal to reduced renal size or asymmetrical increase Normal to reduced bone density
Ultrasonography	Normal to mild increase in renal size	Reduced renal size or asymmetric shape

* Polyuria/polydipsia
† Ethylene glycol toxicity

DYSURIA

Dysuria is difficult urination or straining to urinate. Its presence indicates an abnormality in the bladder or urethra. It is usually associated with frequent attempts to urinate. The amount of urine voided with each attempt is usually small.

Differential Diagnosis

Dysuria is caused by obstruction, irritation, or inflammation of the lower urinary tract (Table 1–4). Urethral obstruction and cystitis are the most common causes. Urethral obstruction can result from urolithiasis, neoplasia, prostatic abscessation or cyst formation, granulomatous inflammation, and fibrosis. Urethral obstruction may also be produced by urethral contraction as the bladder detrusor muscle contracts (bladder–urethral sphincter reflex dyssynergia). Cystitis in dogs is most commonly associated with bacterial infection. In cats, cystitis is usually not bacterial in origin. Of cats with dysuria, 95% have sterile urine cultures.[19,20] Urolithiasis is responsible for dysuria in approximately 33% of these cats, but the cause in the rest of affected cats is unknown.[19]

Other causes of dysuria include intravesicular space occupying masses such as uroliths, neoplasms, polyps (which can be inflammatory in origin), and blood clots. A sterile inflammatory cystitis can be associated with the drug cyclophosphamide.

Diagnostic Plan

A complete history should be taken. What exactly has the owner seen? How long has the problem been noted? Is any urine observed? Is there any evident blood? If so, it is at the beginning, middle, or end of urination? (See Chapter 2.) Is there any possibility of trauma? Are there other signs of illness such as vomiting, anorexia, or lethargy? Has the animal had any previous urinary tract problems?

The physical examination should be sure to include careful palpation of the bladder for degree of distention. If the bladder is not distended, it should be thoroughly palpated for uroliths, soft tissue masses, and wall thickness. If the bladder is overdistended, further palpation is not indicated because it may result in iatrogenic bladder rupture and because overdistention prevents accurate palpation. The urethral orifice should be examined in male dogs and cats. In male dogs, the urethra should be palpated under the skin where accessible behind the os penis and in the perineal area. In both male and female dogs, the pelvic urethra should be palpated per rectum.

Based on the physical examination, animals with dysuria should be subdivided into two groups: those with full or overdistended bladders and those with empty bladders.

Dysuric Animals with Distended Bladders

An attempt should be made to pass a urinary catheter in those animals with full bladders. If an obstruction to passage of the catheter is found, the approximate location and the consistency of the obstruction should be noted. If the obstructing material is hard or gritty, a urolith or unorganized urethral plug is likely. In these cases, survey radiographs of the urethra and abdomen are indicated to determine whether the urolith is radiopaque. If a urolith is visible, the rest of the urinary tract should be carefully examined radiographically for other uroliths. If the obstructing material is soft tissue in nature, a contrast-enhanced urethrogram may be necessary to visualize it further. Relief of urethral obstruction is discussed in Chapters 12 and 15.

Successful passage of a urethral catheter does not eliminate the possibility of a partial urethral obstruction. In fact, small-gauge catheters are often used therapeutically to bypass partial obstructions. All animals unable to urinate with distended bladders, which are neurologically normal, should be considered to have an obstruction to urine outflow until conclusively proved otherwise. Demonstration of a partial obstruction often necessitates very thorough palpation of the urethra and bladder as well as a contrast urethrogram. A mass at the bladder neck, which obstructs urine flow into the urethra, may require a contrast cystogram for visualization. Ultrasonography is especially useful in detecting prostatic abnormalities.

Other diagnostic tests that should be performed include a complete urinalysis; urine culture; CBC; BUN concentration, serum creatinine concentration, or both; and serum electrolyte concentrations. The urine can be collected by cystocentesis or after successful catheterization. The purpose of the CBC is to determine whether there is evidence of systemic inflammation. An inflammatory leukogram suggests renal or prostatic inflammation or the possibility of septicemia. Septicemia can arise in animals with urethral obstruction and urinary tract infection. Ischemic damage to the bladder wall can

---

TABLE 1–4. DIFFERENTIAL DIAGNOSIS FOR DYSURIA

Urethral obstruction
  Urolithiasis
  Neoplasia—prostatic or urethral
  Prostatic abscess or cyst
  Urethral stricture
  Dyssynergia
Urethral inflammation
  Granulomatous urethritis
  Bacterial urethritis
Bladder inflammation
  Bacterial infection
  Drug induced
  Urolithiasis
  Idiopathic (feline urologic syndrome)
Intravesicular space occupying mass
  Urolithiasis
  Neoplasia
  Polyps (polypoid cystitis)
  Blood clots
  Granuloma

allow bacteria in urine to cross into the systemic circulation. The purpose of the BUN, serum creatinine, and serum electrolyte concentrations is to determine the severity of the azotemia and hyperkalemia that develop with urethral obstruction. These tests are especially important if the animal is depressed, anorectic, or vomiting, suggesting uremia.

Dysuric Animals with Empty Bladders

The diagnostic plan should include a complete urinalysis in both dogs and cats. A urine culture is indicated in dogs. Because bacterial infection occurs in only 5% of cats with these signs, urine culture is not indicated, unless bacteriuria or pyuria is evident on urinalysis or unless the cat has been previously catheterized or had a perineal urethrostomy. If bacterial infection is documented, it should be treated with appropriate antibiotics.

If bacterial infection is not present or if the infection proves difficult to eliminate, the diagnostic plan should be expanded to include survey radiographs, ultrasonography, or both of the bladder. If these tests are nondiagnostic, contrast cystography is indicated. In cases difficult to diagnose, exploratory surgery of the bladder with bladder wall biopsy may be indicated.

URINARY INCONTINENCE

Urinary incontinence is defined as lack of voluntary control of urination. It must be distinguished from dysuria, polyuria, nocturia, and behavioral problems in which urination is under voluntary control, but urgency, increased urine production, or behavior make it impossible for the pet to avoid urinating in the "wrong" place.

Physiology of Micturition

To understand the causes of incontinence, an understanding of the basic physiology of micturition is required. Normal micturition requires storage and emptying phases. During the storage phase, the bladder slowly fills via the peristaltic action of the ureters bringing urine from the kidneys. The detrusor muscle of the bladder adjusts to filling by stretching with no increase in intravesicular pressure. The sympathetic system facilitates detrusor relaxation via beta-adrenergic receptors (Fig. 1–4). The external urethral sphincter mechanism (urethral musculature) maintains resting tone, which can increase with sudden increases in intra-abdominal pressure (e.g., coughing). The urethral musculature comprises both striated and smooth muscle. The pudendal nerve innervates the striated muscle, while the sympathetic system via alpha receptors innervates the smooth muscle. Continence is also maintained by an internal sphincter mechanism, which consists of spiralling detrusor muscle fibers at the bladder neck. These fibers are anatomically arranged so that they are pulled closed as the bladder distends.

The emptying phase begins when stretch receptors in

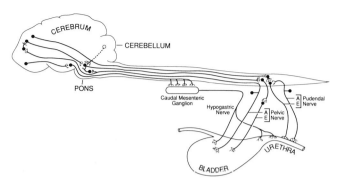

FIG. 1–4. Innervation of the lower urinary tract. The cerebrum controls voluntary micturition through facilitory and inhibitory influences on the brain stem. The cerebellum has an inhibitory influence on the brain stem micturition reflex area. The pelvic nerve carries afferent (A) and efferent (E) fibers between the bladder and sacral spinal cord. The reflex between these fibers is in the brain stem. Efferent fibers are also carried by the sympathetic system (hypogastric nerve). The hypogastric nerve supplies beta-adrenergic fibers to the bladder and alpha-adrenergic fibers to the bladder neck and urethra. The pudendal nerve innervates the striated muscle of the urethra. (Modified from Oliver, J.E., and Osborne, C.A.: Neurogenic urinary incontinence. In Current Veterinary Therapy VII. Edited by R.W. Kirk. Philadelphia, W.B. Saunders, p. 1123, 1980.)

the bladder wall detect bladder fullness. Impulses are relayed via the pelvic nerves to the sacral segments of the spinal cord and up the spinal cord to the brain stem. A reflex occurs at this level back down the spinal cord to the sacral parasympathetic nucleus. Impulses are sent via the pelvic nerve to the detrusor muscle. In the detrusor muscle, excitation spreads via tight junctions between muscle fibers. Contraction pulls the bladder neck open. As the bladder contracts, the fibers spiral toward the bladder neck. For complete bladder emptying in dogs, the bladder neck must be mobile. Simultaneous with bladder contraction, the pudendal motor neurons are inhibited, resulting in relaxation of the external urethral sphincter. Urine is evacuated. After bladder contraction, the afferent discharge from the pelvic nerve stops, the pelvic motor neurons cease their discharge, pudendal motor activity is no longer blocked, and external sphincter tone resumes.

Voluntary control of this reflex pathway is via the cerebral cortex to the brain stem. The cerebellum has an inhibitory effect on the brain stem micturition center.

Differential Diagnosis

Because micturition is a complex process, there are many potential causes of incontinence (Table 1–5). Rather than remembering these with a list, it is easier to group the causes into categories. Two useful subcategories are (1) incontinence associated with other signs of central nervous system dysfunction and (2) incontinence not associated with other central nervous system signs. If other abnormal neurologic signs are present, the diagnostic plan is directed toward localizing

TABLE 1–5. CAUSES OF INCONTINENCE

Neurogenic	Non-neurogenic
Cerebral lesions	Bladder distended
Brain stem lesions	Urethral obstruction
Upper motor neuron spinal cord lesions	Mass in bladder neck
Cervical, thoracic, lumbar spinal cord	Detrusor dysfunction
Lower motor neuron lesions	Detrusor-urethral dyssynergia
Sacral spinal cord	Bladder not distended
Sacral spinal roots	Patent urachus
Pelvic or pudendal nerves	Ectopic ureter(s)
	Other congenital defect
	Urethrovaginal fistula
	Vestibulovaginal stenosis
	Urethral incompetence
	Mass near bladder neck
	Involuntary bladder contractions
	Inflammatory bladder disease
	Noninflammatory (detrusor hyperreflexia)
	Reduced bladder capacity
	After partial cystectomy
	Chronic cystitis
	After radiation therapy

and defining the neurologic lesion. If the animal is neurologically normal, the diagnostic plan is first directed toward abnormalities within the lower urinary tract, although a neurologic lesion affecting only the micturition pathways cannot be excluded.

Abnormalities within the urinary tract that cause incontinence can again be subdivided into those that affect the filling phase and those that affect the emptying phase. With those that affect the filling phase, the animals can empty their bladders. Urine dribbles between urinations, however, and bladder capacity is often reduced. Conditions that affect the filling phase include congenital defects, which allow urine to bypass the urethral sphincter; decreased resting pressure at the bladder neck or within the urethra; and involuntary bladder contractions.

Both a patent urachus and an ectopic ureter cause incontinence by allowing urine to exit the body by bypassing the urethral sphincter. Decreased resting urethral pressures have been associated with neutering in dogs, often referred to as "spay incontinence," although the problem occurs in males as well as females. Approximately 4.5% of spayed bitches developed incontinence in one large survey.[21] A similar condition may occur in juvenile bitches of any breed and in intact bitches, particularly of the Doberman breed.[22] A mass at the bladder neck may interfere with normal closure of the internal bladder sphincter mechanism. Involuntary bladder contractions occur with severe bladder wall irritation as in severe cystitis, either bacterial or drug (cyclophosphamide) induced. Involuntary bladder contractions may also occur in dogs and cats with no evidence of inflammation.[23] Affected cats often test positive for feline leukemia virus, although the exact relationship between the incontinence and the viremia is unknown.[24]

In conditions that affect the emptying phase, urine dribbles constantly, the bladder remains distended, and normal urination cannot occur. The major diagnostic consideration in animals that are neurologically normal is a partial or complete urethral obstruction. Only after a urethral or bladder neck obstruction has been eliminated should other diagnostic possibilities be considered. These include detrusor dysfunction and detrusor–urethral sphincter dyssynergia, in which the urethral musculature fails to relax during detrusor contraction.

Detrusor dysfunction occurs most commonly after loss of tight junctions from prolonged bladder overdistention. Bladder overdistention may result from urethral obstruction, neurologic dysfunction (e.g., intervertebral disk disease), extensive fluid therapy during prolonged anesthesia, and unwillingness to void with forced recumbency (e.g., after pelvic trauma) or with prolonged confinement. One cause of detrusor dysfunction described in Europe in cats and a few dogs is an autonomic polyganglionopathy (Key-Gaskell syndrome).[25,26]

Lack of relaxation of the urethral musculature, preventing micturition despite detrusor contraction, is difficult to confirm in veterinary medicine. There are two possible causes: urethral spasm from inflammation of any cause or dyssynergia, in which the urethra contracts rather than relaxes as micturition is initiated. Dyssynergia has been described only in male dogs to date. The typical history is that the dog initiates urination, but urination ceases immediately thereafter in spite of continued efforts to urinate.

Diagnostic Plan

The diagnostic approach to incontinence should start with a thorough history. The age of onset of the problem, reproductive status of the pet, relationship between the onset of incontinence and neutering, chronologic course of the incontinence, associated urinary tract problems, history of neurologic abnormalities, whether normal micturition occurs, and any drug use or dietary change should be recorded. Any drug or dietary change that stimulates polyuria (e.g., glucocorticoids, diuretics, high salt diet) could precipitate a latent predisposition to incontinence by increasing the volume of urine the bladder must hold.

A complete physical examination should follow. Special attention should be paid to the bladder. Is it distended, contracted, or normal? In male dogs, the prostate should be examined. In both male and female dogs, the urethra should be palpated. A complete neurologic examination should be performed with special attention to anal tone and the integrity of the perineal reflex. A patent urachus can usually be diagnosed on physical examination by observing urine dribbling from the umbilicus.

Micturition should be observed and residual volume determined by palpation or by catheterization. Normal residual volume is considered to be less than 10 ml, although some male dogs may want to mark territory repeatedly before the bladder is completely emptied. The empty bladder should be palpated for calculi, soft tissue masses, and wall thickness. In older male dogs, a yellow fluid dripping from the urethra may originate from a prostatic cyst. For this reason, any yellow fluid from the urethral orifice in male dogs should be compared to urine collected from the bladder to determine whether the fluid is of urinary or prostatic origin.

If the animal has abnormal neurologic signs, the lesion should be localized. The question should then be asked as to whether such a lesion could result in the type of incontinence observed. If the answer is yes, the cause of the neurologic lesion is also the cause of the incontinence. Tests to determine the cause may include skull or spinal radiographs or both, myelography, cerebrospinal fluid analysis, electroencephalography, computed tomography, and nuclear scans.

If the animal's bladder is distended and no neurologic explanation is apparent, an attempt should be made to pass a urinary catheter. (Remember that the urethra and prostate gland should have been palpated.) If an obstruction is encountered, it is characterized as to location and consistency. Survey and contrast contrast radiographs are often necessary to characterize the obstruction further. Laboratory work, including BUN, serum creatinine, and serum electrolyte concentrations, and urinalysis should be obtained to determine the severity of the consequences of obstruction and to evaluate for the presence of urinary tract infection. If a urolith is the cause of the obstruction, survey radiographs of the abdomen are necessary to determine if other uroliths are present in the kidneys, ureters, or bladder.

Ability to pass a urinary catheter to the bladder does not preclude the presence of an anatomic obstruction. An obstruction may prevent urine passage retrograde via bladder contraction but not inhibit passage of a small catheter antegrade. Examples include certain prostatic diseases, masses in the area of the bladder neck, and small uroliths. Retrograde urethrography and contrast cystography are necessary to document such obstructions. Once the obstruction has been localized and characterized, a biopsy may be required to identify precisely the cause.

If the animal has a distended bladder and no cause is evident, sophisticated diagnostic tests such as cystometry, uroflowmetry, and urethral pressure profilometry may be necessary.[27,28] Such tests usually require referral to a specialty center.

If the bladder of an incontinent animal is not distended, the diagnostic plan may vary somewhat with the age of onset of the problem. If the animal is young and the problem was noted with house training, a congenital defect is most likely. A patent urachus can be diagnosed on physical examination. Ectopic ureters can be difficult to diagnose. Excretory urography is used most often because it allows visualization of the course of the ureters. These congenital defects are discussed further in Chapters 24 through 26.

In older animals that are incontinent but whose bladders are not distended, the diagnostic plan should start with a complete urinalysis. Although bacterial infection can cause incontinence by directly stimulating bladder contraction,[29] infection is more likely to be the consequence of whatever urinary tract abnormality is causing the incontinence. In animals with spay incontinence, the animal leaks urine while sleeping or lying down but otherwise urinates normally. The physical examination is usually normal. Urinary tract infection may or may not be present, but therapy for infection does not control the incontinence. Diagnosis requires urethral pressure profilometry[27,28] or response to appropriate medical therapy.[23,30] If a similar type of incontinence is noted in a cat, a feline leukemia test is indicated.

REFERENCES

1. Jackson, O.F., and Tovey, J.D.: Water turnover in cats fed dry rations. Feline Pract., 7:30, 1977.
2. Thrall, B.E., and Miller, L.G.: Water turnover in cats fed dry rations. Feline Pract., 6:10, 1976.
3. Anderson, R.R.: Water balance in the dog and cat. J. Sm. Anim. Pract., 23:588, 1982.
4. Hays, R.E.: Antidiuretic hormone. N. Engl. J. Med., 295:659, 1976.
5. Joles, J.A., Rynberk, A., Van den Brom, W.E., et al.: Studies on the mechanism of polyuria induced by cortisol excess in the dog. Vet. Quart., 2:199, 1980.
6. Tyler, R.D., Qualls, C.W., Heald, R.D., et al.: Renal concentrating ability in dehydrated, hyponatremic dogs. J. Am. Vet. Med. Assoc., 191:1095, 1987.
7. Rutecki, G.W., Cox, J.W., Robertson, G.W., et al.: Urinary concentrating capacity and antidiuretic hormone responsiveness in the potassium-depleted dog. J. Lab. Clin. Med., 100:53, 1982.
8. Hardy, R.M., and Osborne, C.A.: Water deprivation test in the dog: Maximal normal values. J. Am. Vet. Med. Assoc., 174:479, 1979.
9. Ross, L.A., and Finco, D.R.: Relationship of selected clinical renal function tests to glomerular filtration rate and renal blood flow in cats. Am. J. Vet. Res., 42:1704, 1981.
10. Hardy, R.M., and Osborne, C.A.: Repositol vasopressin response

test in clinically normal dogs undergoing water diuresis: Techniques and results. Am. J. Vet. Res., *43:*1991, 1982.

11. Greene, C.E., Wong, P.L., and Finco, D.R.: Diagnosis and treatment of diabetes insipidus in 2 dogs using 2 synthetic analogs of antidiuretic hormone. J. Am. Anim. Hosp. Assoc., *15:*371, 1979.

12. Hardy, R.M., and Osborne, C.A.: Aqueous vasopressin response test in clinically normal dogs undergoing water diuresis: Technique and results. Am. J. Vet. Res., *43:*1987, 1982.

13. Monnens, L., Smulders, Y., Van Lier, H., et al.: DDAVP test for assessment of renal concentrating capacity in infants and children. Nephron, *29:*151, 1981.

14. Zerbe, R.L., and Robertson, G.L.: A comparison of plasma vasopressin measurements with a standard indirect test in the differential diagnosis of polyuria. N. Engl. J. Med., *305:*1539, 1981.

15. Finco, D.R., Rawlings, C.A., Barsanti, J.A., et al.: Kidney graft survival in transfused and nontransfused sibling beagle dogs. Am. J. Vet. Res., *46:*2327, 1985.

16. Finco, D.R., Rawlings, C.A., Crowell, W.A., et al.: Efficacy of azathioprine versus cyclosporine on kidney graft survival in transfused and nontransfused unmatched mongrel dogs. J. Vet. Intern. Med., *1:*67, 1987.

17. Gregory, C.R., Gourley, I.M., Taylor, N.J., et al.: Preliminary results of clinical renal allograft transplantation in the dog and cat. J. Vet. Intern. Med., *1:*53, 1987.

18. Gregory, C.R., Gourley, I.M., and Broadders, T.W.: Clinical renal transplantation in the cat. Vet. Surg., *18:*69, 1989.

19. Osborne, C.A., Kruger, J.M., Johnston, G.R., et al.: Dissolution of feline uroliths with special emphasis on dietary modification. Comp. Anim. Pract., *March:*89, 1987.

20. Barsanti, J.A., and Finco, D.R.: Feline urologic syndrome. Cont. Iss. Sm. Anim. Pract., *4:*43, 1986.

21. Thrusfield, M.V.: Association between urinary incontinence and spaying in bitches. Vet. Rec., *116:*695, 1985.

22. Holt, P.E.: Urinary incontinence in the bitch due to sphincter mechanism incompetence: Prevalence in referred dogs and retrospective analysis of sixty cases. J. Sm. Anim. Pract., *26:*181, 1985.

23. Lappin, M.R., and Barsanti, J.A.: Urinary incontinence secondary to idiopathic detrusor instability: Cystometrographic diagnosis and pharmacologic management in 2 dogs and a cat. J. Am. Vet. Med. Assoc., *191:*1439, 1987.

24. Barsanti, J.A., and Downey, R.: Urinary incontinence in cats. J. Am. Anim. Hosp. Assoc., *20:*979, 1984.

25. Pollin, M., and Sullivan, M.: A canine dysautonomia resembling the Key-Gaskell syndrome. Vet. Rec., *118:*402, 1986.

26. Sharp, N.J.H., Nash, A.S., and Griffiths, I.R.: Feline dysautonomia (the Key-Gaskell Syndrome): A clinical and pathological study of 40 cases. J. Sm. Anim. Pract., *25:*599, 1984.

27. Moreau, P.M., Lees, G.E., and Gross, D.R.: Simultaneous cystometry and uroflowmetry in dogs: Reference values for healthy animals sedated with xylazine. Am. J. Vet. Res., *44:*1774, 1983.

28. Rosin, A.E., and Barsanti, J.A.: Diagnosis of urinary incontinence in dogs: Role of the urethral pressure profile. J. Am. Vet. Med. Assoc., *178:*814, 1981.

29. Abdullahi, S.U., and Amber, E.I.: Isolating the cause of urinary incontinence. Vet. Med., *81:*426, 1986.

30. Richter, K.P., and Ling, G.P.: Clinical response and urethral pressure profile changes after phenylpropanalamine in dogs with primary sphincter incontinence. J. Am. Vet. Med. Assoc., *187:*605, 1985.

2

Abnormalities in Urine Color and on Urinalysis

Abnormal urine may be detected by gross inspection or by complete urinalysis. Changes in color, turbidity, and smell can be determined by observation. Changes in concentration and composition can be confirmed only by measurement of specific gravity, dipstick evaluation, and microscopic examination of the urine sediment.

This chapter focuses on four major abnormalities related by cause or effect to urologic surgery: hematuria, pyuria, bacteriuria, and proteinuria. The purpose of this chapter is to guide the reader from recognition of one of these problems to a list of their potential causes and to a diagnostic plan to determine which cause is responsible in an individual case. The individual causes and their therapy are discussed in the chapters that follow.

ABNORMALITIES IN URINE COLOR

Urine is normally light yellow to amber in color. Depth or urine color is proportional to urine concentration, but intensity of color is not an accurate substitute for measurement of specific gravity. The most frequent abnormal changes in urine color are to red, orange, or brown. Other colors are possible but infrequent and usually related to ingested dyes. Orange urine is usually the result of conjugated bilirubin. This can be confirmed by reagent strips or tablet methods for bilirubin. Brown urine may be caused by bilirubin, myoglobin, or old hemorrhage. Myoglobinuria and hematuria are discussed further under "Red Urine."

Red Urine

There are three major causes of red urine: hematuria, hemoglobinuria (without hematuria), and ingested or injected dyes (e.g., phenolphthalein).[1] After obtaining a complete history and performing a physical examination, the first step in determining the cause is to collect a voided urine sample and perform a complete urinal-

ysis. A voided sample is preferred over a sample collected by cystocentesis or catheterization to avoid the possibility of introducing blood by iatrogenic injury.

Two components of the urinalysis are essential: the occult blood reaction and the examination of the urine sediment for red blood cells (RBCs) (Fig. 2–1). If RBCs are found, the problem is hematuria. The occult blood reaction is usually also positive.

If the occult blood reaction is positive but RBCs are not present, there are three major possibilities: hemoglobinuria with hemoglobinemia, without hemoglobinemia, or myoglobinuria. The first step is to collect a blood sample to determine hematocrit and to examine plasma color. If the plasma is hemolyzed, the cause of the hemoglobinuria is hemoglobinemia. When intravascular hemolysis releases hemoglobin, the hemoglobin is rapidly bound to circulating haptoglobin. The hemoglobin-haptoglobin complex is too large to be filtered through the glomerulus and is cleared by the reticuloendothelial system. Free hemoglobin exists in the plasma only when the haptoglobin binding system is saturated. Free hemoglobin colors the plasma pink and is filtered by the glomerulus, resulting in hemoglobinuria.

If there is no evidence for hemoglobinemia, the positive occult blood reaction may be caused by hemoglobinuria, secondary to complete RBC lysis in urine or secondary to hemoglobin entering voided urine as a contaminant from an external source such as dissolution of flea dirt. RBCs may lyse in dilute or aged urine. Urine must be examined as soon as possible after collection. If urinalysis cannot be conducted immediately, urine should be refrigerated until examined, preferably within a few hours. If hemoglobinuria is present without hemoglobinemia, urine specific gravity, the potential for urine contamination with flea dirt, and the time frame under which the sample was examined should be evaluated.

Myoglobinuria also results in a positive occult blood reaction with no RBCs in the urine sediment. Because myoglobin is relatively small (molecular weight 17,000),

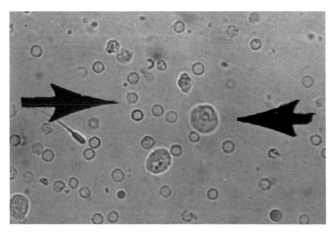

FIG. 2–1. RBCs and WBCs in unstained urine sediment (arrows). The WBCs are larger and more granular than the RBCs. (Courtesy of Dr. Robert Duncan, Department of Pathology, College of Veterinary Medicine, University of Georgia.)

it is rapidly cleared through glomeruli without altering plasma color. Myoglobin generally imparts more of a brown than red color to urine (remember that blood in urine may also appear brown), and there should be clinical evidence of active muscle disease or injury. An ammonium sulfate precipitation test can also be used to distinguish hemoglobinuria from myoglobinuria.[1]

Ingested or injected dyes such as beets or phenolphthalein, respectively, can impart a red color to urine. Both the occult blood reaction and the urine sediment examination for RBCs are negative with such dyes.

Hemoglobinuria and myoglobinuria are not discussed further because the causes of these problems are not directly related to the urinary tract.

Hematuria

Hematuria, by definition, refers to the presence of whole blood in urine. More than 2 to 4 RBCs per high-power field (hpf) is considered abnormal. The patient is usually presented because the owner observes red or brown urine. Significant hematuria can be present, however, even if the urine appears clear. Hematuria in these cases is evident only by urinalysis (microscopic hematuria). Thus, the client may perceive that red urine is intermittent or resolved when hematuria actually is persistent but diminished in severity. Urine normally contains fibrinolysins to prevent the formation of blood clots, which could obstruct the ureters or urethra. The presence of blood clots in the urine indicates hemorrhage severe enough to overwhelm this protective mechanism.

After red urine has been further defined to hematuria as described previously, two major clinical questions need to be answered: Where is the blood from, and what is the cause? In answering these questions, one must first consider how the urine was collected. Cystocentesis, catheterization, and manual expression can result in iatrogenic trauma and mild hemorrhage. To avoid this, voided samples are preferred to establish that hematuria exists. The presence of blood in a voided sample, however, does not localize the bleeding to the urinary tract because the prepuce and prostate gland in the male and the vagina and uterus in the female are other potential sites. Physical examination, which should include rectal examination in males (see Fig. 4–2) and vaginal examination in females (Figs. 2–2, 2–3), is essential to help define the source. Collecting a cystocentesis sample to compare with the previously collected voided sample can also help rule out reproductive tract origin. The exception is the prostate gland in male dogs, which can cause hematuria via reflux of hemorrhagic prostatic fluid into the bladder.

WHERE IS THE BLOOD FROM?

If blood is present in urine collected both by voiding and by cystocentesis, the origin must be kidneys, ureters, bladder, or proximal urethra in females and kidneys, ureters, bladder, proximal urethra, or prostate gland in males. Diseases of the distal urethra may cause a hemorrhagic urethral discharge and blood in voided, but not cystocentesis, urine. To define the site of origin of the blood further, history, physical examination, laboratory evaluation, and radiography may be necessary.

History

An accurate observation of when blood occurs in the urine stream can be helpful in localization. If the blood occurs consistently at the beginning of urination or independent of urination, the urethra, the prostate gland in males, or the reproductive tract in females is most likely. In general, the prostate gland in male dogs is a more likely source of a hemorrhagic urethral discharge than the urethra in dogs without urethral obstruction. Primary urethral diseases are fairly uncommon except for neoplasia in the old dog and urethral urolithiasis. If the blood occurs consistently at the end of urination,

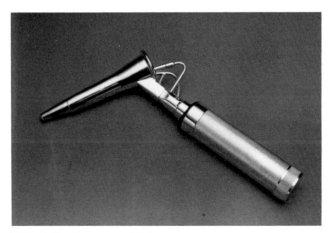

FIG. 2-2. Anoscope (Welch Allen) used for vaginal examination and urethral catheterization in bitches. The scope is passed so that the notch is ventral.

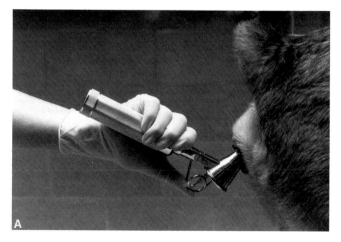

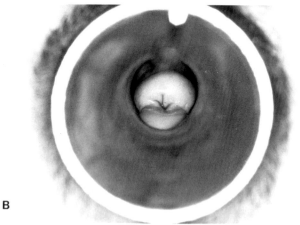

FIG. 2–3. (A) Performance of a vaginal examination in bitches using an anoscope. (B) The urethral papilla is visualized on the ventral floor of the vaginal vault and is accessible for catheterization. A sterile, flexible urethral catheter can be passed without a stylet by using a sterile, needle-nosed forceps.

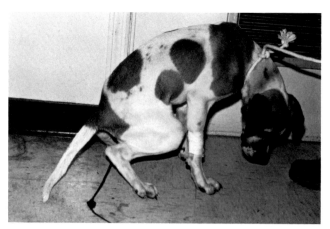

FIG. 2–4. A dog showing dysuria as a result of large blood clots of unilateral renal origin.

the bladder is the most likely origin. If the blood occurs throughout urination, the origin may be kidneys, ureters, bladder, or prostate gland.

If dysuria is an accompanying sign, the lower urinary tract and prostate gland should be considered most highly. An exception to this is that passage of large blood clots of renal origin may cause dysuria (Fig. 2–4). Other important questions include whether the animal has any other sites of bleeding and the possibility of trauma.

Physical Examination

On physical examination, the kidneys should be checked for size, shape, consistency, and symmetry. The bladder should be carefully palpated for wall thickness and the presence of calculi. The prostate gland should be palpated rectally in male dogs. The prepuce should be examined in males and the vagina in females. The animal should be examined for other sites of bleeding.

Urinalysis

A complete urinalysis should always be done. The presence of RBC casts indicates renal bleeding, but they are uncommonly seen and their absence does not exclude a renal origin.

Other Laboratory Tests

Leukocytosis is more common with acute inflammatory diseases or abscessation of the kidneys and prostate gland than with bladder diseases or chronic inflammation anywhere in the urinary tract. Elevations in renal function tests (blood urea nitrogen [BUN] or serum creatinine) suggest a renal origin or a postrenal problem such as obstruction or rupture. Hemorrhage in a semen sample suggests a prostatic, testicular, or epididymal origin. In conjunction with hematuria, a prostatic origin is most likely because it is closely connected to both urinary and reproductive tracts. Worsening hemorrhage after prostatic massage also indicates prostatic or prostatic urethral origin of the bleeding.

Radiography/Ultrasonography

Choice of radiographic study should be based on the most probable site of origin as determined by history and physical examination. Survey abdominal radiographs may indicate an abnormally sized or shaped organ or uroliths. Excretory urography or renal angiography can be used to confirm a renal abnormality. Contrast cystography is used to confirm a bladder disease, and a urethrogram is used to define urethral and prostatic diseases. Ultrasonography can also be useful in defining abnormalities within the urinary tract. See Chapter 6 for further discussion.

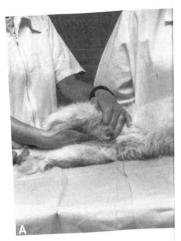
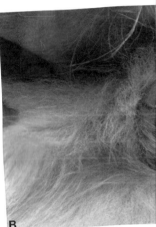

FIG. 2-10. Catheterizati[on]
urine sample. (A) The peni[s]
A sterile, flexible catheter
or by hand wearing sterile

As stated, bacteria in
tract infection. The nex[t]
site of origin of the infe[c]
neys (bacterial pyelonep[hritis]
or chronic cystitis), and [pros]
tatitis). Diagnostic tests t[o]
localize infection include
and complete urinalysis
cated include a comple[te]
tests, survey abdominal
sonography, excretory
thrography, cytologic a[nd]
prostatic fluid, and, occ[asionally]

Proteinuria

To interpret proteinuria
cific gravity and urine
known. Tests for prote[in]
tration in milligrams pe[r]

WHAT IS THE CAUSE OF THE BLEEDING?

Almost every disease of the urinary tract as well as some systemic diseases may result in hematuria. Following the "DAMNIT" scheme can help organize all the possibilities (Table 2-1).

The only degenerative disease of the urinary tract that results in hematuria is cystic prostatic hyperplasia. Prostatic vascularity increases with hyperplasia so that there is an increased tendency for prostatic bleeding.

Common congenital defects such as ectopic ureters and persistent urachus do not cause hematuria unless complicated by secondary infection. Hematuria is the most common clinical finding in telangiectasia of the kidneys in Welsh corgis.

Systemic causes of bleeding should be considered if other sites of bleeding are noted or if other causes of urinary tract bleeding are ruled out. Tests of platelet numbers, platelet function (bleeding time), intrinsic clotting system (activated clotting time, activated partial thromboplastin time), extrinsic system (prothrombin time), common system (thrombin time), von Willebrand's disease, and fibrinolysis (fibrin degradation products, fibrinogen) may need to be performed. Strenuous exercise has also been associated with transient hematuria.[2]

Hematuria frequently accompanies urinary tract neoplasia and may be the major abnormality noted. Neoplasia can affect kidneys, ureters, bladder, urethra, or prostate gland. Radiography may be needed to detect the abnormality in organ size, shape, or contents in the case of the bladder. Abnormal cells may be detected by urine sediment examination, after prostatic massage, or by aspiration or biopsy of the affected organ.

Inflammation is a broad and common category of causes of hematuria. Inflammation can result from neoplasia, urolithiasis, infection, parasitism (*Dioctophyma renale, Capillaria plica*) (Fig. 2-5), or drugs (e.g., cyclophosphamide). As with neoplasia, urolithiasis and infection can affect any urinary tract organ. Autoimmune glomerular diseases have also been associated with hematuria. A complete urinalysis is necessary to determine whether inflammation exists (pyuria) and whether it is associated with infection (bacteriuria) or parasitism

TABLE 2-1. "DAMNIT" SCHEME FOR
REMEMBERING POTENTIAL
CAUSES OF CLINICAL SIGNS

D	=	Degenerative disease
A	=	Anomaly, congenital defect
M	=	Metabolic disorder
N	=	Neoplasm, nutritional disorder
I	=	Inflammatory disease
		Infectious (viral, bacterial, protozoal, fungal)
		Noninfectious (immune-mediated, parasitic, neoplastic, idiopathic)
		Ischemia
		Idiopathic
T	=	Trauma, toxin

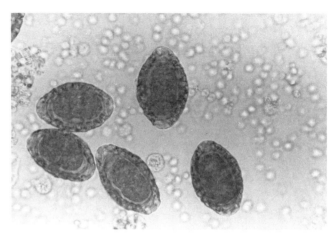

FIG. 2-5. Parasite eggs in urine (*Dioctophyma renale*). (Courtesy of Dr. A. K. Prestwood, Department of Parasitology, College of Veterinary Medicine, University of Georgia.)

(parasite eggs). A marked proteinuria is suggestive of glomerular disease. Survey and contrast radiographs are often necessary to confirm urolithiasis or soft tissue masses. Tissue biopsies and cultures may be needed to determine the cause of inflammation.

Ischemia can also result in hemorrhage. Infarction of the kidney secondary to disseminated intravascular coagulation of any cause (e.g., heat stroke) or secondary to septic emboli as in bacterial endocarditis is the most commonly described cause. Chronic passive congestion of the kidneys of any cause has also been associated with mild hematuria.

There are also numerous idiopathic causes of urinary tract bleeding. The most common is *feline urologic syndrome*, which we define in this text as hematuria of the lower urinary tract of unknown cause. In dogs, "benign essential hematuria" has been described, which is defined as renal bleeding in which no pathologic process can be identified.

Any urinary tract organ can be traumatized resulting in bleeding. Chronic use of cyclophosphamide can be considered toxic to the bladder in that it can result in sterile, hemorrhagic cystitis.

ABNORMALITIES ON URINALYSIS

This section deals with three other abnormalities found on urinalysis that are commonly related to surgical diseases of the urinary tract: pyuria, bacteriuria, and proteinuria.

Pyuria

Pyuria refers to increased numbers of white blood cells (WBCs) in urine (see Fig. 2-1). A few WBCs (<5/hpf) are normal. A greater number is abnormal. If pyuria is found, the first question is to consider how the sample was collected. In a voided sample, the WBCs may have originated from the external genitalia, the reproductive tract, or the urinary tract. The first step in relation to urinary tract disease is to confirm that pyuria is of renal, bladder, or prostatic origin by obtaining a sample of urine directly from the bladder by cystocentesis.

Excessive numbers of WBCs in bladder urine indicates inflammation of the kidneys, ureters, bladder, proximal urethra, or prostate gland (male dogs). Causes of inflammation within the urinary tract include infection, urolithiasis, neoplasia, trauma, toxins (including cyclophosphamide, as described under "Hematuria"), and idiopathic granulomatous diseases. Diagnostic tests to determine the cause include history, physical examination, urinalysis, urine culture, survey and contrast radiography, ultrasonography, and, perhaps, tissue biopsy and culture.

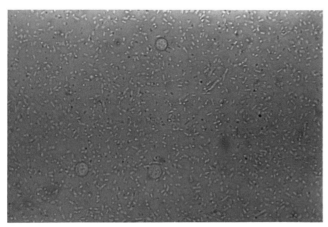

FIG. 2–6. Large numbers of bacteria in urine sediment. (Courtesy of Dr. Robert Duncan, Department of Pathology, College of Veterinary Medicine, University of Georgia.)

Bacteriuri

Bacteriuria refe
Bacteriuria is
amination of ur
teriuria can be
macroscopic (d
bacteriuria sho
cause the micr
number of bac
Some bacteria,
entiate from a
ment. Bacteria
ceed 100,000/m
absence of bact
rule out infecti
urinalysis, but
are that the ob
died before or
usual growth
should always
or transport m

Common a
causes of urina
teus spp., *Pse*
lococci, and s with the animal
bladder urine der back against
be sterile. The
ever, have a n
organisms con
teria in voided
pending on wh
thra, prepuce
The first que
is how the sam
cystocentesis
tion exists, an

the causative organism. Even though the urine
from the bladder, it is not correct to say that cysti
present. The origin of bacteria in bladder urine ca
the kidneys, ureters, or prostate gland as well as
bladder. Cystitis is defined as inflammation of the b
der, not as inflammation in urine collected from the b
der. If the sample was collected by voiding, a sam
should be collected by cystocentesis to exclude ureth
genital, perineal, or environmental contamination.

If urine was collected by catheterization (see Figs.
2, 2-3; Fig. 2–10), a quantitative culture is necessary
determine if the bacteria indicate infection. In male do
and in cats of both sexes, catheterized by aseptic tec
nique and using sterile catheters, greater than 100,0
organisms/ml indicates infection and greater than 10
organisms/ml suggests infection.[8–10] Less than 1000 o
ganisms/ml can be caused by contamination. Thes
guidelines on assessing the results of quantitative cu
tures apply only to samples collected by a single episod
of catheterization.

In bitches, catheterized samples can be contaminated
by greater than 100,000 organisms/ml during the pro
cedure, and there is a risk of inducing infection.[11] For
these reasons, we advise that, for assessment of urinary
tract infection in bitches, only cystocentesis samples be
used. To collect such samples, it may be necessary to
administer a diuretic such as furosemide (1.0 mg/kg, SC)
to cause bladder distention. This should be done only
if other parameters of the urinalysis, such as specific
gravity, which is markedly affected by diuretics, are not
important in the assessment of the individual case.

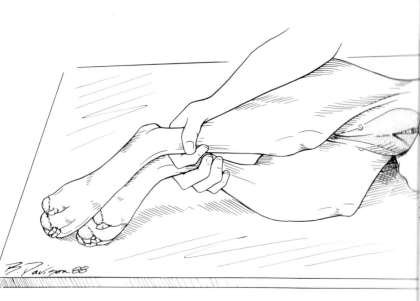

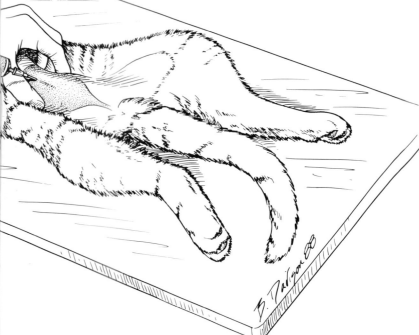

FIG. 2–7. Cystocentesis to collect urine with the animal in lateral recumber
palpating hand is positioned so that the bladder is pushed back toward the th the animal in dorsal recumbency. Again
immobilize it. bladder back against the pelvic brim.

ascites or a large neoplasm that partially obstructs the caudal vena cava. The degree of proteinuria is usually mild to moderate. A mild, transient proteinuria has also been associated with fever, exercise, and exposure to extreme heat or cold.

Both primary glomerular and primary tubular diseases can cause proteinuria. Protein loss with tubular diseases is mild because the protein loss is caused by failure of proximal tubular resorption of the small-molecular-weight proteins in glomerular filtrate. With tubular diseases, other indicators of proximal tubular dysfunction may exist, such as glucosuria with a normal blood glucose concentration. Protein loss with glomerular diseases varies from mild to severe, with severe loss resulting in hypoalbuminemia. Hyaline casts (Fig. 2–11) may be noted in urine from animals with marked proteinuria. These casts are composed of Tamm-Horsfall protein that precipitates in the presence of increased concentrations of albumin.

The diagnostic plan in animals with proteinuria of renal origin should include evaluation of renal function by BUN and serum creatinine concentrations and by complete urinalysis. Serum albumin should be measured to determine if the proteinuria is of sufficient magnitude to cause hypoalbuminemia. The magnitude of proteinuria should be determined by quantitation of protein loss over a known time period (usually 24 hours).[12] Another test that can be used is the urine protein to urine creatinine ratio, in which protein and creatinine are measured in a single random urine sample.[13,14] This ratio corrects for urine concentration changes. A normal ratio is less than 0.2, and an abnormal ratio is greater than 1.0. Values between 0.2 and 1.0 are indeterminate, and a timed collection should be performed. It must be remembered that these determinations are useful only when there is no hemorrhage or inflammation. Significant proteinuria can occur with multiple and varied types of systemic illnesses. When these illnesses resolve, the proteinuria also resolves. In cases of persistent proteinuria with no other definable illness, a renal biopsy, as described in Chapter 5, is often needed to establish an etiologic diagnosis.

REFERENCES

1. Duncan, J.R., and Prasse, K.W.: Veterinary Laboratory Medicine. 2nd Ed. Ames, IA, Iowa State University Press, p. 159, 1986.
2. Crow, S.E.: Hematuria: An algorithm for differential diagnosis. Compend. Contin. Educ. Pract. Vet., 2:941, 1980.
3. Klausner, J.S., Osborne, C.A., and Stevens, J.B.: Clinical evaluation of commercial reagent strips for detection of bacteriuria in dogs and cats. Am. J. Vet. Res., 37:719, 1976.
4. Barlough, J.E., Osborne, C.A., and Stevens, J.B.: Canine and feline urinalysis: Value of macroscopic and microscopic examinations. J. Am. Vet. Med. Assoc., 178:61, 1981.
5. Padilla, J., Osborne, C.A., and Ward, G.E.: Effect of storage time and temperature on quantitative culture of canine urine. J. Am. Vet. Med. Assoc., 18:1077, 1981.
6. Allen, T.A., Jones, R.L., and Purvance, J.: Microbiologic evaluation of canine urine: Direct microscopic examination and preservation of specimen quality for culture. J. Am. Vet. Med. Assoc., 190:1289, 1987.
7. Ling, G.V., and Ruby, A.L.: Aerobic bacterial flora of the prepuce, urethra, and vagina of normal adult dogs. Am. J. Vet. Res., 39:695, 1978.
8. Comer, K.M., and Ling, G.V.: Results of urinalysis and bacterial culture of canine urine obtained by antepubic cystocentesis, catheterization, and midstream voided methods. J. Am. Vet. Med. Assoc., 179:891, 1981.
9. Lees, G.E., Simpson, R.B., and Green, R.A.: Results of analyses and bacterial cultures of urine specimens obtained from clinically normal cats by three methods. J. Am. Vet. Med. Assoc., 184:449, 1984.
10. Carter, J.M., Klausner, J.S., Osborne, C.A., et al.: Comparison of collection techniques for quantitative urine culture in dogs. J. Am. Vet. Med. Assoc., 173:296, 1978.
11. Biertuempfel, P.H., Ling, G.V., and Ling, G.A.: Urinary tract infection resulting from catheterization in healthy adult dogs. J. Am. Vet. Med. Assoc., 178:989, 1981.
12. Barsanti, J.A., and Finco, D.R.: Protein concentration in urine of normal dogs. Am. J. Vet. Res., 40:1583, 1979.
13. Grauer, G.F., Thomas, C.B., and Eicker, S.W.: Estimation of quantitative proteinuria in the dog, using the urine protein-to-creatinine ratio from a random voided sample. Am. J. Vet. Res., 46:2116, 1985.
14. White, J.V., Olivier, N.B., Reimann, K., et al.: Use of protein-to-creatinine ratio in a single urine specimen for quantitative estimation of canine proteinuria. J. Am. Vet. Med. Assoc., 185:882, 1984.

3

Problems of Azotemia and Uremia

Azotemia refers to above-normal concentrations of blood urea nitrogen (BUN) and serum creatinine. Azotemia describes a laboratory abnormality and does not convey any information about presence or absence of clinical signs. An animal is said to be *uremic* when azotemia is associated with any of the typical clinical signs associated with urinary system failure. These clinical signs include anorexia, lethargy, vomition, diarrhea, melena, oral ulceration, and dehydration (Fig. 3–1). A variable number of these signs are present in each uremic patient. Some authors use the term *uremia* only if the cause of the clinical signs is renal disease.[1,2] We use the term in a broader sense to reflect the clinical signs associated with retention of markedly abnormal amounts of urine constituents in blood from postrenal and prerenal causes as well as renal causes.

There is no single BUN or serum creatinine concentration that correlates with the development of clinical signs. This varies with each individual animal. Part of this variability relates to the body's ability to adjust to slow changes in kidney function. For example, signs of

uremia may be evident when the BUN is 100 mg/dl in an animal with acute renal failure, whereas such signs may not occur until the BUN is 200 mg/dl in an animal with chronic renal failure. Another reason for this variability is that neither BUN nor serum creatinine is the cause of the uremic signs. Other waste products that are retained in urinary system failure are the uremic toxins.

CAUSES OF AZOTEMIA

There are two major possibilities whenever blood concentration of a compound increase: increased production or decreased excretion. The source of BUN and serum creatinine is different, but both are excreted primarily in direct proportion to glomerular filtration rate (GFR). There are three major categories of causes of decreased excretion: decreased renal perfusion (prerenal causes), intrinsic renal disease (renal causes), and obstruction to or rupture within the urinary outflow tract (postrenal causes). The purpose of this chapter is to review these various categories of causes of azotemia so that an appropriate diagnostic plan can be formulated.

Increased Production

Blood urea is derived from the metabolism of dietary and endogenous proteins by the liver (Fig. 3–2). Normal values in most laboratories are 10 to 30 mg/dl. Increased nitrogen load to the liver increases BUN concentrations. Causes of increased nitrogen load include a recent high protein meal (within 18 hours),[3-7] gastrointestinal hemorrhage, and increased endogenous protein catabolism (Table 3–1).[1,8] In animals with normal kidneys, the degree of increase is usually mild (<50 mg/dl) with increased dietary protein but may be higher than this with gastrointestinal hemorrhage or extensive tissue injury. In animals with renal failure, such increases can

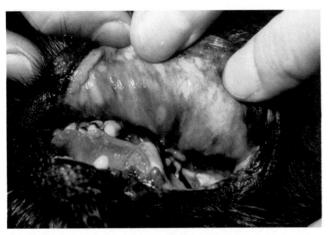

FIG. 3–1. Oral ulcers secondary to uremia.

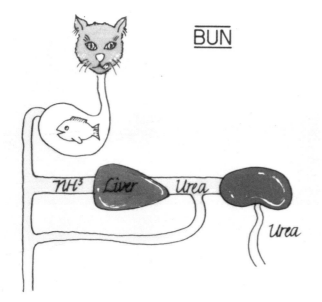

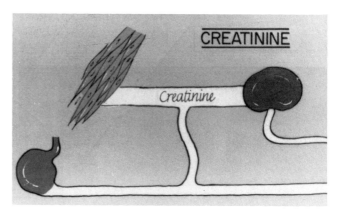

FIG. 3–3. Creatinine is produced from muscle metabolism and excreted in urine. When serum creatinine is chronically increased, some creatinine may be excreted by the gastro-intestinal tract.

FIG. 3–2. Urea is metabolized in the liver from ammonia produced as a result of protein digestion or catabolism. Excess urea is excreted by the kidney.

TABLE 3–1. CAUSES OF INCREASED CONCENTRATION OF BUN

Increased Production	Decreased Excretion
Recent high protein meal	Prerenal
Gastrointestinal	Decreased effective
hemorrhage	blood volume
Increased endogenous	Cardiovascular failure
protein catabolism	Intrinsic renal disease
Fever	Acute renal failure
Extensive tissue injury	Chronic renal failure
Drug-induced	Postrenal
Glucocorticoids	Urinary tract
	obstruction
	Urinary tract rupture

be much greater because of the compounding problem of decreased excretion.

Creatinine is produced in each individual animal at a constant daily rate from creatine in muscle (Fig. 3–3). The value for an individual animal varies from other animals because of variations in muscle mass. The less muscle mass, the less creatinine produced. In general, the normal value in dogs and cats is less than 1.5 mg/dl. Extensive rhabdomyolysis has been reported to elevate serum creatinine concentrations in humans, but such severe muscle injury is extremely rare in dogs and cats. In animals with diabetic ketoacidosis, serum creatinine concentration may be spuriously high as a result of interference of ketones with the laboratory test.[9] The most commonly used tests to measure creatinine also measure noncreatinine chromagens such as ketones.

Thus, the usual clinical problem is determining whether an increase in BUN could be caused by in-

creased production. To eliminate this possibility, one should always evaluate BUN after at least an 18-hour fast, and one should measure serum creatinine in all animals with BUN elevations. If serum creatinine is well within the normal range, considering the animal's muscle mass, increased production of urea becomes a likely possibility. If serum creatinine is also increased above normal, one should proceed to consider decreased excretion.

Decreased Excretion

Blood urea is excreted primarily by the kidney. Because of its small size, it is filtered freely through the glomerulus. About 40 to 50% is passively reabsorbed with water in the proximal tubule independent of urine flow rate. Beyond the proximal tubule, urea excretion is markedly affected by urine flow rates. At slow urine flow rates (0.5 ml/min in humans), an additional 25 to 35% of filtered urea is passively reabsorbed in the medullary collecting ducts. At high urine flow rates (>1.5 ml/min in humans), no further reabsorption of urea occurs. Fluid therapy can thus decrease BUN by increasing urine flow rate, even if GFR is not increased. Urea excretion can be further increased by use of osmotic agents such as hypertonic dextrose to decrease water and thus urea reabsorption in the proximal tubule.

Creatinine is excreted by the kidney via glomerular filtration. It is not reabsorbed by the tubule.[10,11] In male dogs, a small amount of tubular secretion occurs.[12-14] When increases in serum creatinine persist, bowel bacteria can increase metabolism of creatinine and slightly lower serum concentrations.

The clinical usefulness of BUN and serum creatinine concentrations is that, with the aforementioned exceptions, concentrations are directly proportional to GFR, and GFR is the most accurate indicator of overall renal function. For example, a 50% reduction in renal function (GFR) is accompanied by a doubling of serum creatinine and BUN concentrations (Fig. 3–4). Unfortunately, a doubling of BUN or serum creatinine concentration in

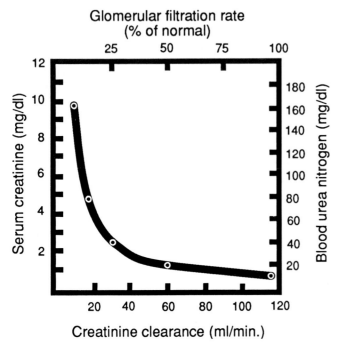

FIG. 3–4. The relationship between GFR and serum creatinine and BUN.

an individual is usually not out of the normal range for the population. For example, a creatinine concentration of 0.8 mg/dl would become 1.6 mg/dl, and a BUN concentration of 12 would become 24 mg/dl. A 75% decrease in GFR is usually required before BUN and serum creatinine consistently increase above the normal range. For this reason, actual measurement of GFR via clearance tests is a more accurate indicator of renal function, particularly when BUN and serum creatinine are within the normal range. (See Chapter 5.)

There are three major groups of causes of decreased excretion of BUN and serum creatinine: prerenal causes, renal causes, and postrenal causes.

Prerenal Causes

Prerenal azotemia occurs even though the kidneys and lower urinary tract are normal. This type of azotemia is usually reversible because the underlying disease can often be successfully treated. Recognition of this cause of azotemia is important. One *never* wants to misdiagnose an animal as having severe kidney disease when the major problem is reversible dehydration from another cause such as gastroenteritis.

The major causes of prerenal azotemia are cardiovascular failure and decreased effective arterial blood volume. Decreased effective blood volume can result from intravascular volume loss, extravascular volume loss, increased vascular capacity, and intravascular to extravascular fluid shifts (Table 3–2). If cardiovascular failure or decreased effective blood volume persist, primary renal dysfunction can develop secondary to nephron damage from poor perfusion.

Differentiation of prerenal azotemia from renal and postrenal azotemia is sometimes difficult. A thorough history and physical examination are extremely important. These help identify cardiovascular failure, hemorrhage, plasma loss, sepsis, ascites, urinary tract obstruction, and urinary tract rupture. Primary gastrointestinal diseases, pancreatitis, and hypoadrenocorticism are difficult to distinguish from primary renal failure because all present with gastrointestinal disturbances. The ratio of BUN to serum creatinine concentration, which is used in human medicine to help differentiate prerenal from renal azotemia, was not reliable in dogs and cats.[15] *The most useful test to differentiate prerenal from renal causes of azotemia is urine specific gravity measured before fluid or drug administration.* Concentrated urine excludes primary renal failure in dogs.

Urine with a specific gravity of 1.035 or greater in dogs is considered to be adequately concentrated in the face of dehydration or poor renal perfusion. A urine specific gravity of <1.030 indicates inadequate concentrating ability in the face of dehydration or azotemia. A urine specific gravity between 1.030 and 1.035 is questionable. A prerenal factor should be pursued first, but consideration should be given to the possibility of renal dysfunction. These figures are based on several research studies in dogs. Most normal dogs with 5% dehydration had urine specific gravities >1.048.[16] A few dogs with experimental reduction of renal mass to 33% of normal could still concentrate their urine to 1.027.[17] Clinical experience to date indicates that animals in renal failure typically have urine specific gravities less than 1.030; the aforementioned guidelines are generally accepted at the present time. Further studies may warrant modifications in the future.

Normal cats concentrate their urine with minimal dehydration to an even greater degree than dogs (> 1.052).[18] Cats lost concentrating ability with experimental reduction in renal mass, but some cats could still concentrate their urine even with azotemia.[18] This has not been a major clinical problem because most sick cats

TABLE 3–2. CAUSES OF PRERENAL AZOTEMIA

Cardiovascular failure
Decreased effective blood volume
    Intravascular volume loss
        Severe hemorrhage
        Plasma loss from severe burns
    Extravascular volume loss
        Vomition
        Diarrhea
        Diabetes insipidus (with limited access to water)
    Increased vascular capacity
        Sepsis
    Intravascular to extravascular fluid shifts
        Ascites
        Pancreatitis
        Peritonitis
        Hypoadrenocorticism (Addison's disease)
        Burns

lose concentrating ability (urine specific gravity < 1.035) by the time clinical signs of renal failure develop. Maintenance of concentrating ability in relatively early chronic renal failure, however, can present a diagnostic dilemma in cats that appear healthy but are azotemic on biochemical profiles. In these cases, one must rely on renal palpation as well as the rest of the physical examination to help differentiate prerenal from renal causes of azotemia. Fortunately, renal palpation in cats is usually much easier than in dogs.

Production of dilute urine requires active reabsorption of more solute than water by the nephron and indicates normal renal function up to the distal tubule. Urine specific gravity values less than 1.006 are not indicative of primary renal failure. The values may be normal or reflect disease within the antidiuretic hormone (ADH) pathway. Examples are pituitary and nephrogenic diabetes insipidus. Occasionally, dogs with polyuric renal failure have mildly hyposthenuric urine (1.006 to 1.007).[19] The mechanism for this is not currently understood.

If urine specific gravity is not determined before fluid therapy, one can only use response to this therapy to differentiate prerenal from renal azotemia. Urine specific gravity decreases with fluid therapy, regardless of whether the cause of the azotemia is prerenal or renal. If azotemia is prerenal in origin, it is usually corrected within 24 hours after successfully reversing the prerenal cause. If the azotemia is renal in origin, BUN and serum creatinine concentrations usually decrease with fluid therapy but at a slower rate. Determining the cause of azotemia by the response to fluid therapy, however, is more likely to be erroneous than by measurement of urine specific gravity before fluid therapy. For example, if a dog has only 30% nephron mass, it will be polyuric but not azotemic. If this dog eats garbage and begins to vomit, it will rapidly dehydrate and become azotemic because of inadequate renal concentrating ability. If the veterinarian measures urine specific gravity before fluid therapy, the loss of concentrating ability will be discovered. If the veterinarian administers fluids, without measuring urine specific gravity, and then notes a rapid resolution of the azotemia with correction of dehydration, the abnormal renal function will be missed.

Although inadequate concentrating ability in the face of dehydration or azotemia indicates renal dysfunction, it does not necessarily indicate intrinsic renal disease. There are many diseases and electrolyte disorders that impair renal concentrating ability. (Review polyuria in Chapter 1 and Table 1–1.) If a prerenal cause of dehydration is superimposed on one of these diseases, azotemia with urine concentration less than 1.030 will result. It is always useful to remember that adequate urine concentrating ability depends not only on adequate nephron numbers and function, but also on ADH and its receptors. For example, if a dog with hyperadrenocorticism develops pancreatitis with profuse vomiting, it will be azotemic from dehydration and have inadequate urine concentration because of hyperadrenocorticism. This points out the importance of thoroughly assessing the history, physical examination, and all laboratory work when determining the probable cause of azotemia.

Distinguishing hypoadrenocorticism from renal failure can also be difficult because presenting signs may be similar and hypoadrenocorticism can prevent adequate urine concentration in the face of dehydration or hypovolemia.[20] The major differentiating factors may be the presence or absence of a stress leukogram and whether hyperkalemia is associated with oliguria or polyuria. In sick animals with renal failure, a stress leukogram is expected, and moderate to marked hyperkalemia is associated with oliguria. (Occasionally, patients with polyuric renal failure have mild hyperkalemia.) In hypoadrenocorticism, a stress leukogram is not present (in spite of stress), and moderate to marked hyperkalemia is associated with normal to increased urine output. Plasma cortisol assays should be used to confirm a diagnosis of hypoadrenocorticism.

Renal Causes of Azotemia

Azotemia of renal origin is caused by renal disease that has resulted in a 75% decrease in GFR. The underlying renal disease may be acute or chronic. (Review the differentiation of these categories in Chapter 1.) In general, moderate increases in BUN and serum creatinine concentrations (e.g., BUN of 100 mg/dl, creatinine of 4 mg/dl) are more likely to be associated with clinical signs of uremia in animals with acute renal failure than in those with chronic renal failure. Animals in chronic renal failure often appear relatively healthy until azotemia is marked (BUN > 150 mg/dl, serum creatinine > 6 mg/dl). Animals with chronic renal failure, however, have lost the renal reserve necessary to respond adequately to sudden changes in water or solute intake. They are much more susceptible than normal animals to dehydration from such causes as fever, vomiting, diarrhea, or restricted access to water. Often, precipitation of a uremic crisis in a previously stable animal with chronic renal failure is caused by the superimposition of a prerenal factor on compensated renal disease.

The judgment that azotemia is caused by primary renal disease should be based on history, physical examination, and findings on the rest of the laboratory work, especially the urinalysis. A postrenal cause of azotemia should be excluded by history, physical examination, and, in some cases, radiographs. A prerenal cause should be excluded by evaluation of history, physical examination, urine specific gravity, and other laboratory work as described in the previous section.

Postrenal Causes of Azotemia

A rupture or obstruction of the urinary tract results in azotemia because urea and creatinine cannot be removed from the body. With a urinary tract rupture, urea and creatinine are reabsorbed into the blood stream because both are relatively small molecules that distribute throughout body water. Because creatinine is a larger molecule than urea, it is redistributed somewhat more slowly. When trying to determine whether an abdominal effusion is urine, one compares concentrations of urea nitrogen or creatinine in abdominal fluid and blood. If the effusion is urine, concentrations of these substances will be higher in the abdominal fluid. In one study in dogs, measurement of abdominal fluid creatinine was more accurate than measurement of urea nitrogen 45 hours after surgically induced bladder rupture.[21] In our clinical experience, however, urea measurements are useful because concentrations of urea in abdominal effusions caused by urine usually exceed serum concentrations.

With urinary tract obstruction, intraurinary tract pressure rises leading to decreased GFR. Urea and creatinine may also be reabsorbed across an ischemic bladder wall. The pathophysiology of obstructive uropathy is more fully covered in Chapters 12 and 15. An atonic, chronically distended bladder can also result in postrenal azotemia.

Because a urinary tract rupture or obstruction requires very specific therapy and because this therapy is usually successful when instituted promptly, this cause of postrenal azotemia should always be considered first, especially when the onset of azotemia or uremia is acute. Urinary tract rupture is usually traumatic, although severe disease of the bladder wall (such as a neoplasm) occasionally results in loss of bladder wall integrity. Diagnosis is usually based on history of definite or possible trauma, physical evidence of other traumatic injuries, presence of abdominal or perineal effusion, and radiographic confirmation of urine leakage. Although many cases are straightforward, some have little historical or physical evidence of trauma and require a high index of suspicion for appropriate tests to be performed. Diagnosis is discussed in further detail in Chapter 21.

Urinary tract obstruction can be caused by uroliths, soft tissue masses such as neoplasms, and strictures. Urethral obstruction is most common, but obstruction may also occur within the bladder at the bladder neck. Unilateral ureteral obstruction would not result in azotemia unless the animal had only one functional kidney.[22] Bilateral ureteral obstruction can occur with masses at the trigone of the bladder and with masses outside the bladder in the area of ureteral insertion into the bladder, most commonly associated with severe prostatomegaly.

Urethral obstruction is diagnosed by history, physical examination, obstruction to catheter passage, and, in some cases, radiography. Affected animals are dysuric and oliguric to anuric. Dribbling of small amounts of urine around the obstruction may occur. On physical examination, the bladder is distended. An obstruction is encountered when attempting to pass a urinary catheter. (See Chapter 1 for diagnostic plans for dysuria, oliguria, and incontinence.) Survey radiographs, contrast-enhanced radiographs, or both can be used to confirm the presence and probable cause of the obstruction. Other sites of urinary tract obstruction require contrast cystography or excretory urography for confirmation. Urethral obstruction is covered further in Chapters12 through 14 and 15 through 17. Other sites of urinary tract obstruction are covered under prostatic diseases and urinary tract neoplasia.

CONCLUSIONS

Whenever an animal is uremic and whenever azotemia is noted on laboratory evaluation, one should always consider the three categories of causes of decreased excretion of urea and creatinine: prerenal, renal, or postrenal. When only BUN is measured and the elevation is mild, one should consider increased urea production as well as decreased excretion. Measuring BUN only after fasting and evaluating serum creatinine in animals with BUN elevations should help eliminate increased urea production as the cause.

One should use the history and physical examination to consider the possibility of urinary tract obstruction or rupture. In questionable cases, survey and contrast-enhanced radiography is often definitive. One should use urine specific gravity collected before therapy to assess renal function in all animals that are dehydrated or azotemic. Normal renal concentrating ability rules out primary renal disease as a cause of azotemia in dogs. In cats, renal palpation should be performed in addition to measuring specific gravity.

If postrenal causes are excluded and urine is not adequately concentrated in spite of demand for water retention, renal dysfunction exists. This dysfunction can be caused by renal disease or by diseases that impair the production or function of ADH in conjunction with a prerenal cause of dehydration. History; physical examination; evaluation of urinalysis, complete blood count, and a biochemical profile; and performance of other laboratory tests and radiography, as indicated by the individual case, should lead to the correct diagnosis.

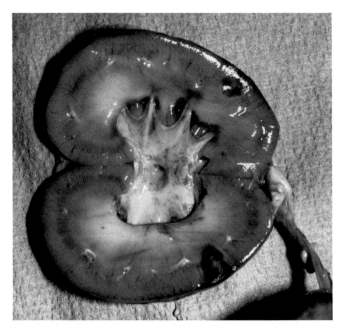

FIG. 3–5. Hydronephrosis secondary to chronic partial urethral obstruction with chronic bladder overdistention.

One must remember that more than one cause of azotemia may be present. As discussed, an animal with chronic renal failure may develop vomiting from gastroenteritis, i.e., prerenal and renal azotemia. Prolonged partial urinary tract obstruction can lead to hydronephrosis, i.e., renal and postrenal azotemia (Fig. 3–5). Animals with urinary tract rupture become uremic, vomit, and become dehydrated, i.e., prerenal and postrenal azotemia. Examples are numerous. In any individual case, one must decide which cause is primary, which causes are reversible, and whether a potentially progressive form of renal disease exists. Serial physical and laboratory evaluations during therapy are often required to make these determinations.

REFERENCES

1. Osborne, C.A., and Polzin, D.J.: Azotemia: A review of what's old and what's new. Part I. Definition of terms and concepts. Compend. Contin. Educ. Pract. Vet., 5:497, 1983.
2. Osborne, C.A., and Polzin, D.J.: Azotemia: A review of what's old and what's new. Part II. Localization. Compend. Contin. Educ. Pract. Vet., 5:561, 1983.
3. Epstein, M.E., Barsanti, J.A., Finco, D.R., et al.: Postprandial changes in plasma urea nitrogen and plasma creatinine concentrations in dogs fed commercial diets. J. Am. Anim. Hosp. Assoc., 20:779, 1984.
4. Watson, A.D.J., Church, D.B., and Fairburn, A.J.: Postprandial changes in plasma urea and creatinine concentrations in dogs. Am. J. Vet. Res., 42:1878, 1981.
5. Vogin, E.E., Skeggs, H.R., Bokelman, D.L., et al.: Liver function: Postprandial urea nitrogen elevation and indocyanine green clearance in the dog. Toxicol. Appl. Pharmacol., 10:577, 1967.
6. Anderson, R.S., and Edney, A.T.B.: Protein intake and blood urea in the dog. Vet. Rec., 84:348, 1969.
7. Street, A.E., Chesterman, H., Smith, G.K.A., et al.: Prolonged blood urea elevation observed in the Beagle after feeding. Toxicol. Appl. Pharmacol., 13:363, 1968.
8. Finco, D.R., Barsanti, J.A., and Rawlings, C.A.: Effects of immunosuppressive drug therapy on blood urea nitrogen concentrations of dogs with azotemia. J. Am. Vet. Med. Assoc., 185:664, 1984.
9. Ward, P.C.J.: Renal dysfunction 1. Urea and creatinine. Postgrad. Med., 69:93, 1981.
10. Eggleton, M.G., and Habib, Y.A.: The mode of excretion of creatinine and insulin by the kidney of the cat. J. Physiol., 112:191, 1951.
11. Finco, D.R., and Barsanti, J.A.: Mechanism of urinary creatinine excretion by the cat. Am. J. Vet. Res., 43:2207, 1982.
12. O'Connell, J.M.B., Romeo, J.A., and Mudge, G.H.: Renal tubular secretion of creatinine in the dog. Am. J. Physiol., 203:985, 1962.
13. Swanson, R.E., and Hakim, A.A.: Stop-flow analysis of creatinine excretion in the dog. J. Physiol., 203:980, 1962.
14. Robinson, T., Harbison, M., and Bovee, K.C.: Influence of reduced renal mass on tubular secretion of creatinine in the dog. Am. J. Vet. Res., 35:487, 1974.
15. Finco, D.R., and Duncan, J.R.: Evaluation of blood urea nitrogen and serum creatinine as indicators of renal dysfunction: A study of 111 cases and a review of related literature. J. Am. Vet. Med. Assoc., 168:593, 1976.
16. Hardy, R.M., and Osborne, C.A.: Water deprivation test in the dog: Maximal normal values. J. Am. Vet. Med. Assoc., 174:479, 1979.
17. Hayman, J.M., Shumway, N.P., Dunke, P., et al.: Experimental hyposthenuria. J. Clin. Invest., 18:195, 1939.
18. Ross, L.A., and Finco, D.R.: Relationship of selected clinical renal function tests to glomerular filtration rate and renal blood flow in cats. Am. J. Vet. Res., 42:1704, 1981.
19. Krawiec, D.R.: Renal failure in immature dogs. J. Am. Anim. Hosp. Assoc., 23:101, 1987.
20. Willard, M.D., Schall, W.D., McCaw, D.E., et al.: Canine hypoadrenocorticism: Report of 37 cases and review of 39 previously reported cases. J. Am. Vet. Med. Assoc., 180:59, 1982.
21. Burrows, C.F., and Bovee, K.C.: Metabolic changes due to experimentally induced rupture of the canine urinary bladder. Am. J. Vet. Res., 35:1083, 1974.
22. Crowell, W.A., Cornelius, L.M., and Barsanti, J.A.: Unusual oliguric urinary failure in a cat. J. Am. Anim. Hosp. Assoc., 18:812, 1982.

4

Prostatomegaly

Prostatomegaly means that the prostate gland is of abnormally large size. This is primarily a problem of male dogs; prostatic diseases have been described only rarely in cats. An animal would not be presented to a veterinarian for the problem of prostatomegaly because prostatomegaly can only be detected by physical examination, radiography, or ultrasonography. Because of the location of the prostate gland (Fig. 4–1), however, animals are presented for problems related to the increase in prostatic size, such as fecal tenesmus or abnormal urination, or for problems related to a concomitant change in prostatic physiology, such as a urethral discharge. Most diseases that affect the prostate gland can result in prostatomegaly. This chapter discusses the

problem of prostatomegaly by briefly reviewing the normal anatomy and physiology of the prostate gland, briefly describing the diseases that result in prostatomegaly, and outlining a diagnostic plan to determine the cause of prostatomegaly. Specific diseases and surgical treatment are discussed in Chapters 27 to 29.

NORMAL ANATOMY OF THE PROSTATE GLAND

The prostate gland is the only accessory sex gland in the male dog. It is a bilobed organ with a median septum on the dorsal surface contiguous with a fibrous capsule.[1]

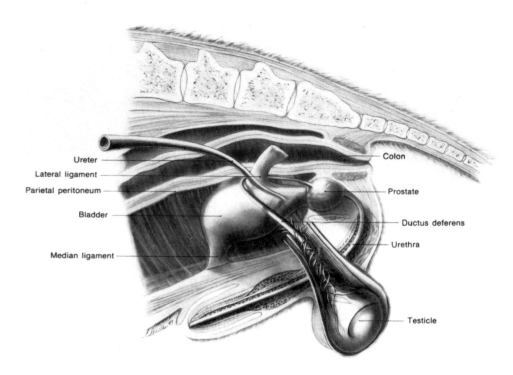

FIG. 4–1. Anatomy of the caudal abdomen of the male dog, showing the relationship of the prostate gland to surrounding structures. (From Barsanti, J.A.: Canine prostatic disease. *In* Veterinary Internal Medicine. Edited by Ettinger, S.J. Philadelphia, W.B. Saunders, pp. 1859–1880, 1989; with permission.)

Ureter

Lateral ligament

Parietal peritoneum

Bladder

Median ligament

Colon

Prostate

Ductus deferens

Urethra

Testicle

It is located predominantly in the retroperitoneal space, just caudal to the bladder neck (see Fig. 4–1). Only the craniodorsal surface is covered by peritoneum. The prostate encircles the proximal urethra at the neck of the bladder with ducts entering throughout the urethra's circumference.[2]

The position of the prostate gland in the caudal abdomen is determined by age, bladder distention, and disease state.[3] In neonates, the prostate is abdominal. After loss of the urachal remnant (at 2 months of age or younger), the prostate resides within the pelvic inlet.[4] With increasing age, the prostate moves cranially so that in intact male dogs over 5 years of age, most of the prostate gland is abdominal.[3]

Histologically, the prostate gland is composed of glandular acini supported by a stroma of connective tissue and smooth muscle, enclosed by a thick fibromuscular capsule. Columnar glandular epithelium is replaced by transitional epithelium in the excretory ducts opening into the urethra. The cells within the prostate gland are of two types: stromal and epithelial.[5] The epithelial cells are of two types: tall columnar secretory epithelium and basal epithelium located sporadically along the basement membrane. The role of the basal epithelial cells is unknown, but they may be precursors of the secretory epithelium.[5,6] The stroma consists of fibroblastic and smooth muscle cells enmeshed in collagen with blood vessels and nerves. The fibromuscular stroma is predominant prior to sexual maturity at 6 months to 1 year of age.[7,8] After this time, the epithelium is predominant.

NORMAL PHYSIOLOGY OF THE PROSTATE GLAND

The purpose of the prostate gland is to produce prostatic fluid as a transport and support medium for sperm during ejaculation. Under parasympathetic stimulation during erection, the prostate increases the rate of fluid production and under sympathetic stimulation ejects the fluid during ejaculation.[9] Basal amounts of prostatic fluid are constantly secreted into the prostatic excretory ducts and prostatic urethra.[10] When neither micturition nor ejaculation is occurring, urethral pressure moves this basally secreted fluid cranially into the bladder (*prostatic fluid reflux*). During micturition, urine enters the prostate gland in men (*intraprostatic urinary reflux*).[11] Whether urine enters the canine prostate gland during micturition is unknown.

Between 4 and 16 months of age in beagles, the prostate grows with a constant doubling time of 0.64 years.[12] This corresponds to the time when serum testosterone is rising to its normal adult level.[12] Once the prostate reaches its normal adult size (12 to 14 g in beagles), growth stops until prostatic hyperplasia develops. If a dog is castrated prior to sexual maturity, normal prostatic growth is completely inhibited.[12] If the dog is castrated as an adult, the prostate will involute to 20% of its normal adult size.[13] Prostatic secretory function, as measured by ejaculate volume, reaches a peak at 4 years of age in beagles and then begins to decline.[8]

Because of the tendency to develop prostatic hyperplasia with aging, prostatic size correlates directly with age; however, this correlation is weak since dogs develop hyperplasia at different ages and to varying degrees.[8,14,15] Prostatic size also correlates weakly in some but not all studies with body weight.[16–18] The Scottish terrier has been reported to have a large prostate gland per body weight compared with eight other breeds.[18] This conclusion was based on only seven dogs, however, whose average age was older than the other breeds and thus needs confirmation.

Apparently there is increased sensitivity of the growth of the prostate gland to testosterone with aging because testosterone secretion decreases with aging.[8] The increase in weight with age is associated with benign prostatic hyperplasia (BPH). BPH has been identified in 40% of beagles by 2.5 years of age, more than 80% of beagles older than 6 years,[8,19,20] and more than 95% of beagles older than 9 years of age.[20] In a few older dogs (>8 years in beagles), another phase of BPH occurs in which the prostate rapidly increases in size again.[20] The reason for this is unknown.

DISEASES THAT CAUSE PROSTATOMEGALY

Prostatic diseases are common in the older male dog. Several result in prostatomegaly (Table 4–1). With aging, the prostate is subject to the development of hyperplasia. In an individual dog, hyperplasia often develops rapidly (within a year).[20] With hyperplasia there is an increase in both glandular and stromal components, although the glandular component is predominant in dogs.[21] There are increases in both epithelial cell numbers and size, so that both hyperplasia and hypertrophy are present. The hyperplastic prostate has a tendency to develop intraparenchymal glandular cysts.[22] Prostatomegaly associated with cystic BPH is symmetrical with normal consistency. Prostatomegaly associated with BPH is also symmetrical, although the consistency may vary from normal to more "cobblestone," with softer and firmer areas.

The prostate is subject to infection from bacteria ascending the urethra. Hematogenous spread of bacteria, spread of bacteria from the kidneys or bladder via urine, or spread from the testicle and epididymis via semen are also possible. Bacterial prostatic infections can be acute or chronic and may lead to abscessation. Decreased secretory function in the aging prostate may

---

TABLE 4–1. DIFFERENTIAL DIAGNOSIS OF PROSTATOMEGALY

Hyperplasia
Metaplasia
Paraprostatic cysts
Neoplasia
Abscessation

increase its susceptibility to infection. In general, acute infection has no or minimal effect on prostatic size. Chronic infection without abscessation also has no effect on size. Development of intraprostatic abscessation, however, does lead to prostatomegaly, which is often asymmetrical. Consistency of the parenchyma is variable with increased or decreased firmness.

The aging prostate gland is also subject to neoplastic transformation, most commonly adenocarcinoma. Transitional cell carcinomas may also arise from distal prostatic ducts or may invade the prostate gland from a tumor originating in the bladder or urethra. Other neoplasms, such as lymphosarcoma, squamous cell carcinoma, and leiomyosarcoma may occasionally affect the prostate as a primary or metastatic site.[18,23] Prostatomegaly associated with neoplasia is often asymmetrical with increased firmness.

In the presence of excess estrogens, either endogenous or exogenous, the prostatic epithelium undergoes squamous metaplasia.[24,25] Squamous metaplasia can lead to prostatic fluid stasis and predispose to infection with abscessation.[18,26,27] Stromal hypertrophy also occurs in the estrogen-stimulated prostate gland. Prostatomegaly associated with squamous metaplasia is symmetrical unless complicated by abscessation.

Paraprostatic cysts, which may or may not be of prostatic origin, are usually associated with the prostate and may be detected as severe asymmetrical prostatomegaly. Such cysts may ossify (osteocartilaginous cysts) and thus feel very firm.[28,29]

DIAGNOSTIC APPROACH TO PROSTATOMEGALY

Determining the cause of prostatomegaly involves obtaining a complete history and performing a thorough physical examination. The prostate gland is best palpated by concomitant rectal and abdominal palpation (Fig. 4–2). The hand palpating the caudal abdomen can both evaluate the cranial aspects of the gland and push the prostate into or near the pelvic canal for better palpation per rectum. The dorsal median groove, which is the division between the two lobes, is palpable per rectum and is a guide to determining symmetry. The prostate should be evaluated for size, symmetry, surface contour, consistency, movability, and pain. The size in 2- to 5-year-old, 25-pound dogs was found to vary from ovoid, 1.7 cm in length by 2.6 cm transverse by 0.8 cm dorsoventral, to spheroid, 2 cm in diameter.[30] Size varies with age, body size, and breed, however, so that judging whether size is normal or not is subjective. Estimated size should always be recorded so that changes can be followed.

Additional tests required to determine the cause of prostatomegaly are a complete blood count, complete

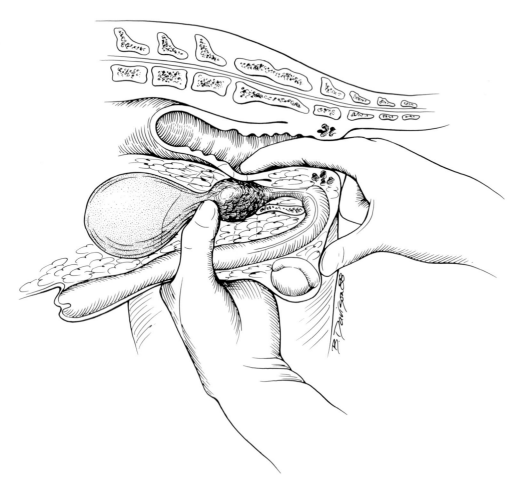

FIG. 4–2. Rectal palpation of the prostate gland in male dogs. One hand should apply pressure on the caudal abdomen while the other palpates rectally. The prostate gland, when enlarged, can be palpated in the caudal abdomen as well as per rectum.

urinalysis, and urine culture. Evaluation of prostatic fluid obtained by ejaculation or after prostatic massage is often necessary. Ultrasonography and survey and contrast-enhanced radiography are required in some cases. Prostatic biopsy is considered the definitive test. The performance and interpretation of these tests is reviewed in Chapter 5. The use of these tests to arrive at a specific diagnosis is discussed in Chapter 27.

REFERENCES

1. Neumann, F., Tunn, U., and Funke, P.J.: Male accessory sex glands: Experimental basis and animal models in prostatic tumor research. *In* Animal Models in Human Reproduction. Edited by M. Serio and L. Marteni. New York, Raven Press, pp. 249–282, 1980.
2. Christensen, G.E.: The urogenital apparatus. *In* Miller's Anatomy of the Dog. 2nd ed. Edited by H.E. Evans and G.E. Christensen. Philadelphia, W.B. Saunders, pp. 544–601, 1979.
3. Gordon, N.: Position of the canine prostate gland. Am. J. Vet. Res., *22*:142, 1961.
4. Stead, A.C., and Borthwick, R.: The canine urinary bladder and prostate. J. Sm. Anim. Pract., *17*:629, 1976.
5. Isaacs, W.B.: Structural and functional components in normal and hyperplastic canine prostates. Prog. Clin. Biol. Res., *145*:307, 1984.
6. Merk, F.B., Ofner, P., and Kwan, P.W.L.: Ultrastructural and biochemical expressions of divergent differentiation in prostates of castrated dogs treated with estrogen and androgen. Lab. Invest., *47*:437, 1982.
7. Leav, I., and Cavazos, L.F.: Some morphologic features of normal and pathologic canine prostate. *In* Normal and Abnormal Growth of the Prostate. Edited by M. Goldand. Springfield, Ill., Charles C. Thomas, pp. 69–101, 1975.
8. Berry, S.J., Coffey, D.S., and Ewing, L.L.: Effects of aging on prostate growth in Beagles. Am. J. Physiol., *250* (Regulative Integrative Comp. Physiol. 19):R1039, 1986.
9. Bruschini, H., Schmidt, R.A., and Tanagho, E.A.: Neurologic control of prostatic secretion in the dog. Invest. Urol., *15*:288, 1978.
10. Farrell, J.I.: The newer physiology of the prostate gland. J. Urol., *39*:171, 1938.
11. Kirby, R.S., Lowe, D., and Bultitude, M.I.: Intra-prostatic urinary reflux: An aetiological factor in abacterial prostatitis. Br. J. Urol., *54*:729, 1982.
12. Isaacs, J.T.: Common characteristics of human and canine benign prostatic hyperplasia. Prog. Clin. Biol. Res., *145*:217, 1984.
13. Huggins, C., and Clark, P.G.: Quantitative studies of prostatic secretion II. The effect of castration and of estrogen injection on the normal and on the hyperplastic prostate glands of dogs. J. Exp. Med., *72*:747, 1940.
14. Brendler, C.B., Berry, S.J., and Ewing, L.L.: Spontaneous benign prostatic hyperplasia in the Beagle. J. Clin. Invest., *71*:1114, 1983.
15. James, R.W., and Heywood, R.: Age-related variations in the testes and prostate of Beagle dogs. Toxicology, *12*:273, 1979.
16. Schlotthauer, C.F.: Observations on the prostate gland of the dog. J. Am. Vet. Med. Assoc., *81*:645, 1932.
17. Zuckerman, S., and McKeown, T.: The canine prostate in relation to normal and abnormal testicular changes. J. Pathol. Bacteriol., *46*:7, 1938.
18. O'Shea, J.D.: Studies on the canine prostate gland. J. Comp. Path., *72*:321, 1962.
19. Ewing, L.L., Thompson, D.L., and Cochran, R.C.: Testicular androgen and estrogen secretion and benign hyperplasia in the Beagle. Endocrinology, *114*:1308, 1984.
20. Berry, S.J., Strandberg, J.D., and Saunders, W.J.: Development of canine benign prostatic hyperplasia with age. Prostate, *9*:363, 1986.
21. Zirkin, B.R., and Strandberg, J.D.: Quantitative changes in the morphology of the aging canine prostate. Anat. Rec., *208*:207, 1984.
22. DeKlerk, D.P., Coffey, D.S., and Ewing, L.L.: Comparison of spontaneous and experimentally induced canine prostatic hyperplasia. J. Clin. Invest., *64*:842, 1979.
23. Leav, I., and Cavazos, L.F.: Some morphologic features of normal and pathologic canine prostate. *In* Normal and Abnormal Growth of the Prostate. Edited by M. Goland. Springfield, Ill., Charles C. Thomas, pp. 69–101, 1975.
24. Mulligan, R.M.: Feminization in male dogs: A syndrome associated with carcinoma of the testes and mimicked by the administration of estrogen. Am. J. Pathol., *20*:865, 1944.
25. Barrach, E.R., and Berry, S.J.: DNA synthesis in the canine prostate: Effects of androgen and estrogen treatment. Prostate, *10*:45, 1987.
26. Jacobs, G., Barsanti, J., and Prasse, K.: Colliculus seminalis as a cause of a urethral filling defect in two dogs with Sertoli cell testicular neoplasms. J. Am. Vet. Med. Assoc., *192*:1748, 1988.
27. Spackman, C.J.A., and Roth, L.: Prostatic cyst and concurrent Sertoli cell tumor in a dog. J. Am. Vet. Med. Assoc., *192*:1096, 1988.
28. Akpavie, S.O., and Sullivan, M.: Constipation associated with calcified cystic enlargement of the prostate in a dog. Vet. Rec., *118*:694, 1986.
29. Sisson, D.D., and Hoffer, R.E.: Osteocollagenous prostatic retention cyst: Report of a canine case. J. Am. Anim. Hosp. Assoc., *13*:61, 1977.
30. Christensen, G.S.: The urogenital system and mammary glands. *In* Anatomy of the Dog. Edited by M.E. Miller, G.C. Christensen, and H.E. Evans. Philadelphia, W.B. Saunders, p. 762, 1964.

Section Two

Performance and Interpretation of Diagnostic Tests

5

Diagnostic Tests

This chapter reviews laboratory tests commonly used in the diagnosis of urinary tract diseases. The methodology of the tests and general interpretation of their results are briefly summarized. More information relating specifically to disease states is included in the chapters that follow.

BLOOD TESTS

Serum Urea Nitrogen

Urea nitrogen concentrations in whole blood and in serum are the same; thus, the terms *blood urea nitrogen* (BUN) and *serum urea nitrogen* (SUN) are used interchangeably. Blood urea is derived from dietary protein via hepatic metabolism (see Fig. 3–2). Blood urea is excreted primarily by the kidney. BUN concentrations can be normal, increased, or decreased.

Normal blood urea concentrations have a range (approximately 10 to 30 mg/dl for dogs and cats in many laboratories) of values that reflect differences in dietary protein intake. This threefold variation in normal values and the variability in protein intake prevent detection of significant changes in glomerular filtration rate (GFR). As an example, GFR can decrease by 50% and, although BUN concentration would double from 10 to 20, the clinician would still find a BUN within normal laboratory ranges (see Fig. 3–4). As a general rule, GFR must decrease by 75% for an animal to have consistently elevated BUN concentrations. To reduce fluctuations from protein intake, samples collected after a 12-hour fast should be used. An increased blood urea concentration is referred to as *azotemia*. An approach to azotemia has been reviewed in Chapter 3.

Decreased BUN concentrations can be caused by a very low protein intake, hepatic insufficiency, or urea cycle enzyme abnormalities. In relation to urinary tract diseases, decreased concentrations are much less relevant than increased concentrations. Low protein diets

used for medical dissolution of struvite uroliths, however, often induce lower than normal BUN concentrations.

Urea nitrogen concentrations are usually determined on serum by standard spectrophotometric methods. Although less accurate, test strips (Azostix, Miles Laboratories Inc., Elkhart, IN 46515) are available for rapid evaluation as to whether urea nitrogen concentrations are increased or not. The test strips contain urease and a dye indicator system. Recommended use involves covering the test strip with fresh whole blood, rinsing, and matching the resulting color with color blocks, which range from BUN concentrations of 10 to 60 mg/dl. Although test strip results correlate with results from spectrophotometric methods, the actual numerical results are not the same.[1] Thus, results from test strips should be considered estimates only.

Serum Creatinine

Creatinine is a byproduct of muscle metabolism (see Fig. 3–3). In any individual, the production and excretion of creatinine is constant each day. Between individuals, serum concentrations vary directly with variations in muscle mass. The normal range in dogs and cats is generally less than or equal to 1.5 mg/dl. Creatinine concentrations are determined in serum or plasma and may be normal or increased.

As with BUN, normal serum creatinine (SC) concentration encompasses a wide range. Thus, a substantial decrease in GFR may not increase the SC concentration above the normal range. As with BUN, GFR must decrease by 75% to increase SC concentrations consistently (see Fig. 3–4). Serum creatinine concentrations are generally not affected by diet.[2]

An increase in SC concentration above the normal range usually parallels an increase in BUN and is referred to as azotemia. Chapter 3 discusses the causes for elevations in SC concentration. In uremia, SC concentration does not increase in exact proportion to the decrease in GFR because intestinal bacterial degradation of creatinine increases in a uremic animal (see Fig. 3–3).

Serum creatinine concentration is usually measured spectrophotometrically using the Jaffe (alkaline picrate) procedure. This reaction measures noncreatinine chromagens (such as ketones) as well. Noncreatinine chromagens account for almost 50% of the creatinine measured in serum of normal animals. As renal dysfunction develops and worsens, leading to an increase in SC, noncreatinine chromagens do not increase. Thus, SC concentration measured by alkaline picrate becomes progressively more accurate as the degree of renal dysfunction increases. The influence of noncreatinine chromagens has two important clinical considerations. First, spuriously high SC concentrations can occur in ketoacidotic diabetics. Second, measurement of endogenous creatinine clearance is affected by noncreatinine chromagens as described next under GFR measurements. Newer methods of measuring SC concentration use enzymatic hydrolysis of creatinine, which has fewer false-positive interactions.[3]

MEASUREMENT OF GLOMERULAR FILTRATION RATE

As already noted above, BUN and SC concentrations are used as indicators of GFR. When both are increased above normal, one can assume that GFR is significantly decreased. When BUN and SC are within normal limits, however, one cannot be sure that GFR is normal. Accurate measurement of GFR is the most precise determinant of renal function, but GFR itself is not easily determined. The most reliable measurement of GFR is inulin clearance. This is the standard test with which all other measures of GFR are (or should be) compared. Inulin clearance has not been widely used in clinical small animal medicine. The most widely used measure of GFR in clinical medicine has been endogenous or exogenous creatinine clearance. A radioisotope method, technetium 99m (Tc 99m) diethylene-triaminepentaacetic acid clearance, has been found to correlate well with inulin clearance in dogs.[4,5] This method requires access to nuclear medicine facilities, however.

Endogenous Creatinine Clearance

Endogenous creatinine clearance involves collection of all urine produced during a specific time period, usually 24 hours. It is important that the bladder be empty at the beginning of the test and that all urine produced be collected. The animal is allowed to eat and drink normally during the collection. The volume of urine produced, concentration of creatinine in a mixed aliquot of this urine, and concentration of SC during the collection time (measured either at the midpoint or as an average of samples collected at the beginning and end of urine collection) are used to calculate GFR. Because dogs vary so much in size, the result in milliliters per minute is often divided by body weight (ml/min/kg) or by body surface area (ml/min/m^2). An example of calculating GFR by this method is given in Table 5–1.

Because SC concentration, but not urine creatinine concentration, may be affected by noncreatinine chromagens (depending on the test used to measure creatinine), endogenous creatinine clearance often underestimates GFR, especially in animals whose SC concentrations are normal.[6] Male dogs have a weak secretory mechanism for excretion of creatinine. This is more important in dogs with reduced renal mass than in normal dogs,[7] but the change is not enough to affect interpretation of results in most clinical cases.

A normal value for 24-hour clearance in dogs in one study was 3.7 + 0.77 ml/min/kg.[8] A normal value for a 20-minute clearance test was reported to be 2.98 + 0.96.[7] Normal values for cats have ranged from 2.31 + 0.47 ml/min/kg (24-hour collection)[9] to 2.70 + 1.12 (20-minute collection).[10] These values are consistently lower than inulin clearance in cats (3.5–3.8 ml/min/kg),[10,11] even though creatinine is excreted solely by glomerular filtration in normal cats.[12]

TABLE 5–1. EXAMPLE CALCULATION OF GLOMERULAR FILTRATION RATE USING ENDOGENOUS CREATININE CLEARANCE

A 20-kg dog produces 1200 ml of urine over 24 hours (0.83 ml/min). The urine creatinine concentration is 120 mg/dl and the serum creatinine concentration is 1.4 mg/dl. The dog's creatinine clearance would be:

$$\text{Creatinine clearance (ml/min)} = \frac{\text{urine volume (ml/min)} \times U_c}{S_c}$$

$$U_c = \text{urine creatinine concentration (mg/dl)}$$

$$S_c = \text{serum creatinine concentration (mg/dl)}$$

$$\text{Creatinine clearance (ml/min)} = \frac{0.83 \times 120}{1.4} = 71 \text{ ml/min}$$

$$\text{Creatinine clearance (ml/min/kg)} = \frac{71}{20} = 3.6 \text{ ml/min/kg}$$

Exogenous Creatinine Clearance

Exogenous creatinine clearance involves injection of creatinine and then timed urine collections. One method involves subcutaneous injection of creatinine followed by collection of urine from 40 to 60 minutes and 60 to 80 minutes after injection[6,13] (Table 5–2). Calculations are the same as for endogenous creatinine clearance (see Table 5–1). This method correlates well with inulin clearance in dogs. By increasing SC concentrations, the effect of noncreatinine chromogens in serum is reduced, and clearance values are more accurate than with endogenous creatinine clearance. The method also avoids 24-hour urine collections, which are often difficult to obtain in a practice setting. Normal values in dogs are 4.0 + 0.5 ml/min/kg.[6] Normal values in cats have not been determined for subcutaneous injection of creatinine, but are 2.94 + 0.32 ml/min/kg with 20-minute intravenous infusions.[12]

Plasma Clearance Tests

Because of the inconvenience of collecting timed urine samples, several different types of timed blood tests have been evaluated in dogs and cats. Although useful in some situations, these tests are considered less reliable than clearance tests. One plasma clearance test involves intravenous injection of 0.2 ml/kg 5% sodium sulfanilate with collection of heparinized blood samples at 30, 60, and 90 minutes. The plasma half-life is calculated. Excretion of sodium sulfanilate was shown to correlate with GFR in cats.[11] Normal half-life in cats is 40 to 50 minutes.[11] Although the test was sufficiently accurate to detect unilateral nephrectomy in dogs,[14] it was not superior to loss of concentrating ability as an indicator of renal dysfunction in clinically ill dogs. Normal values in dogs are 50 to 80 minutes.[15]

URINE TESTS

As discussed previously, knowledge of the method of urine collection is of utmost importance in interpreting the results of a urinalysis or urine culture. The results of these tests should *always* include the method by which the sample was collected. The results of tests on urine may be affected by diagnostic tests such as contrast-enhanced radiography[16] and by therapy, for example, with fluids, diuretics, or antibiotics. For these reasons, urine should be collected for urinalysis and urine culture before therapy or contrast-enhanced radiography, unless the animal's condition precludes such collection.

Urinalysis

A complete urinalysis, including observation of color and turbidity, measurement of urine specific gravity, qualitative chemical analysis by reagent strip (dipstick) or tablets, and microscopic examination of urine sediment, is essential in evaluating the dog or cat with suspected urinary tract disease. In one survey of dogs with suspected urinary tract disease and with negative dipstick evaluations, 38% had abnormal urine sediments.[17] Thus, a normal urine dipstick evaluation does not indicate that the urine is necessarily normal.

Urine should be examined as soon as possible after collection. If urine cannot be examined within 30 minutes, the sample should be refrigerated and examined within 6 hours. If refrigerated, urine should be allowed to return to room temperature before dipstick analysis. Dipstick reactions can change with temperature, and crystals are more likely to precipitate at lower temperatures. Formed elements deteriorate after storage for more than several hours.

Normal urine color is yellow. The depth of urine color varies with concentration and presence of urine pigments. Normal urine varies in turbidity, depending on concentration and type of suspended particles.

Urine Specific Gravity

Urine specific gravity is used as a measure of urine concentration. Water intake and urine output are directly related, unless a substantial nonrenal source of water loss exists (such as severe diarrhea). Any urine specific

---

TABLE 5–2. DIRECTIONS FOR MEASUREMENT OF GLOMERULAR FILTRATION RATE BY EXOGENOUS CREATININE CLEARANCE IN THE DOG*

1. Fast dog for 8 to 12 hours. Allow free access to water
2. Weigh dog to the nearest 0.1 kg
3. Administer 2 ml/kg creatinine solution (50 mg/ml) SQ for dogs up to 20 kg and 1.5 ml/kg SC for dogs over 20 kg; 10 ml is injected per site. Start timer. (Creatinine solution is prepared by mixing 10 g of creatinine powder [Sigma Chemical Company, St. Louis, MO 63178] with 200 ml of distilled water. The solution should be sterilized)
4. Immediately after the injection of creatinine, pass a stomach tube, and give a volume of water equal to 3% of body weight (e.g., a 10-kg dog would receive 0.3 kg or 300 ml)
   Urine collection—Two 20-min collection periods (40–60 and 60–80 min after creatinine injection)
5. At about 30 min after creatinine injection, pass a urinary catheter so that urine collection can begin at 40 min after creatinine injection. To ensure the bladder is empty before beginning urine collection, remove all urine, and rinse the bladder with 50 ml sterile saline at least twice. Discard urine and rinses. The rinses should occur at about 38–40 min
6. At 40 min, timed urine collection begins
7. Collect a blood sample at 40 min
8. At 58 min, begin emptying the bladder. Use one 50-ml rinse of saline. Complete urine collection at 60 min. Combine and save all urine and flushes collected from 40–60 min
9. Collect a blood sample at 60 min
10. Repeat urine collection as in No. 8 from 60–80 min
11. Collect blood sample at 80 min
12. Measure creatinine in serum collected at 40, 60, and 80 min. Measure creatinine in urine collected 40–60 min and 60–80 min. Calculate creatinine clearance for the two 20-min collection periods

* Derived from references 6 and 13.

gravity value can be normal, depending on degree of hydration. If the animal is dehydrated, urine should be concentrated (urine specific gravity > 1.035 for dogs and cats). If the animal is overhydrated, urine should be dilute (<1.008). Another measure of urine concentration is osmolality. Osmolality is related only to the number of particles in solution and is unaffected by particle size and molecular weight, which do influence specific gravity. Urine osmolality is more difficult to measure than specific gravity. Thus, specific gravity is the standard clinical measure of urine concentration, with osmolality reserved for in-depth study of animals with unusual or difficult to solve disorders of urine concentration or dilution.

Urine pH

Normal urine pH varies from 5.0 to 8.5. The more carnivorous the diet, the more acidic the urine pH (except for the few hours after eating). Cat and dog urine is usually acidic when the cat or dog is consuming a meat-based diet. Urine becomes alkaline after eating (*postprandial alkaline tide*). The degree of alkalinity varies directly with the amount of vegetable protein consumed.

Urine Protein

Normal urine protein varies with degree of urine concentration. In concentrated urine (>1.035), a protein of trace to 1^+ is considered normal. In nonconcentrated urine, any amount of protein may be significant. Measurement of urine protein by reagent strip is qualitative only and is subject to observer variability. Reagent strips are more sensitive to albumin than globulins. Thus, proteinuria caused by myeloma, which is mostly globulins, may not be detected by reagent strips. Because of this and because of variability in reading the reagent strips for protein, many laboratories use qualitative turbidometric methods for proteinuria, such as the sulfosalicylic acid test or the nitric acid ring test. Confirmation of significant proteinuria may require protein quantitation (see later), especially when the degree of proteinuria is marginal.

Other Urine Dipstick Tests

Other useful urine dipstick tests include those for glucose, ketones, bilirubin, and blood. The dipstick test for glucose is highly specific for glucose, although numbers printed on the various color results do not correlate well with spectrophotometric methods. The sticks are better read as "trace, 1^+, 2^+, 3^+" rather than by the numbers listed. Only highly oxidizing contaminants, such as chlorine, result in false-positive tests. Glucose is not present in normal canine or feline urine. If glucose is found, either the renal threshold for reabsorption of glucose has been exceeded or a defect in proximal tubular reabsorption of glucose exists. Measurement of blood glucose concentration would be the first step in approaching the problem of glucosuria. In dogs, the renal threshold for glucose reabsorption is exceeded when the plasma concentration of glucose exceeds 180 mg/dl. In cats, the renal threshold for glucose reabsorption is not exceeded until the plasma concentration of glucose exceeds 300 mg/dl.[18]

The reagents on the dipstick for ketones react with acetoacetic acid primarily. Ketonuria is primarily associated with diabetes mellitus. Ketonuria is uncommon in urinary tract diseases except in association with severe anorexia.

The reagent strip for bilirubin detects conjugated urine bilirubin. The test must be conducted on fresh urine (less than 30 minutes after collection), which has not been excessively exposed to light. Normal canine urine can contain trace to 2^+ bilirubin, depending on urine specific gravity (the more concentrated the sample, the higher the normal dipstick reading). Normal feline urine does not contain bilirubin. Abnormal bilirubinuria usually reflects the problem of icterus. Icterus is uncommonly related to urinary tract disease except in association with sepsis. In septicemia, normal hepatic excretion of bilirubin may be impaired.

The reagent strip test for "blood" detects hemoglobin, either free or within red blood cells (RBCs), or myoglobin. A finding of positive occult blood should first prompt a close examination of the urine sediment for RBCs. The presence of more than 5 to 20 intact RBCs gives at least a "trace" positive reaction. Lysed RBCs release hemoglobin, also resulting in a positive test. If RBCs are not present, the serum should be examined for hemolysis. Hemoglobinuria follows the development of hemoglobinemia, visible as red discoloration of plasma. Myoglobinuria is derived from myoglobinemia caused by muscle disease or injury. Muscle injury that is severe enough to result in myoglobinemia is uncommon in dogs and cats. Myoglobinemia does not change the serum color. An ammonium sulfate precipitation test on urine can also be used to differentiate hemoglobin from myoglobin. Myoglobin is soluble in 70 to 80% ammonium sulfate, but hemoglobin precipitates.

Dipstick tests for bacteria and leukocytes are inaccurate for dogs and cats. A recently introduced dipstick test for specific gravity has yet to be evaluated in companion animals. It measures only urine specific gravities less than 1.030 and is pH dependent; both factors may limit its usefulness in dogs and cats.[19]

Sediment Examination

The purpose of the sediment examination is to identify cells, microorganisms, renal tubular casts, and crystals. The sediment examination of urine is generally performed on a wet mount of unstained, centrifuged urine. Ten milliliters of urine is centrifuged for 5 to 10 minutes at 350 × g. Lesser speeds can be used for longer times.[20] The urine is decanted and the sediment resuspended in the remaining drop of urine. The method is not quantitative because of variations in volume of initial urine, amount of urine decanted, and volume of sediment placed on the slide.

The sediment is generally examined for cells on high power (40× objective). The numbers of RBCs and white blood cells (WBCs) are counted per field and reported per high-power field (hpf; see Fig. 2–1). Normal numbers are less than 5 RBC/hpf and less than 5 WBC/hpf. RBCs may be introduced into urine by trauma during catheterization or cystocentesis. Although numbers of RBCs introduced during these procedures are usually low (<50/hpf), larger numbers are possible.[21] Dipstick tests for pyuria are not accurate in dogs.[22]

The number of bacteria are also usually determined on high-power microscopic examination (see Fig. 2–6). Urine collected from the bladder by cystocentesis should contain no bacteria. Urine collected by catheterization, voluntary voiding, or bladder expression may be contaminated by the normal bacterial flora of the distal urethra, reproductive tract, and skin. Bacteria are usually reported as trace (occasional bacteria but not in all fields), 1^+ (1 to 10 organisms/hpf), 2^+ (11 to 100 organisms/hpf), 3^+ (>100 organisms/hpf), and 4^+ (too numerous to attempt to count).[20] Many attempts have been made to correlate these estimates with quantitative urine culture results. In general, sensitivity and specificity for urine microscopy in estimating quantitative urine culture results have been variable.[20] One major problem has been accurately distinguishing cocci from random brownian movement of particles within urine. Fairly large numbers of bacteria (>10^4/ml) must be present in urine to be detected by microscopic examination. Thus, any bacteria observed in urine collected by cystocentesis are considered significant (although the possibility of contamination from the skin or gastrointestinal tract or during sample handling must be considered). If bacteria are seen in urine collected by catheterization, the sample must be quantitatively cultured to assess significance of the observed bacteria. If bacteria are seen in urine collected by voluntary voiding or midstream expression, another sample collected by cystocentesis should be evaluated to distinguish infection from contamination.

The presence of bacteria can be more accurately determined by the use of Gram-stained smears of centrifuged urine and an oil immersion lens, although occasional false-negative and false-positive results still occur.[20,23] Use of Gram stains has the added advantage of identifying the causative organism as gram-positive or gram-negative to assist in antibiotic choice, pending urine culture results.

The most commonly seen renal tubular cast is the granular cast, composed of renal tubular cell debris as a result of renal tubular cell turnover (Fig. 5–1). A low number (<2/low-power field (lpf), <6/hpf) of granular casts are found in normal urine. Higher numbers of casts indicate ongoing renal tubular injury. Hyaline casts, which are composed of Tamm-Horsfall protein, are occasionally seen in low numbers in normal urine (<1/lpf; see Fig. 2–11). Higher numbers are often associated with glomerular diseases, since Tamm-Horsfall protein tends to precipitate in the presence of albumin. Waxy and broad casts (Fig. 5–2) are usually associated with slow urine flow rates (oliguria). Cellular casts (RBC and WBC casts) are rare but are always abnormal and indicate renal hemorrhage or inflammation, respectively.

Struvite crystals are commonly seen in normal dog and cat urine and, by themselves, do not indicate urinary tract disease. The number of crystals seen is affected by urine temperature, urine concentration, and urine pH. Urate crystals can be seen normally in Dalmatians. In other breeds, urate crystals may indicate hepatic failure. Cystine crystals are abnormal and indicate abnormal cystine reabsorption. The major significance is to indicate a predisposition to the formation of cystine calculi. Oxalate crystals are occasionally seen normally, but when present in large numbers or in association with acute renal failure suggest ethylene glycol toxicity (Fig. 5–3). Bilirubin crystals are occasionally seen normally in dogs or in association with bilirubinuria in dogs or cats. Color prints to assist in identification of urine crystals in animals have been published.[24]

Other findings on urine sediment examination can include parasitic ova (*Capillaria*, *Dictyophyma*; see Fig. 2–5). Occasionally, hyperplastic or neoplastic epithelial cells may be identified.

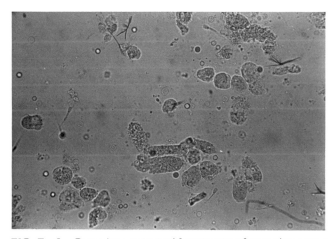

FIG. 5–1. Granular casts and fragments of granular casts in urine. (Courtesy of Dr. R. Duncan, Department of Pathology, College of Veterinary Medicine, University of Georgia.)

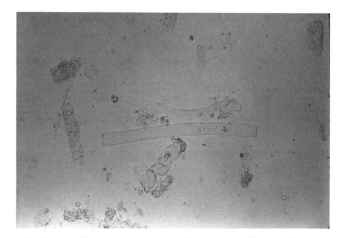

FIG. 5–2. Waxy cast in urine. (Courtesy of Dr. R. Duncan, Department of Pathology, College of Veterinary Medicine, University of Georgia.)

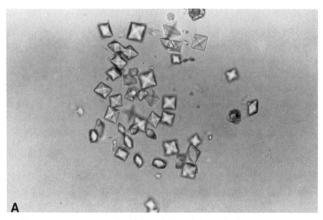

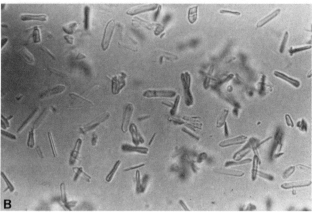

FIG. 5–3. Oxalate crystals in urine of a dog that had ingested ethylene glycol. (A) Calcium oxalate dihydrate; (B) calcium oxalate monohydrate. (Courtesy of Drs. R. Duncan, K. Prasse, K. Lattimer, E. Mahaffey, and W. Crowell, Department of Pathology, College of Veterinary Medicine, University of Georgia.)

Urine Bacterial Culture

The definitive test for the presence of urinary tract infection is urine culture. In general, quantitative cultures are preferred. Quantitative cultures are essential for samples collected by catheterization because of possible contamination from the normal distal urethral flora. Collection of urine for culture by voluntary voiding or manual expression is discouraged because of the high probability of sample contamination.

Following collection, urine should be cultured within 6 hours to prevent change in bacterial numbers. Urine should always be stored at refrigeration temperatures (4°C) following collection. If urine cannot be cultured within 6 hours, it should be placed in a preservative such as boric acid–glycerol–sodium formate (Methyl-p-hydroxybenzoate, Eastman Kodak Co., Rochester, NY 14850) and maintained at refrigeration temperatures until cultured within 72 hours.[23]

Protein Quantitation

In an animal with proteinuria and normal urine sediment examination, which excludes hemorrhage or inflammation as sources of urine protein, the origin of the urine protein is usually renal. Small amounts of excessive protein loss are associated with renal tubular diseases, whereas low to very high amounts of protein loss are found with glomerular diseases. As described for urinalysis, an estimate of urine protein loss can be obtained by comparing the dipstick estimate of proteinuria with urine specific gravity. More precise determination of the severity of urine protein loss, however, requires quantitation of urine protein.

The most accurate measure of urine protein is measurement over at least 24 hours. More than a single 24-hour collection is optimal because day to day variation can be substantial.[9] With this method, all urine is collected for 24 hours. Urine protein is measured (usually by a spectrophotometric method for small quantities of protein such as Coomassie Brilliant Blue). Urine volume is also measured. Results are returned from the laboratory as milligrams per deciliter of protein. This value is then multiplied by urine volume to determine milligrams per 24 hours. For example, a dog produced 1200 ml of urine over 24 hours. An aliquot of this urine has 200 mg/dl protein. The dog thus lost 2400 mg (2.4 g) protein/24 hours. Normal values are <200 mg/24 hours in dogs[25] and <120 mg/24 hours in cats.[9] An association of urine protein loss with body weight in normal dogs has been shown.[26] The correlation is statistically significant, but a wide variation occurs. These authors have recommended a maximal normal value of 22 mg/kg/day. Others have recommended 10 mg/kg/day.[27]

An estimate of urine protein loss can be obtained by determining a urine protein to urine creatinine ratio.[28] Because creatinine is excreted at a constant rate each day in each individual (unless renal function is changing), urine creatinine concentrations primarily fluctuate with urine concentration. Use of urine creatinine concentration provides a control for urine protein changes caused by changes in urine concentration. The urine protein to urine creatinine ratio in most normal dogs is <0.2. A value of >1.0 is abnormal, with values in between indeterminate. Urine protein to urine creatinine ratio works well as a screening test for abnormal proteinuria. Whether this ratio can be used repeatedly to evaluate an animal for changes in severity of renal disease remains unanswered.

Urine Concentration Tests

Dogs and cats with polydipsia and polyuria may have a renal defect in urine concentrating ability or may have a nonrenal disease that prevents the kidneys from concentrating urine. An example of such a nonrenal disease is pituitary-origin diabetes insipidus, a deficiency of antidiuretic hormone (ADH).

There are two types of tests used to evaluate urine concentrating ability: water deprivation test and ADH response test. A test of ability to concentrate urine is indicated for the clinical problems of polyuria/polydipsia or specific gravity values consistently <1.030 with the following reservations.

A complete serum biochemical profile should be performed first to identify a potential cause of the decreased urine concentration. Water deprivation testing is contraindicated in animals that are unequivocally azotemic. Diagnostic efforts should focus on the cause of azotemia. Water deprivation tests should *never* be performed on an animal that is already dehydrated. The test is needless in such cases because stimulus to concentrate is already present. It is also dangerous because it imposes additional dehydration on an already compromised animal. Water deprivation testing is also contraindicated when laboratory evaluation reveals a cause of polyuria such as diabetes mellitus, hypercalcemia, or electrolyte disorders (see Table 1–1). Water deprivation tests are difficult to perform in cats.

The water deprivation test acts by inducing endogenous secretion of ADH. Endogenous secretion of ADH should be stimulated with loss of 3% of body water. The test is performed by abruptly or gradually withholding water. Gradual withdrawal of water has been advocated by some clinicians because of concern that any cause of polyuria may cause medullary washout of solute and decreased concentrating ability. Dogs with induced diabetes insipidus, however, maintained some medullary hyperosmolality, and dogs with induced and spontaneous diabetes insipidus responded to pitressin tannate within 24 hours, indicating medullary hypertonicity is not lost from severe polyuria alone.[29,30] Certain drugs such as furosemide, however, can result in medullary washout. Thus, whether medullary washout exists or not may vary with the underlying disease process. We generally perform abrupt water deprivation testing.

The abrupt water deprivation test is described in Chapter 1. The test is always performed under hospital conditions so that the animal can be closely monitored. The test should not be performed by having the owner withhold water at home, risking severe dehydration and interfering with adequate interpretation of test results.

The other commonly used test of urine concentration is to administer exogenous ADH. Regardless of hydration status, concentrated urine should be produced by a normal kidney. The test can be used in cats. Aqueous pitressin, pitressin tannate in oil, or synthetic preparations of ADH can be used. We usually use pitressin tannate in oil. Tests of responsiveness to ADH are described in Chapter 1.

KIDNEY BIOPSY

Kidney biopsies are performed to determine the precise cause of abnormalities in renal structure or function. Indications for kidney biopsy are problems such as persistent abnormal proteinuria of renal origin or renal failure in which the results of the biopsy might alter prognosis or therapy. The clinician should perform noninvasive diagnostic tests, such as complete blood count, biochemical profile, urine tests, radiography, and ultrasonography, first. On the basis of these tests, the problem should be clearly defined (such as chronic, azotemic, renal failure) and a list of differential diagnoses formulated. The clinician should determine whether making a precise diagnosis via biopsy would alter treatment or prognosis. If the answer to that question is yes, a biopsy is indicated.

Kidneys are highly vascular organs, each receiving 10% of cardiac output,[31] and significant hemorrhage is a potential complication of any biopsy procedure. To reduce the chances of severe hemorrhage, coagulation tests should be performed before the biopsy. These should include at least a platelet count and activated clotting time. If coagulopathy is suspected, more extensive coagulation testing is indicated, including measurement of partial thromboplastin time, prothrombin time, thrombin time, and bleeding time. Also, to minimize hemorrhage, the biopsy should be taken from the renal cortex rather than medulla, where large blood vessels are located.[32] The degree of renal damage caused by a biopsy needle is primarily dependent on the size and number of renal vessels damaged.[32,33] Although macroscopic hematuria is rare after renal biopsy (approximately 3% of properly performed biopsies in dogs and cats), self-limiting microscopic hematuria is common for 2 to 3 days.[33,34] Mortality following properly performed renal biopsies is uncommon (<1%) even in severely uremic animals.[33]

To decrease the possibility of blood clots forming within the renal tubules or renal pelvis, which can cause hydronephrosis,[33,34] intravenous fluids should be administered for several hours before and after needle biopsy. Quantity of fluids administered should induce a diuresis. Animals with macroscopic hematuria should be followed closely for the development of acute anemia. Most do not require transfusion, but blood transfusion should be available if hypotension or severe anemia develops. Severe hemorrhage requiring such therapy has been found to occur in about 3% of biopsies in dogs.[33–35]

Kidney biopsies can be performed either percutaneously or via laparotomy. No comparisons have been made in veterinary medicine, but in human medicine the complication rate is similar.[31] The advantages of percutaneous biopsy are shorter anesthetic time and minimal healing time. As a general rule in small animal practice, percutaneous biopsies are preferred for the same reasons. If a laparotomy is being performed for another reason, however, this is an excellent time to obtain a renal biopsy if abnormalities in renal function or structure have been noted.

Contraindications to renal biopsy include coagulopathies (as already discussed), a single functional kidney, marked hydronephrosis, markedly contracted kidneys, large cysts, suspected abscessation, and acute pyelonephritis.[31] Biopsies are usually unrewarding in cases of chronic, end-stage renal disease because the lesion is irreversible and only symptomatic therapy is available at this stage.

Once a biopsy specimen is obtained, it should be placed immediately into the desired fixative. Neutral buffered formalin is recommended for routine histopathology. Kidney samples may also be placed in special fixatives, however, for immunologic evaluation or electron microscopic examination. If renal infection is suspected, the tip of the biopsy needle may be twirled in a tube of culture medium, or a small piece of fresh tissue can be placed in a sterile Petri dish or whirlpack and submitted immediately to a laboratory for bacterial culture.

Percutaneous Kidney Biopsy

Percutaneous kidney biopsies can be performed with guidance by palpation, ultrasonography, or laparoscopy, using a biopsy needle (Tru-Cut biopsy needle, Travenol Laboratories, Inc., Deerfield, IL 60015). We perform most renal biopsies by palpation in cats and by ultrasonography in dogs because feline kidneys are readily palpable, whereas canine kidneys are difficult to immobilize by palpation.[33] If a renal biopsy cannot be obtained under ultrasound guidance in dogs, a ''keyhole'' type percutaneous biopsy is our second choice.[33] Laparoscopy is also acceptable,[35] but in one study, it did not improve the quality of the biopsy specimen or decrease the potential complications, compared with the standard keyhole biopsy.[36]

In cats, a renal aspirate can often be performed with little or no sedation. The side of the cat over the kidney is clipped and scrubbed as for surgery. The kidney is immobilized by palpation (Fig. 5–4). A 21- or 22-gauge needle attached to a syringe or other aspiration device is inserted and aspiration performed. This technique is useful for rapid diagnosis of renomegaly caused by lymphosarcoma or renal cysts, although ultrasonography, where available, is preferable for renal cystic disease. If ultrasonography is unavailable, an aspirate should always be performed before biopsy of enlarged kidneys in cats because of the possibility of polycystic renal disease or perirenal cysts (Fig. 5–5).

A renal biopsy is performed in the same way as a renal aspirate in cats except that the cat is given a short-acting general anesthetic. The purpose of anesthesia is analgesia plus muscle relaxation to permit renal immobilization by palpation. The cat's hair is clipped before in-

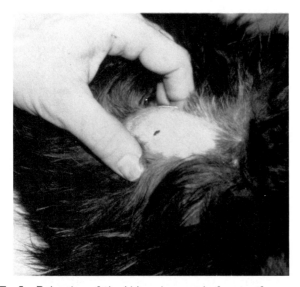

FIG. 5–4. Palpation of the kidney in a cat before performing a renal aspirate.

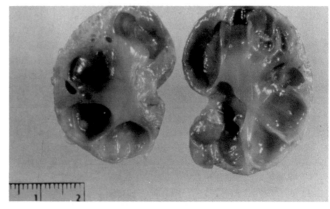

FIG. 5–5. Polycystic renal disease in a cat. A needle biopsy is contraindicated, but such cases can be diagnosed by ultrasonography or renal aspiration. (Courtesy of Dr. W. Crowell, Department of Pathology, College of Veterinary Medicine, University of Georgia.)

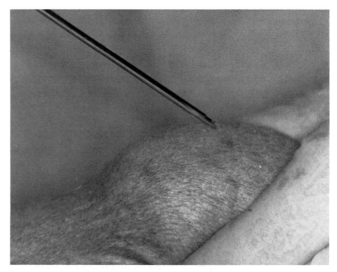

FIG. 5–6. Percutaneous kidney biopsy in the cat. The kidney is immobilized by one hand while the other manipulates the biopsy needle.

ducing anesthesia, anesthesia is induced, and the cat's skin is aseptically prepared. The kidney is palpated and immobilized with one hand, while the other hand inserts the biopsy needle through a small (2 to 4 mm) nick in the skin made with a scalpel blade (see Fig. 5–4; Fig. 5–6). The needle is directed across the cranial or caudal pole of the kidney, avoiding the area around the renal pelvis and the renal medulla (Figs. 5–7, 5–8). The biopsy needle is positioned at the surface of the kidney but not inserted into the kidney before obtaining the biopsy specimen. The Tru-Cut biopsy needle has a solid needle tip, which extends beyond the specimen notch. If this tip is positioned into the kidney, the renal cortex may not be sampled owing to the small size of the kidney.[33] A method of shortening the Tru-Cut biopsy needle to avoid these problems has been described.[37] A sample of renal cortex is essential for proper interpretation of most biopsy specimens to examine glomeruli and tu-

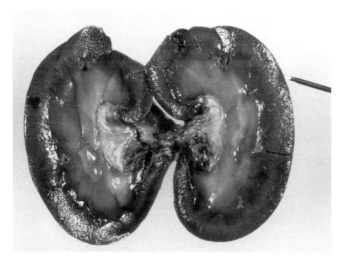

FIG. 5–7. The biopsy needle should be directed across the cranial or caudal pole of the kidney, avoiding the renal pelvis. The needle should be positioned at the surface but not into the kidney. (Courtesy of Dr. D. Finco, Department of Physiology and Pharmacology, College of Veterinary Medicine, University of Georgia.)

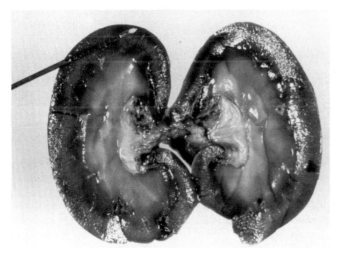

FIG. 5–8. Performance of a renal biopsy, obtaining a sample of the renal cortex across one pole. (From Barsanti, J.A.: Diagnostic procedures in urology, Vet Clin North Am [Sm Anim Pract] 14:3, 1984, with permission.)

sound guidance, if available, using probes with channels for biopsy needle insertion. At least mild sedation and local anesthesia are usually required.

If ultrasound-directed biopsy is unavailable or unsuccessful, a keyhole biopsy can be performed in anesthetized dogs. The right kidney is generally preferred for biopsy if the disease process is thought to affect both kidneys because the right kidney is less mobile. A 7.5- to 10-cm incision is made in the flank, bisecting the angle between the last rib and the edge of the lumbar musculature (Fig. 5–9). The muscle fibers are separated along muscle planes and the peritoneum incised (Fig. 5–10). The incision is made large enough for easy insertion of one index finger. The finger holds the kidney against the edge of the lumbar musculature. The size and conformation of the kidney should be noted. The other hand inserts the biopsy needle through a separate incision. This incision requires only a 2- to 4-mm nick in the skin. The biopsy needle is directed into the peritoneal cavity and positioned at the surface of the kidney so that the needle is directed across the cranial or caudal pole of the kidney[33] (see Fig. 5–5). As in the cat, the needle should not be positioned in the kidney before biopsy. Often an additional person is needed to operate

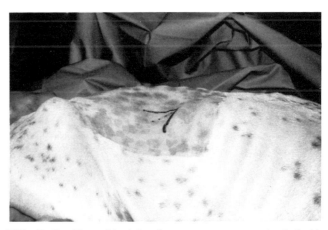

FIG. 5–9. Site of incision for a percutaneous keyhole biopsy in the dog.

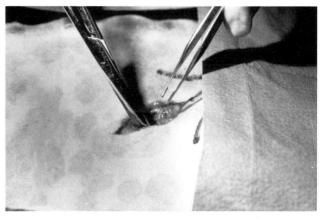

FIG. 5–10. Making the incision for insertion of a finger for percutaneous renal biopsy in the dog.

bules. Also, hemorrhage may be more severe when the corticomedullary junction is penetrated.[32] To obtain a good biopsy specimen, the needle must be thrust rapidly into the kidney. Otherwise the kidney may be pushed away from the needle and only a small specimen obtained. An assistant is usually required to assist in manipulation of the biopsy needle by holding the specimen notch in position as the cutting section is thrust over it. If one individual operates the needle, this person often has difficulty holding the specimen notch in position while thrusting forward with the cutting section. After the biopsy is completed, digital pressure is exerted over the kidney for approximately 5 minutes.

In dogs, renal biopsy can be performed under ultra-

the biopsy needle (see previously under biopsy in the cat). More than one biopsy specimen can be obtained if necessary. After the biopsy is completed, digital pressure is applied over the kidney for approximately 5 minutes. The incision is closed in two layers: subcutaneous tissue and skin.

Surgical Kidney Biopsy

A surgical biopsy specimen of the kidney can be obtained through a paracostal incision or a cranial midline abdominal incision, as described in Chapter 10 (see Figs. 10-1, 10-2, 10-5). The paracostal incision is used when only one kidney requires examination and biopsy, as determined by preoperative evaluation. The cranial midline incision enables the clinician to examine and obtain a biopsy specimen of either or both kidneys.

After the kidney has been immobilized with thumb and forefinger, a wedge-shaped incision is made through the capsule and cortex (Fig. 5–11A). The incision extends into the medulla but not the pelvis. Tissue forceps are used to lift the biopsy sample gently, while any remaining attachments are severed with the scalpel blade (Fig. 5–11B). The biopsy site is closed with a 4–0

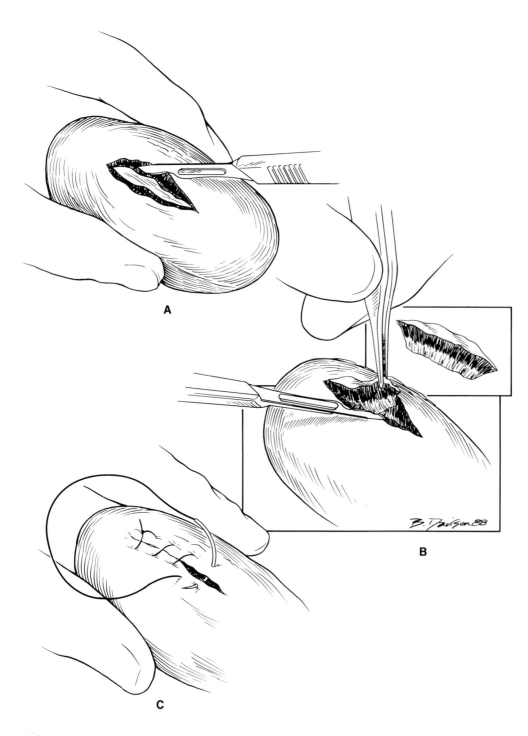

FIG. 5–11. Surgical kidney biopsy. (A) The kidney is immobilized between thumb and forefinger. A wedge-shaped incision is made through the capsule and cortex. (B) Tissue forceps are used to lift the biopsy sample gently. Any remaining attachments are severed with the scalpel blade. (C) The biopsy site is closed with 4–0 monofilament absorbable suture material through the capsule. Pressure is applied with thumb and forefinger to appose the edges during suturing.

monofilament, absorbable suture material in a simple continuous pattern through the capsule (Fig. 5–11C). The thumb and forefinger compress the edges together during suturing.

TESTS FOR PROSTATIC DISEASE

Examination of Urethral Discharge

Examination of a urethral discharge is useful in the diagnostic plan for prostatic disease in dogs because the most common cause of a urethral discharge is disease of the prostate gland. One must also consider urinary incontinence and urethral diseases, however, as potential causes of a urethral discharge. Urinary incontinence can be ruled out by comparing the appearance and microscopic characteristics of the urethral discharge with urine collected from the bladder. Primary urethral diseases are relatively uncommon in dogs with the exceptions of urolithiasis and neoplasia. These are generally accompanied by dysuria, which is uncommon with prostatic disease in the absence of severe prostatomegaly. In some dogs, however, a thorough radiographic or endoscopic evaluation of the urethra may be needed to exclude the possibility of urethral disease.

If urethral discharge is present, it should be examined microscopically. The penis is extruded from the sheath. Any preputial exudate is gently removed with lightly moistened gauze sponges. The discharge is collected on a microscope slide, dried, stained, and examined.

In general, a urethral discharge is not cultured for bacteria because of potential contamination by the normal resident bacterial flora of the distal urethra and prepuce. Samples collected by ejaculation are preferred for culture. If the discharge is purulent and attempts at ejaculate collection are unsuccessful, however, a urethral discharge can be cultured. The penis is extruded from the sheath and gently cleansed with dilute hexachlorophene soap or chlorhexidine solution. The penis is gently dried with a sterile gauze sponge. The discharge is allowed to drip freely into a sterile container (such as a sterile urine cup or syringe case) without the container touching the penis. Quantitative bacterial culture should always be performed because of the presence of normal urethral flora.[38] Any organism isolated by culture is considered significant only if it is present in large numbers (>100,000/ml of urine). Finding the same organism in urine collected by cystocentesis increases the likelihood that the isolated organism is causing infection and is not merely a contaminant.

Examination of Ejaculate

An ejaculate is valuable in assessing prostatic disease because prostatic fluid is the largest component of semen volume (>95% in dogs).[39,40] The prostatic fluid is the last fraction of the ejaculate, following the sperm-rich fraction.

To evaluate a dog for prostatic disease using an ejaculate, first remove any preputial discharge from the penis with gentle, minimal cleansing using gauze sponges and warm water. If any soap is used, it must be rinsed off carefully and the penis dried. Contamination of the sample with detergents can invalidate the quantitative bacterial culture.[41] The ejaculate is collected using a sterile funnel and test tube, a sterile large plastic syringe case, or a sterile urine cup. If the dog does not ejaculate by manual stimulation alone, a teaser is used. The bitch may be one in estrus or an anestrus bitch with the dog phermone, methyl-p-hydroxybenzoate (Eastman Kodak Co.), applied to the vulva.[42] Part of the ejaculate is used for microscopic examination and part for quantitative bacterial culture. Quantitative culture is essential because the distal urethra has a normal bacterial flora.[38]

Both ejaculate cytology and culture must be assessed for accurate interpretation. Normal dogs have occasional WBCs and positive bacterial cultures.[43] In normal ejaculates, bacterial numbers are less than 100,000/ml and are usually gram-positive. High numbers (> 100,000/ml) of gram-negative organisms indicate infection. High numbers of gram-positive organisms with large numbers of WBCs probably also indicate infection if preputial contamination did not occur. Lower numbers of gram-negative or gram-positive organisms must be correlated with clinical signs, results of urinalysis and urine culture, and ejaculate cytology to determine significance.[44] Blood may be found in ejaculates in dogs with bacterial infection, prostatic cysts, prostatic neoplasia, and possibly hyperplasia.

An abnormality in the ejaculate does not localize the problem to the prostate because the testicles, epididymides, deferent ducts, and urethra also contribute to or transport the ejaculate. Collection and comparison of the early fraction of the ejaculate, which is of testicular origin, with a late fraction of prostatic origin may help to localize an abnormal finding. If the ejaculate is milky and uniform throughout, evaluation of the testicles, epididymides, and urethra by palpation and ultrasonography and radiography is indicated.

Use of a urethral swab (Calgiswab Type IV, American Can Co., Glenwood, IL 60425) has been advocated to rule out urethral contamination as a cause of a positive ejaculate culture.[40] With this technique, the sterile swab is advanced several centimeters into the distal urethra after cleansing and drying the penis. The swab is placed in 3 ml of sterile saline and agitated. The saline is then cultured quantitatively. Larger numbers of organisms in the ejaculate than from the urethral swab by a factor of 10^2 is reported to be diagnostic of prostatic infection. In dogs with experimental prostatitis, however, some dogs without prostatic infection had higher numbers of gram-positive organisms in the ejaculate than in the urethral swab, and some dogs with urinary tract infection and prostatic infection had high numbers of the same organism in the urethral swab sample.[44] In men as well, contamination with urethral organisms may be greater in the prostatic fluid than the urethral specimen.[45] Both these problems indicate that results from urethral swabs may be misleading in some dogs. We use urethral swabs primarily in dogs without urinary tract infection and with questionable numbers of organisms in the ejaculate to determine the distal urethral flora of that particular dog for comparison to the suspected infecting agent.

Examination of Prostatic Massage

Because of a dog's pain, inexperience, or temperament, it is not possible to collect semen on all dogs with suspected prostatic disease. An alternative technique for collection of prostatic fluid is prostatic massage.[43] First, the dog is allowed to urinate to empty the bladder. A urinary catheter is then passed to the bladder using aseptic technique. The bladder is emptied, residual urine volume determined, and a sample of urine saved for urinalysis and urine culture. The bladder is flushed several times with sterile saline to ensure that it is empty. The last flush of 5 to 10 ml is saved as the preprostatic massage sample. The catheter is then retracted distal to the prostate as determined by rectal palpation. The prostate is massaged rectally, per abdomen, or both for 1 to 2 minutes. Sterile physiologic saline (5 to 10 ml) is injected slowly through the catheter to prevent reflux of the fluid out the urethral orifice. The catheter is slowly advanced to the bladder with repeated aspiration, especially from the area of the prostate as determined by rectal palpation. The majority of the fluid is aspirated from the bladder. The urine and both the premassage and postmassage samples are examined microscopically and by quantitative culture. It is important to compare the postmassage sample with the premassage sample to be sure any abnormality was caused by prostatic fluid and not diseases of the bladder or urethra. Prostatic massage in normal dogs produces only a few RBCs and transitional epithelial cells.[43] Cytologic evidence of inflammation in the massage sample highly correlates with prostatic infection[44] and is often helpful in determining whether inflammatory prostatic disease exists.

Disadvantages of prostatic massage include the necessity for cytology and culture of two samples (premassage and postmassage) and the difficulty in detecting increased bacterial numbers in prostatic fluid when urine is infected.[41,44] In dogs with urinary tract infection, we have administered antibiotics that enter the urine but do not enter prostatic fluid (e.g., ampicillin)[41,46,47] for 1 day before massage.[44] The samples obtained must be cultured immediately so that the antibiotic in the urine does not kill any bacteria in the prostatic fluid after collection.[41] In experimental infection, this method identified three of six dogs with prostatic infection, but in two of six dogs all cultures became negative in spite of continuing prostatic infection.[44] Whenever antibiotics are being given, even low counts of bacteria may be significant.[41]

In dogs in which involvement of the prostatic urethra is suspected, e.g., in the presence of dysuria or suggestive radiographic findings, a urinary catheter biopsy technique[48] can be combined with prostatic massage. This can be especially useful in cases of neoplasia of either prostatic or transitional epithelial cell origin.[48] A catheter is placed in the urethra with the tip in the prostatic urethra as determined by rectal palpation. A syringe with a small amount of sterile saline is attached

to the catheter. As negative pressure is applied, the catheter is moved rapidly back and forth. Negative pressure is maintained and the catheter quickly withdrawn. Slides for cytology are prepared from the material collected. Normal prostatic epithelial cells are cuboidal and uniform with central, round to oval nuclei and moderate, lightly basophilic cytoplasm.[49] A few large transitional cells are often seen, which may be binucleate.

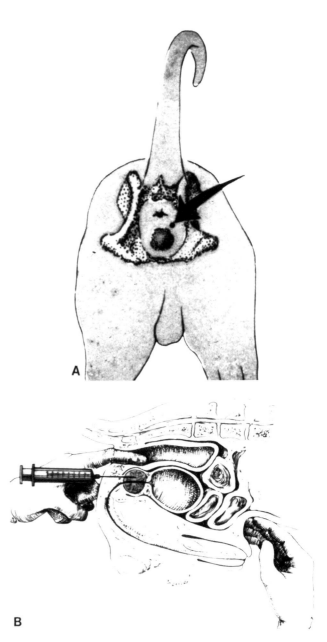

FIG. 5–12. (A) Site of needle insertion for aspiration of the prostate gland via the perirectal approach. (B) Schematic of perirectal aspiration of the prostate gland. The needle is guided into the prostate gland via digital rectal palpation. (From Barsanti, J.A. Canine prostatic disease. *In* Veterinary Internal Medicine. Edited by Ettinger, S. Philadelphia, W.B. Saunders, pp. 1859–1880, 1989; with permission.)

Prostatic Aspirate

Diagnosis of prostatic disease can be aided by needle aspiration. Needle aspiration is most easily done in the dog by the perirectal or transabdominal routes, depending on the location of the prostate gland. The procedure is done aseptically using a long needle with a stylet, such as a spinal needle. In the perirectal approach, the needle is guided by rectal palpation (Fig. 5–12). In the transabdominal approach, the needle can be guided by palpation or ultrasonography.[50] The procedure can be performed in most dogs with mild tranquilization.

Needle aspiration is avoided in dogs with abscessation because large numbers of bacteria may be seeded along the needle tract, or localized peritonitis may develop. In dogs with fever, leukocytosis, or purulent prostatic fluid, aspiration should be performed only after examining fluid obtained by ejaculation or massage, only if it is deemed necessary for case management, and only if potential adverse effects are recognized. Occult abscesses may be present in dogs without fever and leukocytosis. Ultrasonography may help identify such abscesses as cystic lesions and may help guide needle as-

piration. If an abscess is suspected on the basis of laboratory work and ultrasonography but an aspirate is still deemed necessary, the aspirate is performed only after results of urine or prostatic fluid culture are known. The dog is placed on appropriate intravenous antibiotic therapy before, during, and for 24 hours after aspiration. If an abscess is aspirated inadvertently, intravenous antibiotics should be administered immediately and continued for at least 24 hours, followed by oral antimicrobial therapy.

PROSTATIC BIOPSY

Percutaneous Prostatic Biopsy

Percutaneous (closed) prostatic biopsy can be performed perirectally or transabdominally,[43,51,52] using tranquilization and local anesthesia. The biopsy needle (Travenol Laboratories Inc.) can be guided by palpation (Fig. 5–12) or ultrasonography.[50] Because of the possibility of an occult abscess, aspiration should always be performed before a percutaneous biopsy. Parenchymal cystic lesions, identifiable by ultrasonography,

FIG. 5–13. Surgical prostatic biopsy. (A) A wedge-shaped incision is made into the prostatic parenchyma. (B) After the biopsy specimen is removed, the biopsy incision is apposed with 4–0 absorbable suture material in a mattress pattern through the parenchyma.

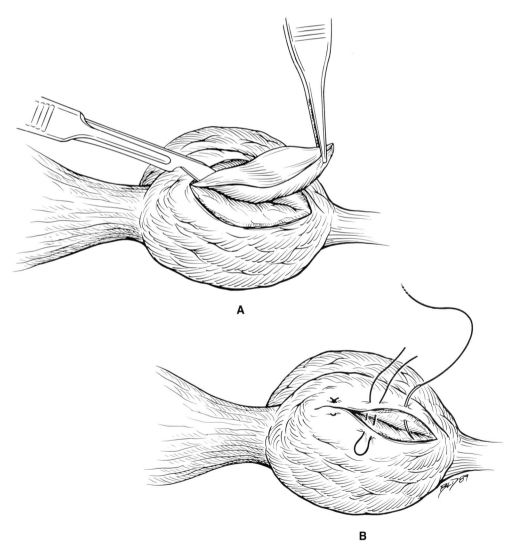

A

B

should be aspirated rather than biopsied. If purulent material is obtained, biopsy should not be performed. Acute, septic inflammation is also considered a contraindication to biopsy. With these precautions, the most common complication reported from biopsy in dogs is mild hematuria,[43,53] although significant hemorrhage is possible as with any biopsy procedure. Orchitis and scrotal edema were reported in one dog.[51] Dogs should be observed closely for several hours after biopsy. Biopsy samples can be used for bacterial culture as well as for histologic examination.

Surgical Prostatic Biopsy

The surgical approach for prostatic biopsy is through a parapreputial abdominal incision, as described in Chapter 10 (see Fig. 10–3). Cystic or abscessed areas should be aspirated before the biopsy specimen is taken. A wedge-shaped incision is made into the prostatic parenchyma (Fig. 5–13A). If the location of the urethra is obscure, a urethral catheter should be placed before the biopsy to identify the urethra. The biopsy site is apposed with 4–0 absorbable suture material in a mattress pattern through the parenchyma (Fig. 5–13B). Additional sites may be biopsied to diagnose diverse disease processes within the prostate.

ELECTRODIAGNOSTIC TESTS

The ability of the lower urinary tract to store and expel urine can be evaluated by electrodiagnostic testing. Cystometry and urethral profilometry are most frequently indicated in animals with incontinence in which the cause is difficult to determine. See Chapter 1 for help in diagnosing incontinence. Such testing requires specialized equipment, generally confined to referral centers. The techniques are only briefly described to assist the reader in determining in which animals referral for these procedures would be useful.

Cystometry

Cystometry is used to evaluate the ability of the bladder to relax and store appropriate urine volumes and its ability to contract when full.[54] Cystometry is generally performed under xylazine restraint to minimize movement artifact and to reduce the incidence of voluntary inhibition of the detrusor reflex.[55,56] Cystometry is most useful to determine whether the bladder is capable of contracting or to determine whether bladder storage capacity is normal (Fig. 5–14).

Urethral Profilometry

The function of the urethra can be evaluated by measuring pressure throughout the entire urethra at rest (resting urethral pressure profile, Fig. 5–15)[57,58] or by measuring urine flow through the urethra (urethral flowmetry).[59,60] Electromyography (EMG) of the urethra can be performed simultaneously.

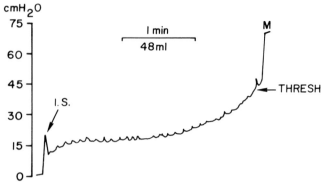

FIG. 5–14. Cystometrogram from a normal dog under xylazine restraint. The vertical axis indicates intravesicular pressure. The horizontal axis indicates intravesicular volume. In this animal, CO_2 was infused at approximately 50 ml/min. The initial spike is an artifact of the gas filling the catheter. Note that there is little change in pressure as the bladder fills until the bladder contracts. When the bladder contracts, the intravesicular pressure rises rapidly and then falls as the CO_2 is expelled. (From Barsanti, J.A.: Diagnostic procedures in urology. Vet Clin North Am [Sm Anim Pract] 14:3, 1984, with permission.)

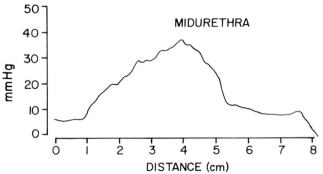

FIG. 5–15. A urethral pressure profile from a normal female dog under xylazine restraint. Pressure is recorded on the vertical axis and urethral length on the horizontal axis. The tracing begins at resting bladder pressure. When the catheter is withdrawn from the bladder and enters the urethra, pressure begins to increase. Maximal pressure is exerted in the midurethra in female dogs. (From Rosin, A.E., and Barsanti, J.A.: Diagnosis of urinary incontinence in dogs: Role of the urethral pressure profile. J Am Vet Med Assoc 178:814, 1981; with permission.)

The urethral pressure profile has been more frequently used in dogs and cats than urethral flowmetry. The urethral pressure profile can be performed with or without xylazine restraint. Xylazine restraint results in lower urethral pressures and eliminates or markedly attenuates the EMG response.[61] The urethral pressure profile is used to determine whether resting pressure is normal or reduced and whether areas of increased pressure, associated with possible partial urethral obstruction, are detectable.

ENDOSCOPY

The mucosal surface of the lower urinary tract can be examined by endoscopy. Endoscopes can be passed through the urethra to the bladder in dogs[62] or can be inserted into the bladder percutaneously.[63]

A small (3 Fr) flexible endoscope can be passed through the urethra of most male dogs. This allows visualization of the urethral lumen and mucosa. Endoscopes of this small size generally do not have biopsy capability. Such endoscopes often do not permit adequate visualization of the bladder lumen. Visualization of the bladder in these cases requires cystotomy or percutaneous endoscopy.

Larger, rigid cystoscopes can be used to see the mucosal surfaces of the urethra and bladder of female dogs. Biopsies can be obtained through these instruments.

REFERENCES

1. Watson, A.D.J., and McDonald, P.J.: Comparison of several laboratory tests for quantifying azotemia in dogs. Aust. Vet. J., 57:407, 1981.
2. Epstein, M.E., Barsanti, J.A., Finco, D.R., et al.: Postprandial changes in plasma urea nitrogen and plasma creatinine concentrations in dogs fed commercial diets. J. Am. Anim. Hosp. Assoc., 20:779, 1984.
3. Mitchell, E.K.: Flucytosine and false elevation of serum creatinine level. Ann. Intern. Med., 101:278, 1984.
4. Krawiec, D.R., Twardock, R., Badertscher, R.R., et al.: Use of 99mTc diethylenetriaminepentaacetic acid for assessment of renal function in dogs with suspected renal disease. J. Am. Vet. Med. Assoc., 192:1077, 1988.
5. Krawiec, D.R., Badertscher, R.R., Twardock, A.R., et al.: Evaluation of 99mTc diethylenetriaminepentaacetic acid nuclear imaging for quantitative determination of the glomerular filtration rate of dogs. Am. J. Vet. Res., 47:2175, 1986.
6. Finco, D.R., Coulter, D.B., and Barsanti, J.A.: Simple, accurate method for clinical estimation of glomerular filtration rate in the dog. Am. J. Vet. Res., 42:1874, 1981.
7. Robinson, T., Harbison, M., and Bovee, K.C.: Influence of reduced renal mass on tubular secretion in the dog. Am. J. Vet. Res., 35:487, 1974.
8. Bovee, K.C., and Joyce, T.: Clinical evaluation of glomerular function: 24 hour creatinine clearance in dogs. J. Am. Vet. Med. Assoc., 174:488, 1979.
9. Russo, E.A., Lees, G.E., and Hightower, D.: Evaluation of renal function in cats, using quantitative urinalysis. Am. J. Vet. Res., 47:1308, 1986.
10. Osbaldison, G.W., and Fuhrman, W.: The clearance of creatinine, inulin, paraminohippurate, and phenosulphothalein in the cat. Can. J. Comp. Med., 24:138, 1970.
11. Ross, L.A., and Finco, D.R.: Relationship of selected renal function tests to glomerular filtration and renal plasma flow in cats. Am. J. Vet. Res., 42:1704, 1981.
12. Finco, D.R., and Barsanti, J.A.: Mechanism of urinary excretion of creatinine by the cat. Am. J. Vet. Res., 43:2207, 1982.
13. Finco, D.R., Coulter, D.B., and Barsanti, J.A.: Procedure for a simple method of measuring glomerular filtration rate in the dog. J. Am. Anim. Hosp. Assoc., 18:804, 1982.
14. Carlson, G.P., and Kaneko, J.J.: Sulfanilate clearance in clinical renal disease in the dog. J. Am. Vet. Med. Assoc., 158:1235, 1971.
15. Maddison, J.E., Pascoe, P.J., and Jansen, B.S.: Clinical evaluation of sodium sulfanilate clearance for the diagnosis of renal disease in dogs. J. Am. Vet. Med. Assoc., 185:961, 1984.
16. Feeney, D.A., Walter, P.A., and Johnston, G.R.: The effect of radiographic contrast media on the urinalysis. In Current Veterinary Therapy IX. Edited by R.W. Kirk. Philadelphia, W.B. Saunders, pp. 1115–1118, 1986.
17. Fettman, M.J.: Evaluation of the usefulness of routine microscopy in canine urinalysis. J. Am. Vet. Med. Assoc., 190:892, 1987.
18. Kruth, S.A., and Cowgill, L.D.: Renal glucose transport in the cat. In American College of Veterinary Internal Medicine, Scientific Proceedings, p. 78, 1983.
19. Jackson, J.A., and Conrad, M.E.: Technical aspects of urine dipstick reagent areas. Am. Clin. Prod. Rev., Dec:10, 1985.
20. Jenkins, R.D., Fenn, J.P., and Matsen, J.M.: Review of urine microscopy for bacteriuria. J.A.M.A., 255:3397, 1986.
21. Comer, K.M., and Ling, G.V.: Results of urinalysis and bacterial culture of canine urine obtained by antepubic cystocentesis, catheterization, and the midstream voided methods. J. Am. Vet. Med. Assoc., 179:891, 1981.
22. Vail, D.M., Allen, T.A., and Weiser, G.: Applicability of leukocyte esterase test strip in detection of canine pyuria. J. Am. Vet. Med. Assoc., 189:1451, 1986.
23. Allen, T.A., Jones, R.L., and Purvance, J.: Microbiologic evaluation of canine urine: Direct microscopic examination and preservation of specimen quality for culture. J. Am. Vet. Med. Assoc., 190:1289, 1987.
24. Osborne, C.A., Davis, L.S., Sanna, J., et al.: Urine crystals in domestic animals: A Laboratory Identification Guide. Vet. Med., 85:18, 1990.
25. Barsanti, J.A., and Finco, D.R.: Protein concentration in urine of normal dogs. Am. J. Vet. Res., 40:1583, 1979.
26. DiBartola, S.P., Chew, D.J., and Jacobs, G.: Quantitative urinalysis including 24-hour protein excretion in the dog. J. Am. Anim. Hosp. Assoc., 16:537, 1980.
27. Biewenga, W.J., Gruys, E., and Hendriks, H.J.: Urinary protein loss in the dog: Nephrological study of 29 dogs without signs of renal disease. Res. Vet. Sci., 33:366, 1982.
28. White, J.V., Olivier, N.B., Reimann, R., et al.: Use of protein-to-creatinine ratio in a single urine specimen for quantitative estimation of canine proteinuria. J. Am. Vet. Med. Assoc., 185:882, 1984.
29. Appelboom, J.W., Brodsky, W.A., and Scott, W.N.: Effect of osmotic diuresis on intrarenal solutes in diabetes insipidus and hydropenia. Am. J. Physiol., 208:38, 1965.
30. Greene, C.E., Wong, P.L., and Finco, D.R.: Diagnosis and treatment of diabetes insipidus in two dogs using two synthetic analogs of antidiuretic hormone. J. Am. Anim. Hosp. Assoc., 15:371, 1979.
31. Gault, M.H., and Muehrcke, R.C.: Renal biopsy: Current views and controversies. Nephron, 34:1, 1983.
32. Nash, A.S., Boyd, J.S., Minto, A.W., et al.: Renal biopsy in the normal cat: An examination of the effects of a single needle biopsy. Res. Vet. Sci., 34:347, 1983.
33. Osborne, C.A.: Clinical evaluation of needle biopsy of the kidney and its complications in the dog and cat. J. Am. Vet. Med. Assoc., 158:1213, 1971.
34. Jeraj, K., Osborne, C.A., and Stevens, J.B.: Evaluation of renal biopsy in 197 dogs and cats. J. Am. Vet. Med. Assoc., 181:367, 1982.
35. Grauer, G.F., Twedt, D.C., and Mero, K.N.: Evaluation of laparoscopy for obtaining renal biopsy specimens from dogs and cats. J. Am. Vet. Med. Assoc., 183:677, 1983.
36. Wise, L.A., Allen, T.A., and Cartwright, M.: Comparison of renal biopsy techniques in dogs. J. Am. Vet. Med. Assoc., 195:935, 1989.
37. Nash, A.S.: Renal biopsy in the normal cat: Development of a modified disposable biopsy needle. Res. Vet. Sci., 40:246, 1986.

38. Ling, G.V., and Ruby, A.C.: Aerobic bacterial flora of the prepuce, urethra, and vagina of normal adult dogs. Am. J. Vet. Res., 39:695, 1978.

39. Huggins, C., Masina, M.H., Eichelberger, L.E., et al.: Quantitative studies of prostatic secretion. J. Exp. Med., 70:543, 1939.

40. Ling, G.V., Branam, J.E., Ruby, A.L., et al.: Canine prostatic fluid: Techniques of collection, quantitative bacterial culture, and interpretation of results. J. Am. Vet. Med. Assoc., 183:201, 1983.

41. Fair, W.R.: Diagnosing prostatitis. Urology, Suppl 24:6, 1984.

42. Goodwin, M., Gooding, K.M., and Regnier, F.: Sex phermone in the dog. Science, 203:559, 1979.

43. Barsanti, J.A., Shotts, E.B., Prasse, K., et al.: Evaluation of diagnostic techniques for canine prostatic diseases. J. Am. Vet. Med. Assoc., 177:160, 1980.

44. Barsanti, J.A., Prasse, K.W., Crowell, W.A., et al.: Evaluation of various techniques for diagnosis of chronic bacterial prostatitis in the dog. J. Am. Vet. Med. Assoc., 183:219, 1983.

45. Fowler, J.E., and Mariano, M.: Difficulties in quantitating the contribution of urethral bacteria to prostatic fluid and seminal fluid cultures. J. Urol., 132:471, 1984.

46. Winningham, D.G., Nemoy, N.J., and Stamey, T.A.: Diffusion of antibiotics from plasma into prostatic fluid. Nature, 219:139, 1968.

47. Stamey, T.A., Meares, E.M., and Winningham, D.G.: Chronic bacterial prostatitis and the diffusion of drugs into prostatic fluid. J. Urol., 103:187, 1970.

48. Melhoff, T., and Osborne, C.A.: Catheter biopsy of the urethra, urinary bladder, and prostate gland. In Current Veterinary Therapy VI. Edited by R.W. Kirk. Philadelphia, W.B. Saunders, pp. 1173–1175, 1977.

49. Thrall, M.A., Olson, P.N., and Freenmyer, F.G.: Cytologic diagnosis of canine prostatic disease. J. Am. Anim. Hosp. Assoc., 21:95, 1985.

50. Smith, S.: Ultrasound-guided biopsy. Vet. Clin. North Am. [Sm. Anim. Pract.], 15:1249, 1985.

51. Weaver, A.D.: Transperineal punch biopsy of the canine prostate gland. J. Sm. Anim. Pract., 18:573, 1977.

52. Finco, D.R.: Prostate gland biopsy. Vet. Clin. North Am., 4:367, 1974.

53. Leeds, E.B., and Leav, I.: Perineal punch biopsy of the canine prostate gland. J. Am. Vet. Med. Assoc., 154:925, 1969.

54. Oliver, J.E., and Young, W.O.: Air cystometry in dogs under xylazine-induced restraint. Am. J. Vet. Res., 34:1433, 1973.

55. Oliver, J.E., and Young, W.O.: Evaluation of pharmacologic agents for restraint in cystometry in the dog and cat. Am. J. Vet. Res., 34:665, 1973.

56. Johnson, C.A., Beemsterboer, J.M., Gray, P.R., et al.: Effects of various sedatives on air cystometry in dogs. Am. J. Vet. Res., 49:1525, 1988.

57. Rosin, A., Rosin, E., and Oliver, J.: Canine urethral pressure profile. Am. J. Vet. Res., 41:1113, 1980.

58. Rosin, A.E., and Barsanti, J.A.: Diagnosis of urinary incontinence in dogs: Role of the urethral pressure profile. J. Am. Vet. Med. Assoc., 178:814, 1981.

59. Moreau, P.M., Lees, G.E., and Gross, D.R.: Simultaneous cystometry and uroflowmetry for evaluation of the caudal part of the urinary tract function in dogs: Reference values for healthy animals sedated with xylazine. Am. J. Vet. Res., 44:1774, 1983.

60. Moreau, P.M., Lees, G.E., and Hobson, H.P.: Simultaneous cystometry and uroflowmetry for evaluation of micturition in two dogs. J. Am. Vet. Med. Assoc., 183:1084, 1983.

61. Richter, K.P., and Ling, G.V.: Effects of xylazine on the urethral pressure profile of healthy dogs. Am. J. Vet. Res., 46:1881, 1985.

62. Brearley, M.J., and Cooper, J.E.: The diagnosis of bladder disease in dogs by cystoscopy. J. Sm. Anim. Pract., 28:75, 1987.

63. McCarthy, T.C., and McDermaid, S.L.: Prepubic percutaneous cystoscopy in the dog and cat. J. Am. Anim. Vet. Med. Assoc., 22:213, 1986.

6

Radiographic and Ultrasonographic Evaluation of the Urinary Tract

MARY B. MAHAFFEY
DON L. BARBER

Radiography and ultrasonography provide additional information to that obtained by physical examination and laboratory analysis. Radiography is useful in evaluating urinary tract abnormalities. The kidneys and urinary bladder are usually visible on survey radiographs, but the ureters and urethra are not. For optimum evaluation, animals should be fasted and given an enema before radiography to ensure gastrointestinal evacuation. Ingesta and feces may obscure urinary tract structures. Calculi can be masked by overlying ingesta and feces. Mineral dense material within the bowel can be misinterpreted as renal or bladder calculi. Thus, animals should be fasted 12 to 24 hours; withholding food overnight is usually adequate. Soapy water enemas are administered about 2 hours before radiography so that there is adequate time for the patient to evacuate fluid and gas after the enema. Gastrointestinal preparation may be avoided in animals with anorexia, vomition, or diarrhea. Gastrointestinal preparation is not performed in emergencies or if medically contraindicated. Both lateral and ventrodorsal (VD) views are made routinely. Because inherent abdominal contrast is usually poor, relatively high mAs and low kVp exposure techniques are used. Radiographic lesions are described according to their radiographic signs, i.e., changes in density, geometry, and function. These descriptions are used to formulate a "rule-out" list. The radiographic sign approach is used throughout this chapter to describe radiographic findings.

Ultrasonography is used with increasing frequency in animals and is an excellent adjunct to radiography, providing detailed information about the internal architecture of structures. Ultrasonography is especially valuable for evaluation of the kidneys and prostate. In this chapter, descriptions of ultrasonographic findings are included where appropriate. In ultrasound terminology, *anechoic* structures appear black, and *hyperechoic* structures appear white or light gray. Information concerning ultrasound physics, artifacts, and techniques is available elsewhere.[1-4]

EXAMINATION OF THE KIDNEYS

Kidneys are located within the retroperitoneal space. They appear as bean-shaped, soft tissue dense structures with smooth, sharp margins (Fig. 6-1). Fat within the retroperitoneal space usually provides sufficient contrast for identification of renal margins. Cats tend to have more retroperitoneal fat than do dogs, and thus kidneys in cats are usually better visualized. Cat kidneys are rounder than dog kidneys (Fig. 6-2). The right kidney is usually located at the level of lumbar vertebra (L) 1 and 2, and the left kidney is usually located farther caudally at the level of L2 and L3. The cranial pole of the right kidney is nestled within the renal fossa of the caudate lobe of the liver and is, therefore, frequently obscured. The left kidney can usually be more completely visualized on survey radiographs, whereas identification of the right kidney is less consistent. The right kidney is relatively fixed in its position, whereas the left kidney is more mobile. Cat kidneys are more mobile than dog kidneys. In lateral recumbency, the dependent kidney tends to shift cranially.[5] As a result, there is less superimposition of the two kidneys on the right lateral view than on the left lateral view. Normal renal length is 2.5 to 3.5 times the length of the body of L2 in the dog[6] and 2.4 to 3.0 times the length of the body of L2 in the cat.[7] These measurements should be made on the VD view because the kidneys are a similar distance from the film as the vertebrae and because this was the view in which the normal comparative measurements were made. On the lateral view, there is unequal and inconsistent magnification of the kidneys relative to the spine

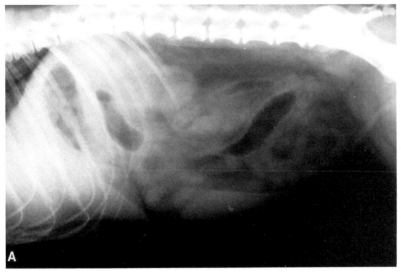
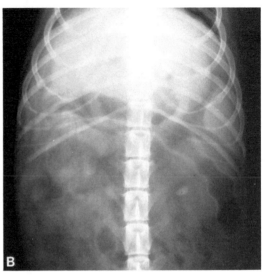

FIG. 6–1. (A and B) Lateral and VD views of the abdomen of a normal dog. The left kidney is located slightly caudal and ventral to the right kidney. The cranial pole of the left overlaps the caudal pole of the right on the lateral view. The cranial pole of the right kidney is not well identified because it is nestled in the renal fossa of the liver. The focal opacity near the hilus of the left kidney on the VD view is a nipple.

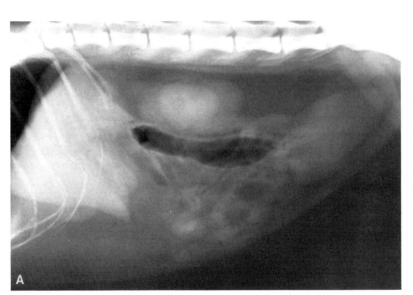
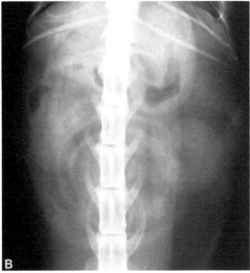

FIG. 6–2. (A and B) Lateral and VD views of the abdomen of a normal cat. Both kidneys can be easily identified because of abundant fat in the retroperitoneal space. Fat is visible in the renal sinus of the left kidney.

and to each other. Ureters are not normally visualized on survey radiographs because of their small diameter.

On ultrasound examination, the renal cortex is hypoechoic and can be differentiated from the less echogenic medulla, which is anechoic to slightly hypoechoic (Fig. 6–3). As a general rule, the normal renal cortex is less echogenic than the spleen or liver. Increased renal cortical echogenicity can be used as a rough indication of renal disease.[8,9]

Intravenous Urography

Intravenous urography (IU) is a radiographic contrast-enhanced procedure used to enhance visualization of the renal parenchyma and to provide visualization of structures not normally identified on survey radiographs, i.e., pelvic recesses (diverticulae), renal pelves, and ureters. Sequential radiographs are made following intravenous injection of a radiopaque contrast medium, which is ex-

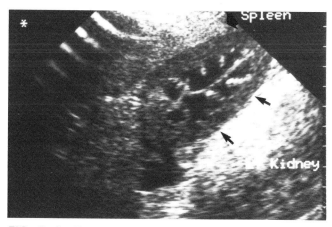

FIG. 6—3. Sagittal sonogram of the left kidney (arrows) and spleen (arrowhead) of a normal dog. The renal cortex is less echogenic than the spleen and is seen as a hypoechoic (dark gray) band around the nearly anechoic (black) medulla.

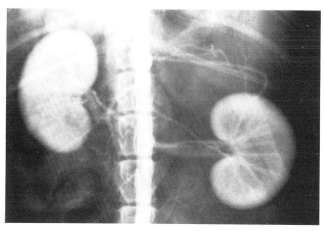

FIG. 6—4. VD view of the vascular nephrogram phase made during an IU of a normal dog. Contrast medium opacifies the aorta, renal vessels, and renal parenchyma. The more opaque renal cortex can be differentiated from the medulla.

creted by the kidneys. Aqueous, organically bound, triiodinated contrast medium injected intravenously is excreted by glomerular filtration with essentially no tubular resorption. Contrast medium is concentrated by tubular resorption of water, providing greater radiopacity to allow visualization of the renal collecting system. Synonyms for IU include *excretory urography* (EU) and *intravenous pyelography* (IVP).

The basic phases of IU are the excretory nephrogram, from opacification of renal parenchyma, and the pyelogram, from opacification of pelvic recesses, pelves, and ureters. In dogs with normal renal function, pyelographic opacity is more radiopaque than the excretory nephrogram. An additional nephrographic phase is the vascular nephrogram that can be visualized following rapid bolus injection of contrast medium.[10] The vascular nephrogram is visualized on a radiograph exposed as a bolus of contrast medium circulates through the renal vessels for the first time, approximately 7 to 15 seconds after rapid intravenous injection. Renal opacification is primarily caused by contrast medium within the renal arteries, capillaries, and veins. The appearance varies considerably depending on the nature of the bolus injection and the progression of the bolus at the instant of radiographic exposure. A relatively early exposure may show only major renal arteries. A slightly later exposure may show the cortex with greater opacity than the medulla (Fig. 6–4). A later exposure may show more uniform opacification of the entire kidneys owing to a diffuse capillary phase. Renal veins are usually poorly visualized if at all. Note that these vascular subphases are not separate but lead one into the other with much overlap. Later opacification of renal parenchyma is primarily caused by contrast medium within renal tubules and subsequent recirculation of contrast medium through renal vessels. Renal parenchyma, which has a uniform appearance on the excretory nephrogram (Fig. 6–5), decreases in opacity with time. Renal pelves may

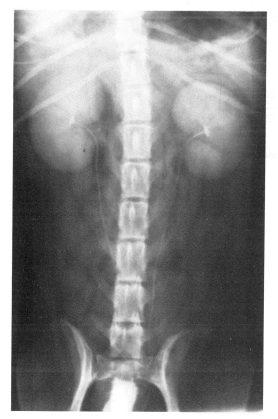

FIG. 6—5. VD view of a normal dog made 5 minutes after intravenous injection of contrast medium for an IU. Opacity of the renal parenchyma is uniform. Contrast medium can be seen in the renal pelves, ureters, and bladder. The entire ureters are not visualized because of peristalsis.

be opacified as early as 1 minute after injection but are usually seen best as a thin curved line 20 and 40 minutes after injection. Pelvic recesses are also seen best at those times and appear as paired thin lines radiating from the pelvis into the medulla (Fig. 6–6). Specific measurements for these structures have been described[11] but are not used routinely. IU does not quantitate renal function, but in general, the poorer the renal function, the poorer the opacification of the nephrogram and pyelogram.[12,13] In addition, the function of one kidney can be compared with the other kidney, especially if one is normally opacified and the other is not.

Technique

Survey radiographs should always be made before IU. Survey radiographs (1) may obviate the need for contrast study, i.e., be diagnostic; (2) allow evaluation of exposure technique and abdominal preparation before injection of contrast medium; and (3) help determine the procedure of choice if more than one is available. In most cases, radiographic exposure for the intravenous urogram should be increased over that used for survey radiographs to enhance contrast between opacified kidneys and surrounding soft tissues and to allow for greater opacification of the entire body created by the systemically distributed contrast medium. This can be accomplished by increasing either the mAs by 50% or increasing the kVp by 10%. Unless patient motion owing to long exposure times is a concern, it is best to increase the mAs. If possible, kVp should not exceed 80.

Any commonly used aqueous, organic, tri-iodinated contrast medium approved for intravenous injection may be used for IU. Most economical are the ionic media, which are either iothalamate or diatrizoate anions with sodium or meglumine cations. Many contrast media are combinations of these substances. Newer nonionic contrast media may also be used, but these are much more expensive and in veterinary medicine are usually reserved for myelography. The dosage for excretory urography is 400 mg iodine (I)/0.45 kg (400 mg I/lb).[14] In dogs with poor renal function, the dosage may be doubled to obtain adequate opacification of the kidneys.[15] The iodine concentrations of several contrast media are listed in Table 6–1.

It is best to place a catheter within the cephalic vein for contrast medium injection. This lessens the likelihood of contrast medium extravasation, allows rapid injection if desired, and provides rapid venous access for treatment of systemic reactions.

If a vascular nephrogram is desired, contrast medium is injected rapidly as a bolus so that it will reach the kidneys as a bolus and give maximum opacification of renal vessels. A contrast medium bolus is difficult to administer in large dogs because of the large volume required. The animal is placed in dorsal recumbency during injection so that it will be properly positioned for the exposure to be made 7 to 15 seconds after the end of injection. One of the best indications for the correct time to make the exposure is when the patient begins to react to the contrast medium. Contrast medium pro-

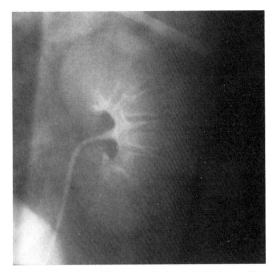

FIG. 6–6. Close-up of a VD view of the left kidney of a normal dog made 20 minutes after injection of contrast medium for an IU. The pelvic recesses are seen as thin lines radiating from the renal pelvis. Parenchymal opacity is uniform and less than that seen earlier in an IU.

TABLE 6–1. CONTENT OF ORGANIC TRI-IODINATED CONTRAST MEDIA FOR URINARY CONTRAST-ENHANCED PROCEDURES

Trade	Generic	Manufacturer	mg Iodine/ml
Hypaque sodium 50%	Na diatrizoate	Winthrop*	300
Hypaque sodium 25%	Na diatrizoate	Winthrop	150
Hypaque meglumine 60%	Meglumine diatrizoate	Winthrop	282
Renovist	Na and meglumine diatrizoate	Squibb†	370
Renografin-76	Meglumine and Na diatrizoate	Squibb	370
Renografin-60	Na and meglumine diatrizoate	Squibb	292
Conray	Meglumine iothalamate	Mallinckrodt‡	282
Conray-400	Na iothalamate	Mallinckrodt	400

* Withrop Laboratories, New York, NY 10016
† Squibb Laboratories, New Brunswick, NJ 08903
‡ Mallinckrodt Chemical Works, St. Louis, Missouri 63160

vides a metallic taste that may cause the animal to lick and causes a warm sensation when it reaches the systemic circulation. Unfortunately, many animals begin to move at this time. Unless there are reasons to evaluate the renal vessels, it is better to make the first exposure at 1 minute after injection to avoid the difficulty of making the exposure at an earlier time without motion artifact.

Recommended views and exposure sequencing following injection are as follows: VD views at 7 to 15 seconds, 1 minute, or both after injection and at 5, 20, and 40 minutes and a lateral view at 5 minutes. This protocol is not absolute and is modified to meet the diagnostic requirements.

Complications

Because contrast medium is hypertonic, accidental injection into perivascular tissues causes swelling, which resolves within a few days. Injection of lidocaine and saline solutions in the affected area may relieve any immediate irritation and dilute the contrast medium. Preplacement of a cephalic catheter helps prevent extravascular injection of contrast medium.

Adverse reactions to intravenous injection of contrast media in dogs and cats are uncommon but can be life-threatening. Mechanisms of these reactions are not fully understood and are beyond the scope of this text. The most common adverse reactions are nausea and vomiting, which usually occur within the first 1 to 2 minutes after injection, last only a few minutes, and do not require treatment. One should be aware of the potential for vomiting, so that a muzzle, if applied, may be rapidly removed. Transitory decrease in renal function may occur[16] but is not considered clinically significant. Dehydration may increase the risk of adverse renal reactions[17]; thus, animals should be adequately hydrated prior to IU. Idiosyncratic "allergic" reactions, resulting in systemic hypotension, shock, and rarely death, may occur. Such reactions occur within the first few minutes after injection but are uncommon. A more complete discussion of contrast medium reactions and treatment may be found elsewhere.[18]

Contrast medium in the urine may cause erroneous results of urinalysis[19] and inhibit growth of some bacteria.[20] Therefore, urine samples for analysis and culture should be collected before any urinary contrast-enhanced study.

Interpretation of Abnormal Findings

Size and Shape

Increased kidney size is characterized as parenchymal or collecting system enlargement and as symmetrical (normal shape) or asymmetrical. IU is especially valuable in determining whether enlargement is from parenchymal or collecting system disease. Symmetrical renal enlargement is associated with acute nephritis, compensatory hypertrophy, some types of neoplasia (usually diffusely infiltrative, e.g., lymphosarcoma), hydronephrosis, and feline infectious peritonitis. In cats with unilateral or bilateral symmetrical renal enlargement, lymphosarcoma should be the primary differential diagnosis (Fig. 6–7). Primary renal neoplasia usually affects only one kidney (Fig. 6–8) but may be bilateral. Differential diagnoses for asymmetrical or irregularly shaped enlarged kidneys include neoplasia, cyst (Fig. 6–9), abscess, hematoma, and polycystic renal disease.

Symmetrically small kidneys may be caused by hypoplasia, end-stage renal disease, and renal dysplasia. Differential diagnoses for small, irregularly shaped kidneys include healed renal infarcts, chronic pyelonephritis, end-stage kidneys, and renal dysplasia.

Normal renal size does not rule out renal disease. The kidneys may appear radiographically normal in size and shape with interstitial nephritis, acute pyelonephritis, glomerulonephritis, and amyloidosis.

On ultrasound examination, the kidneys of dogs with diffuse renal disease, such as glomerulointerstitial nephritis, renal tubular necrosis, and nephrocalcinosis, may have hyperechoic renal cortices or have a diffuse increase in echogenicity with poor corticomedullary differentiation (Fig. 6–10).[8] Such ultrasonographic findings are not disease specific; therefore, biopsy is needed for a definitive diagnosis. Hyperechoic renal cortices have been reported as a normal finding in cats with abundant fat vacuoles in the renal cortex.[21] Cysts appear as rounded anechoic structures with distal acoustic enhancement (Fig. 6–11).

Large renal pelves on IU may be caused by either hydronephrosis or pyelonephritis. IU can be used to differentiate hydronephrosis from other diseases that primarily affect the parenchyma. In mild to moderate hydronephrosis, the renal pelvis and pelvic recesses are dilated (Fig. 6–12). In later stages, pelvic recesses are stretched and may be incorporated with the dilated pelvis (Fig. 6–13). Eventually only a thin shell of parenchyma may remain. In pyelonephritis, pelvic recesses are poorly identified or not seen at all (Fig. 6–14).[22] IU can be very useful for diagnosis of pyelonephritis, but

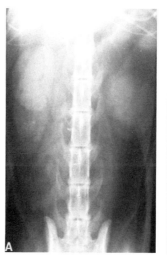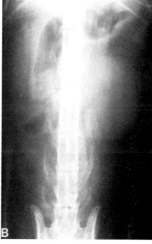

FIG. 6–7. VD views of a cat made before (A) and after (B) symmetrical renal enlargement caused by lymphosarcoma. The view in (B) was made 2 months after (A).

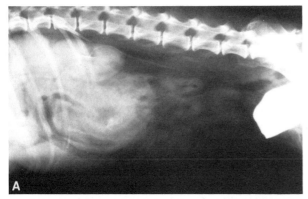

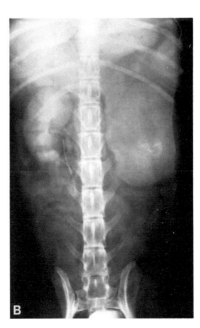

FIG. 6–8. IU of a dog with renal carcinoma ([A] lateral, [B] VD). The left kidney is enlarged and irregularly shaped and contains dystrophic mineralization. (C) Sonogram of a different dog with a renal carcinoma. Normal renal architecture is not visible; the kidney (cranial and caudal borders marked by cursors) appears as a mixed echogenic mass.

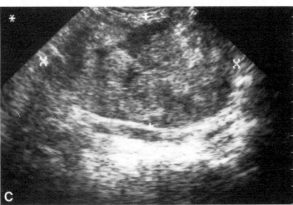

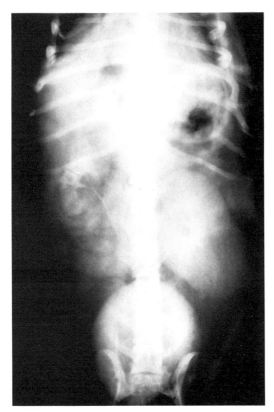

FIG. 6–9. Asymmetrical renal enlargement caused by a cyst in the caudal pole of the left kidney of a dog. On an IU, the cyst is less opaque than the adjacent parenchyma.

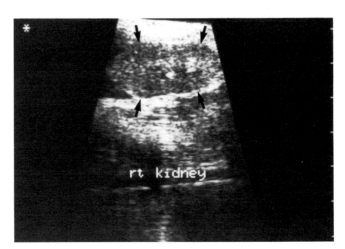

FIG. 6–10. Sagittal sonogram of the right kidney (arrows) of a dog with poor renal function. The kidney is more echogenic than the liver (dark gray structure adjacent to the cranial pole of the kidney), and there is poor differentiation between the cortex and medulla. Cranial is to the left, and ventral is at the top.

normal appearing kidneys do not rule out this diagnosis. Ultrasonography also can be used to detect enlargement of the renal pelvis, which appears as a centrally located anechoic area within the kidney (Fig. 6–15).

Location

An abdominal mass such as an adrenal tumor may displace a kidney from its normal location. An enlarged kidney may shift in position. Renal masses usually dis-

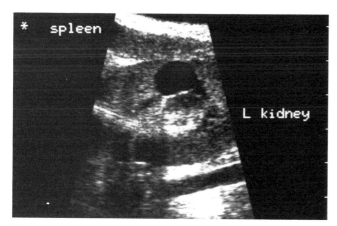

FIG. 6–11. Sagittal sonogram of the left kidney of a dog with a renal cyst. The cyst is seen as a rounded anechoic (black) structure in the renal cortex. Acoustic enhancement (bright echoes) is seen distal to the cyst. Cranial is to the left, and ventral is at the top.

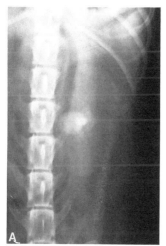 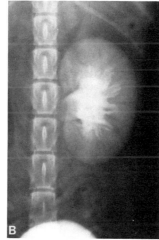

FIG. 6–12. Survey film (A) and IU (B) of the left kidney of a dog with a calculus in the proximal ureter and renal pelvis. The calculus is opaque on the survey film but radiolucent on the IU because it is surrounded by the more opaque (metal dense) contrast medium. The renal pelvis and pelvic recesses are dilated on the IU, indicating hydronephrosis, and the kidney is enlarged (greater than 3.5 times the length of L2).

place the colon and small intestines ventrally (see Fig. 6–8A,B). IU or ultrasonography can be used to confirm or exclude the origin of the mass as kidney. A less common cause of abnormal kidney location is ectopia.

Density

Decreased renal density is uncommon. Occasionally, in animals with vesicoureteral reflux, gas may ascend into the ureters and into the renal collecting system during pneumocystography.

Increased renal opacity may result from parenchymal mineralization or calculus formation within the pelvis. Diffuse renal mineralization may be seen in dogs with chronic renal failure. In such animals, radiographically detectable mineralization may be found elsewhere, such as the stomach wall, vasculature, and footpads.[23] Dystrophic mineralization of the kidney is found in renal tumors, abscesses, or healed infarcts. Osseous metaplasia of a hydronephrotic kidney was reported in a dog.[24] Linear mineral dense radiopacities in the wall of the renal pelvis and pelvic recesses may be seen in dogs with or without active renal disease (Fig. 6–16).[25] These are seen most often in older dogs. These radiopacities must be distinguished from calculi because they cannot be removed.[26] Radiographic detection of renal calculi is dependent on mineral content and size of calculi. Calculi are frequently associated with infection, and it is not uncommon for pyelonephritis to be present concurrently. Large calculi may obstruct pelvic outflow, causing hydronephrosis (see Fig. 6–12). Opaque calculi on survey radiographs commonly appear as radiolucent filling defects on IU because of the greater relative opacity of the contrast medium (see Fig. 6–12). On ultrasound examination, calculi appear as echogenic foci with acoustic shadowing (Fig. 6–17).

Margination

Indistinct renal margins may be a result of decreased retroperitoneal fat, perirenal inflammation, or, more commonly, retroperitoneal fluid accumulation. Fluid within the retroperitoneal space silhouettes with kidneys and obscures their margins. Hemorrhage from trauma or urine accumulation following urinary tract

FIG. 6–13. (A and B) Hydronephrosis and hydroureter caused by transitional cell carcinoma in the bladder trigone (arrow), resulting in ureteral obstruction. The renal pelvic recesses are dilated and are being incorporated with the greatly enlarged renal pelves, indicating chronic obstruction. The ureters are dilated and tortuous. The lucent round filling defect in the center of the bladder is an air bubble introduced during previous catheterization.

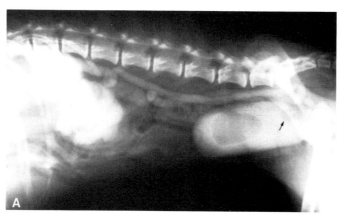 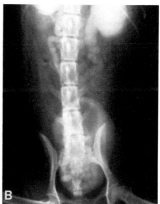

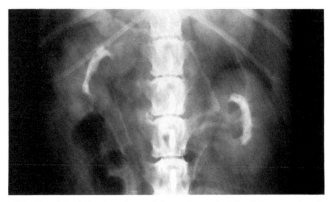

FIG. 6–14. IU of a dog with pyelonephritis. The renal pelves are dilated, and the pelvic recesses are poorly identified. Flattened areas on the renal cortices are probably healed infarcts.

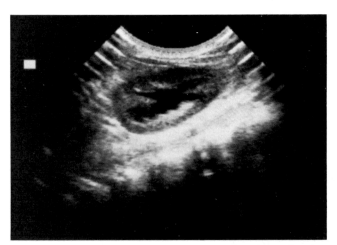

FIG. 6–15. Sagittal sonogram of the left kidney of a dog with hydronephrosis. The enlarged renal pelvis appears as a centrally located anechoic area within the kidney. Cranial is to the left, and ventral is at the top.

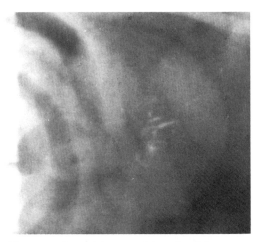

FIG. 6–16. Linear radiopacities overlying the kidney represent mineralization of the wall of the renal pelvis and pelvic recesses.

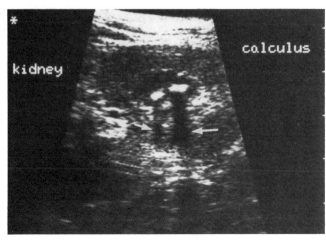

FIG. 6–17. Sagittal renal sonogram of a dog with two renal calculi. Calculi appear as bright echogenic foci with acoustic shadowing (arrows) distally.

rupture are the most likely types of retroperitoneal fluid. Because retroperitoneal urine accumulation may result from a ruptured kidney, ureter, or urethra, an IU should be performed whenever retroperitoneal fluid is identified (Fig. 6–18).

EXAMINATION OF THE URETERS

IU is used to evaluate ureters because they are too small to visualize on survey radiographs. Ureters are seen as thin opaque lines approximately 1 to 2 mm in diameter that extend caudally from the renal hilus to the urinary bladder. They normally have a cranioventral course just before entering the bladder wall (Fig. 6–19). Ureters are not normally identified throughout their entire length on a single radiograph because of peristaltic emptying of the radiopaque urine (see Fig. 6–5).

Interpretation of Abnormal Findings

Size and Shape

Increased ureteral diameter is most often a result of obstruction. Ureters may become convoluted if obstruction is prolonged or nearly complete. Neoplasia of the bladder trigone is the most common cause of ureteral obstruction (see Fig. 6–13). Calculi may lodge in the ureter causing obstruction (Fig. 6–20). Surgical manipulation, such as ureterotomy, repair of rupture,[27] or transplantation,[28,29] can produce stricture. Temporary obstruction owing to postoperative edema is an expected finding but should subside within a few weeks (Fig. 6–21).[30,31] Ureteral inflammation causes dilatation and may be secondary to pyelonephritis or ascending infections from the urinary bladder or urethra (if the ureter is ectopic). Congenital anomalies such as ectopic ureter and ureterocele may be associated with ureteral dilatation. A ureterocele is focal dilatation of the intramural portion of the ureter.

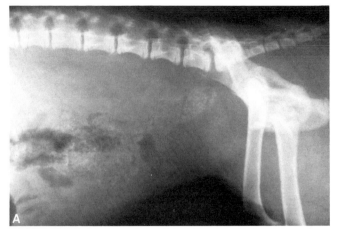

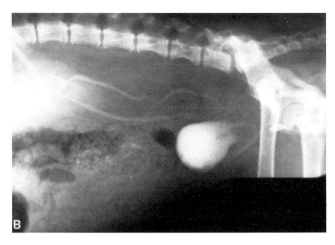

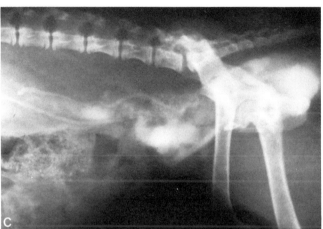

FIG. 6–18. (A) Survey abdominal film of a dog that had been hit by a car. Increased soft tissue density within the retroperitoneal space that silhouettes with the kidneys is indicative of free fluid. The colon is displaced ventrally. One acetabulum is displaced cranially; pelvic fractures were seen on other views. (B) Film made 5 minutes after start of IU. No leakage of contrast medium is identified. (C) Film made 20 minutes after start of IU. Extravasation of contrast medium primarily into the pelvic canal and retroperitoneal space is consistent with urethral rupture. At surgery, a urethral tear was found near the bladder neck.

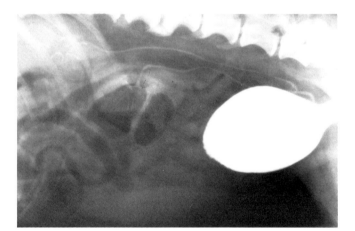

FIG. 6–19. Lateral view of an excretory urogram made 40 minutes after the start of an IU. Notice the normal cranioventral course of the ureters as they enter the bladder trigone.

Density

A ureteral calculus is suspected if a focal mineral opacity is found in the retroperitoneal space. IU is performed for confirmation. The ureter is dilated proximal to the calculus (see Fig. 6–20). Occasionally, the cross-section view of the deep circumflex iliac arteries, which lie ven-

tral to L6 and L7, may be misinterpreted as ureteral calculi (Fig. 6–22) on a lateral abdominal radiograph.[12]

Location

An ectopic ureter may terminate in the urethra or vagina (Fig. 6–23). The ureter may enter the bladder wall in a normal location and then remain intramural until it opens into the urethra or vagina.[32] Occasionally, the ectopic ureter also opens into the bladder, making diagnosis difficult. IU helps determine the diagnosis and if one or both ureters are affected. Simultaneous pneumocystography and IU enhances contrast between the ureters and bladder by outlining the terminal portions of the ureters and increases the accuracy of ureteral evaluation.[32] Oblique lateral views are made 2 to 5 minutes after injection of contrast medium. Dilatation of the ectopic ureter is a frequent finding. A straightening of the terminal portion of the ureter, with a loss of its cranioventral course, is suggestive of an intramural ectopic ureter.[32] Positive contrast vaginourethrography may also be used to identify the terminal portion of an ectopic ureter.[33,34] This technique is described in the following discussion on the urethra. An advantage of IU over positive contrast vaginourethrography is that it allows evaluation of the kidneys for concurrent pyelonephritis or dysplasia. Radiographic techniques are not always diagnostic. In one report, radiographic studies failed to

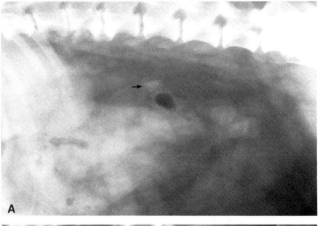

A

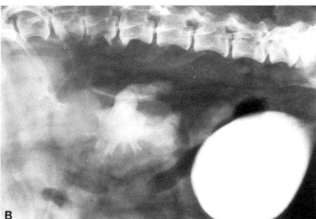

B

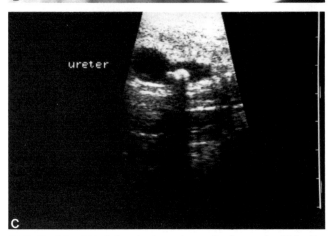

C

FIG. 6—20. (A) A focal mineral opacity (arrow) within the plane of the retroperitoneal space is suggestive of a ureteral calculus. (B) An IU confirmed the presence of a ureteral calculus causing obstruction. The left ureter and renal pelvis are dilated proximal to the calculus. (C) Sonogram of the dilated anechoic left ureter and the echogenic calculus with acoustic shadowing distally.

define accurately termination of ectopic ureters in approximately 25% of dogs with ureteral ectopia.[33]

Function

After ureteral rupture, urine usually leaks into the retroperitoneal space. Avulsion of the ureter from the blad-

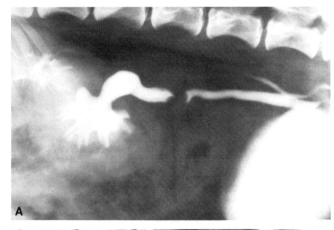

A

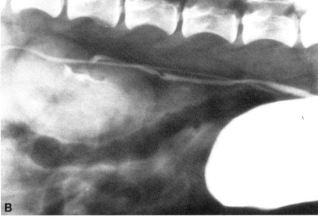

B

FIG. 6—21. (A) Ureteral stricture following repair of a ruptured left ureter. Hydronephrosis and hydroureter proximal and distal to the stricture are present. (B) On films made 10 months later, the stricture is less severe, and hydronephrosis and hydroureter have dissipated. (This case was discussed in detail in reference 27.)

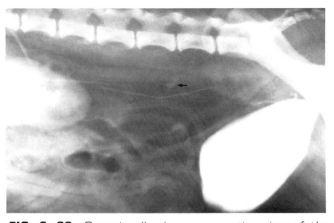

FIG. 6—22. Occasionally the cross-section view of the deep circumflex iliac arteries (arrow) may appear similar to a ureteral calculus. If necessary, an IU can be used to rule out a calculus.

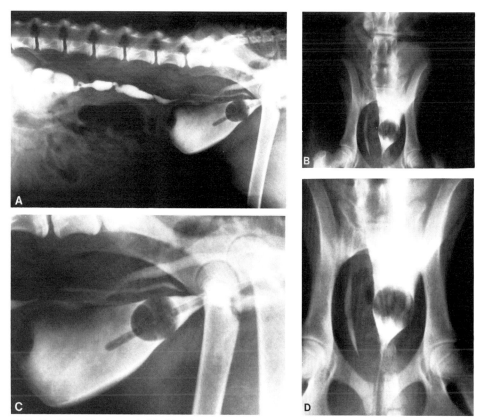

FIG. 6–23. (A through D) Simultaneous pneumocystography and IU in a 6-month-old bitch with ureteral ectopia. The right ureter and renal pelvis are dilated. The right ureter is tortuous, and its terminal portion completely bypasses the bladder neck (see close-up [C and D]). The left ureter appears to terminate at the bladder trigone, but the terminal portion does not course in a typical cranial and ventral direction. Thus, the left ureter may also be ectopic, and its opening should be examined carefully during a ventral cystotomy.

der may also leak urine into the peritoneal cavity. As already noted, diffuse increased fluid, dense opacity within the retroperitoneal space following trauma is compatible with blood or urine accumulation. Therefore, IU is indicated for differentiation.

EXAMINATION OF THE URINARY BLADDER

The urinary bladder is not visible radiographically when empty. When not empty, the urinary bladder is seen as a soft tissue dense, pear-shaped structure in the caudoventral abdomen. Because urine and bladder wall are the same density, mucosal margins cannot be identified on survey radiographs. Normal bladder size and shape are variable, depending on the degree of distention. When nearly empty, the bladder can be indented by adjacent intestine and does not assume the characteristic oval shape until intravesical pressure is increased (Fig. 6–24). The location is also variable. In dogs, the majority of the bladder may be located within the pelvic canal when the bladder is empty. With increasing distention, the bladder tends to move cranially. Because

of the geometry of image projection, even when distended, the bladder is often projected over the pelvis on the VD view and is thus more difficult to visualize. In most dogs, the bladder neck is located near the pelvic brim when the bladder is full, but as much as 35% of the bladder length may be located within the pelvic canal of normal dogs, even when the bladder is full.[35] In cats, the bladder is almost always located within the abdominal cavity even when empty. On the VD view, the bladder may fall to one side or the other. Bladder wall thickness and mucosal margins are identified with cystography. Normal wall thickness is 1 to 2 mm circumferentially even when the bladder is incompletely distended.[36,37]

Cystography

Cystography is the preferred contrast procedure to evaluate the urinary bladder. Urine is removed from the bladder, and contrast medium is injected so that bladder wall and luminal content can be evaluated. In instances in which the urethra cannot be catheterized, limited bladder evaluation can be obtained on 20-minute or 40-

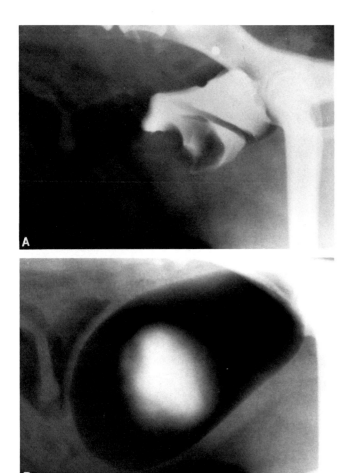

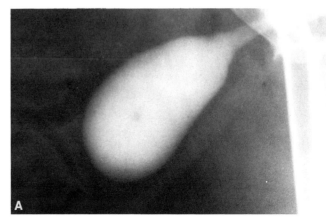

FIG. 6–24. Double-contrast cystogram in a normal dog. (A) When the bladder is incompletely distended, it is indented by adjacent intestine, giving the appearance of a mass lesion. (B) With more complete distention, the bladder shape is oval.

ily seen within the peritoneal space if a rupture is present (Fig. 6–26), even if small. Conversely, free gas within the peritoneal space from a pneumocystogram is much more difficult to detect. If only a small amount leaks out with most of the gas retained in the bladder, hori-

minute radiographs during IU. This is not preferred, however, because there is little control of bladder opacity and distention during IU.

The three types of cystography are positive-contrast (Fig. 6–25A), double-contrast (Fig. 6–25B), and negative-contrast (pneumocystography; Fig. 6–25C). Positive-contrast cystography is performed using water-soluble, organically bound, tri-iodinated contrast media. Most of the commercially available contrast media manufactured for intravenous use are acceptable (Table 6–1) but need to be diluted with sterile saline or water if not specifically formulated for cystography. Double-contrast cystography is performed using a combination of positive-contrast and negative-contrast media. A small amount of the positive-contrast medium forms a puddle in the dependent portion of the bladder, while the bladder is further distended with a negative-contrast medium such as carbon dioxide, nitrous oxide, or room air. Negative-contrast cystography is performed using negative-contrast medium only.

Positive-contrast cystography is the procedure of choice for detecting a ruptured bladder and for evaluating bladder location. Positive-contrast medium is eas-

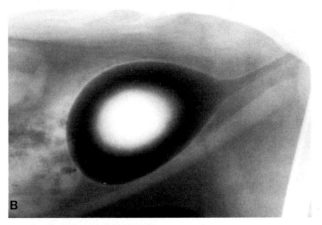

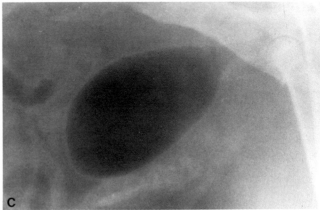

FIG. 6–25. Normal cat cystograms. (A) Positive-contrast cystogram. The mucosal surface is identified, but the serosal surface is not. Therefore, the wall thickness cannot be evaluated. The round lucent filling defect in the center of the bladder is an air bubble. (B) Double-contrast cystogram. Positive-contrast medium forms a puddle in the dependent portion of the bladder. Bladder wall thickness is uniform and can be clearly identified. (C) Negative-contrast cystogram. Wall thickness can be identified.

zontal beam radiography may have to be used to confirm the presence of free gas in the peritoneal cavity definitely (Fig. 6–27).

Bladder wall thickness, mucosal margination, and luminal content are better defined with double-contrast cystography (see Fig. 6–25; Fig. 6–28).[37] Positive-contrast media may adhere to mucosal erosions making them visible (Fig. 6–28). Calculi and blood clots are seen as filling defects within the positive-contrast medium puddle (Figs. 6–28, 6–29). Although very small calculi may be missed with any cystographic technique, they are less likely to be missed with double-contrast cystography than with positive-contrast or negative-contrast cystography. Small calculi may be obscured on a positive-contrast cystogram or an intravenous urogram because of the greater opacity of the media within the lumen. Gas used in negative-contrast cystography may not provide enough contrast to detect small radiolucent calculi.

The only advantage of negative-contrast cystography is availability and low cost if room air is used as the contrast agent. Negative-contrast cystography is not advised because the other two techniques are diagnosti-

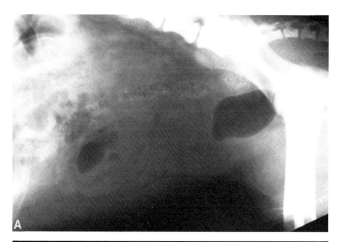

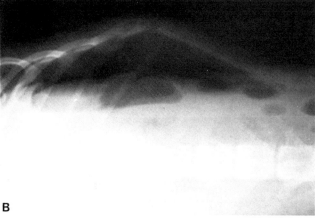

FIG. 6–27. Pneumocystogram in a dog with a ruptured urinary bladder. (A) Poor intra-abdominal contrast enhancement is compatible with free peritoneal fluid. The bladder is partially distended with CO_2. (B) Free intra-abdominal gas indicating bladder rupture was not positively identified until a horizontal beam, VD radiograph was made with the dog in left lateral recumbency.

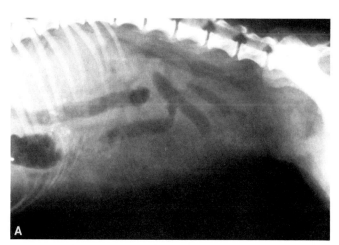

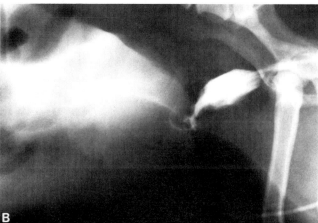

FIG. 6–26. Ruptured urinary bladder in a dog that had been hit by a car. (A) On a survey radiograph, serosal margins of intra-abdominal organs are obscured by free peritoneal fluid. (B) Bladder rupture is easily confirmed by positive-contrast cystography.

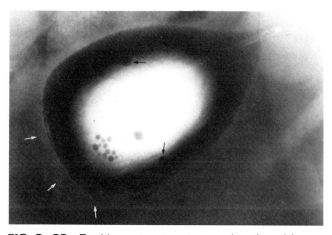

FIG. 6–28. Double-contrast cystogram in a dog with cystitis and urinary bladder calculi. The bladder wall is thickened cranioventrally (white arrows), and contrast medium adheres to the mucosal surface cranioventrally, indicating erosion. Round, lucent filling defects at the periphery of the contrast puddle (black arrows) are air bubbles. Rounded filling defects located more centrally within the contrast puddle are calculi.

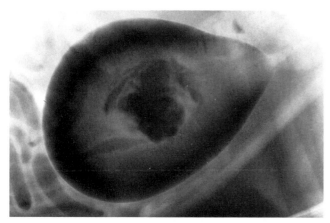

FIG. 6—29. Double-contrast cystogram in a dog with hematuria. A large, irregularly shaped filling defect with indistinct margins is a blood clot outlined by the positive-contrast puddle.

cally superior. Negative-contrast cystography may be adequate, however, for detection of most mass lesions of the bladder if the film is not overexposed.

Technique

Standard abdominal preparation is essential so that the bladder will not be obscured by overlying bowel contents or deformed by a fecal-filled colon. Radiopaque calculi that could be seen on survey radiographs could be missed if superimposed over fecal material in the colon. Lateral and VD survey radiographs should be made to confirm intestinal evacuation and proper radiographic exposure technique.

Chemical restraint is usually needed for cystography. The urinary bladder should be aseptically catheterized and emptied. If blood clots are present, the bladder is flushed with sterile saline. A rubber urethral catheter may be used in males and females, but a Foley catheter is preferred in females to prevent reflux of contrast medium around the catheter (see Chapter 7 for a discussion of catheters). Infusion of lidocaine into the urinary bladder has been recommended to eliminate bladder spasm that might prevent complete bladder distention.[38] A study of cystography in cats showed that lidocaine had no effect on bladder distention in normal cats. In cats with cystitis, bladder distention increased after intravesical lidocaine application, but cystographic evidence of cystitis became more subtle in some cats.[39]

Positive-Contrast Cystography

If the purpose of cystography is to evaluate the bladder for rupture or for change in location, as with a perineal hernia, the contrast medium is diluted to approximately 50 mg/ml with sterile saline or water. If the bladder is ruptured, contrast medium will usually be seen within the peritoneal space. A small volume of contrast medium (approximately 1.5 ml/kg body weight) is infused into the bladder initially so that an excessive amount does not leak into the peritoneal space through

a large rupture. Small tears may be temporarily sealed, however, and may not be detected unless the bladder is more fully distended (Fig. 6–30). Thus, if a rupture is not seen on the initial radiograph, a second radiograph should be made after the bladder is more completely distended. Sufficient bladder distention is achieved when the bladder is palpably taut, contrast medium refluxes around the catheter, or increased back pressure is felt on the syringe plunger. Approximately 10 ml/kg body weight should be sufficient contrast medium to achieve adequate distention.

If a positive-contrast cystogram is to be used to evaluate bladder conditions other than rupture or abnormal location, the contrast medium should be diluted to a concentration of 30 mg I/ml. This dilution lessens the chance of obscuring mucosal lesions or calculi. Cystographic exposure depends on the exposure density of the survey radiographs, but the exposure is usually increased by 50%. This can be done by either increasing the kVp by 10% or by increasing the mAs by 50%.

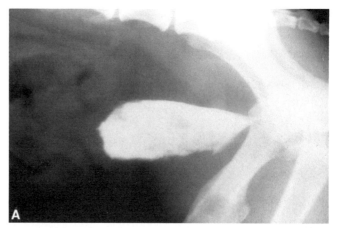

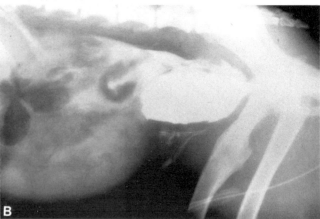

FIG. 6—30. Positive-contrast cystogram in a dog with a bladder rupture that had temporarily sealed. (A) With the bladder mildly distended, there is no leakage of contrast medium from the bladder. Mucosal margins are irregular. Ill-defined filling defects more centrally located are blood clots. (B) Additional contrast medium further distended the bladder and confirmed the bladder tear. A healed femoral fracture from a previous traumatic incident can be seen.

Double-Contrast Cystography

Infuse 0.44 to 0.88 ml/kg body weight of undiluted positive-contrast medium (280 to 300 mg I/ml) into the bladder, then further distend the bladder with carbon dioxide (CO_2). False-positive findings of bladder disease (such as mucosal irregularity and pseudomasses caused by indentation of the bladder by adjacent bowel) may occur if the bladder is inadequately distended (see Fig. 6–24A). It is not necessary to distend the bladder completely to eliminate such false-positive findings, however.[36] In addition, mucosal irregularity and bladder wall thickening seen in dogs with mild cystitis may be more obvious when the bladder is mildly distended than when the bladder is fully distended[37] (Fig. 6–31). Fifty to 100 ml of CO_2 eliminate mucosal irregularity in most normal dogs weighing less than 20 kg. A dose of 5 ml/kg should be adequate for larger dogs. If at that dose, bladder indentation mimics a wall mass, the bladder should be further distended. A total dose of 11 ml/kg CO_2 in addition to the positive-contrast medium should adequately distend a normal bladder. Because the bladder is usually less distensible in dogs with cystitis, the amount of contrast medium required to distend the blad-

der adequately may be less. The bladder should always be palpated during infusion of contrast medium, and infusion should be stopped whenever the bladder is palpably taut or increased back pressure is felt on the syringe plunger. The dosages given here are approximate and based on a study of normal dogs.[36] The amount of CO_2 needed to distend the bladder adequately is variable, and there is no standard dosage that is adequate for all dogs.

Both right and left lateral and right and left VD oblique views should be obtained because lesions not visible on one view are visible on another. Depending on survey radiographic exposure, the kVp should be decreased 8 to 10%.

Complications

A rare complication of double-contrast and negative-contrast cystography is air embolization, which can cause death.[40–43] CO_2 and nitrous oxide are much more soluble in blood than is air and are considered safer to use. Excessive bladder distention may cause hematuria, cystitis, and rupture.[44,45] For this reason, mild to moderate instead of complete distention should be used in cystography. A catheter can form a knot within the urinary bladder if excessive length is passed into the bladder. Stiff catheters can be forced through the bladder wall, especially if the wall is diseased. Bacteria can be introduced into the bladder by catheterization; aseptic techniques reduce the risk of urinary tract infection.

Interpretation of Abnormal Findings

Location

Cranial displacement of the bladder occurs with prostatic enlargement or with avulsion of the bladder from the urethra (Fig. 6–32). Paraprostatic cysts can displace the bladder in any direction. The bladder may herniate ventrally through the inguinal canal or caudally into a perineal hernia (Fig. 6–33). Intrapelvic location of the bladder neck may be normal in dogs without urinary incontinence,[35,46] but an intrapelvic location of the bladder neck may contribute to incontinence[47] in bitches with incompetent urethras.

Free Intraluminal Filling Defects Seen on Cystography

Three causes of free intraluminal filling defects are calculi, blood clots, and air bubbles. In double-contrast cystography, calculi usually create sharply marginated radiolucent filling defects in the dependent portion of the bladder, which is the central area of the positive-contrast medium puddle (see Fig. 6–28). Calculi may be round or irregularly shaped. Air bubbles are located at the periphery of the positive-contrast medium puddle owing to the meniscus effect at the edge. They appear as sharply marginated, rounded radiolucent filling defects (Fig. 6–28). Blood clots may be located anywhere within the bladder and are usually variable in size and

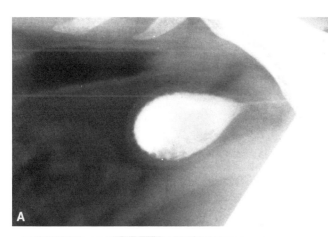
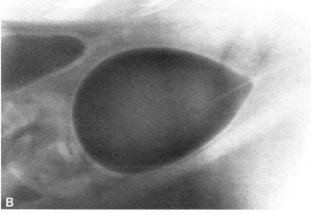

FIG. 6–31. Double-contrast cystogram in a cat with cystitis. (A) The bladder wall is thickened, and the mucosa is irregular when the bladder is mildly distended. (B) The lesions are masked when the bladder is more completely distended. Only slight wall thickening remains in the cranioventral region.

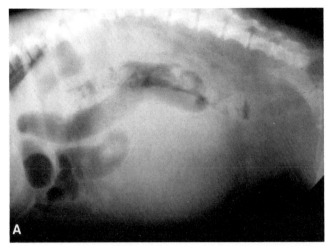

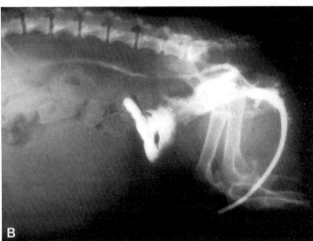

FIG. 6–32. Avulsion of the urinary bladder from the urethra in a dog that had been hit by a car. (A) A large, soft tissue dense mass is located in the midventral abdomen. Pelvic and femoral fractures can be seen on the edge of the film. (B) On a urethrogram, contrast medium is free in the peritoneal space and has been taken up by the pelvic veins. The abdominal mass is the avulsed urinary bladder with a competent urethral sphincter. (Courtesy of Dr. Royce E. Roberts, College of Veterinary Medicine, University of Georgia.)

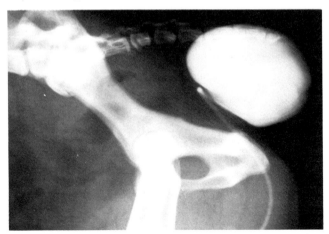

FIG. 6–33. Positive-contrast cystogram demonstrating caudal displacement of the urinary bladder into a perineal hernia.

irregularly shaped with indistinct margins (see Fig. 6–29).

Density

Decreased density of the bladder is caused by gas within the bladder lumen or bladder wall. Intraluminal gas can be differentiated from intramural gas in that intraluminal gas rises to the uppermost portion of the lumen and thus is centrally located (see Figs. 6–13, 6–25A), round in shape, and sharply marginated. Intraluminal gas may be introduced during catheterization or cystocentesis. Gas within the bladder wall (emphysematous cystitis) usually has an irregular bubbly appearance, and increased bladder wall thickness is seen on survey radiographs as the x-ray beam strikes the bladder wall tangentially (Fig. 6–34). Emphysematous cystitis is an uncommon condition caused by gas-producing bacterial infections. Secondary bacterial bladder infections associated with diabetes mellitus are the most common cause of emphysematous cystitis.[48]

Opacity of the bladder increases with intraluminal calculi (Fig. 6–35) or mineralization of the bladder wall.

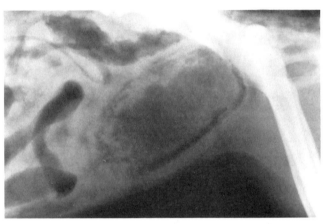

FIG. 6–34. Emphysematous cystitis in a dog with diabetes mellitus. Gas within the bladder wall has a bubbly appearance. The thickened bladder wall can be identified because of submucosal gas.

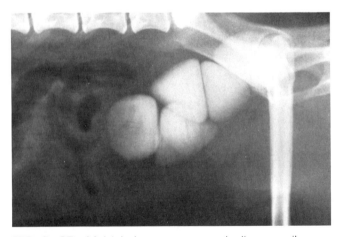

FIG. 6–35. Multiple large, opaque calculi are easily seen in the urinary bladder of this dog.

Calculi vary in size and shape; density of calculi is dependent on mineral content. Phosphate and oxalate calculi are usually radiopaque, whereas the radiopacity of cystine calculi is variable. Urate calculi are usually radiolucent. If radiolucent calculi are suspected, a double-contrast cystogram should be performed. Ultrasonography can also be used to detect bladder calculi. Calculi appear as echogenic structures in the dependent portion of the bladder with acoustic shadowing distal to the calculi (Fig. 6–36). Dystrophic mineralization of the bladder wall is uncommon but may occur with neoplasia or inflammation.[26]

Wall Thickness and Mucosal Margination

Increased thickness of the bladder wall and irregular mucosal margination may occur with cystitis, neoplasia, or polyps. Cystitis is usually characterized by gradual, relatively diffuse thickening and mucosal irregularity of the cranioventral aspect of the bladder wall (see Fig. 6–28). Mucosal irregularity can also be seen at the periphery of the positive-contrast medium puddle. Degree of wall thickening and mucosal irregularity increase with severity and chronicity of cystitis. Mucosa is often eroded in both cystitis and neoplasia. Positive-contrast medium may adhere to the eroded areas (Fig. 6–28). In chronic cystitis in cats, wall thickening may involve the majority of the bladder (see Fig. 6–31A). Most neoplastic lesions are located at the trigone and are characterized by irregularly shaped filling defects that protrude from the wall into the lumen (Fig. 6–37). The transition between normal and thickened wall is usually more abrupt than with inflammation. Rarely, tumors are more diffuse and located in the cranioventral aspect of the bladder, making them difficult to differentiate from cystitis. Tumors at the trigone frequently obstruct ureters, causing hydroureter and hydronephrosis (see Fig. 6–13). Polyps may be located anywhere within the bladder and tend to appear as discrete, sharply marginated,

small masses protruding abruptly into the lumen (Fig. 6–38). Bladder wall lesions must be biopsied for definitive diagnosis.

Function

Bladder rupture and vesicoureteral reflux are functional changes that can be evaluated radiographically. Following urinary bladder rupture, serosal margins of abdominal organs are indistinct or obscured by urine in the peritoneal space (see Fig. 6–26A). Depending on the amount of peritoneal fluid, the size of the tear, and whether the tear has sealed, the bladder may or may not be visible. As noted previously, positive-contrast cystography is the preferred contrast procedure for evaluating ruptures of the urinary bladder. Vesicoure-

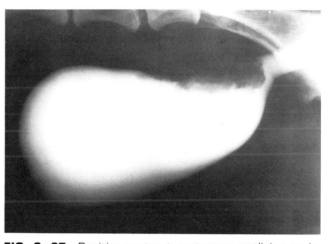

FIG. 6–37. Positive-contrast cystogram outlining an irregularly shaped filling defect in the urinary bladder trigone. The appearance and location of the filling defect are characteristic of a bladder neoplasm.

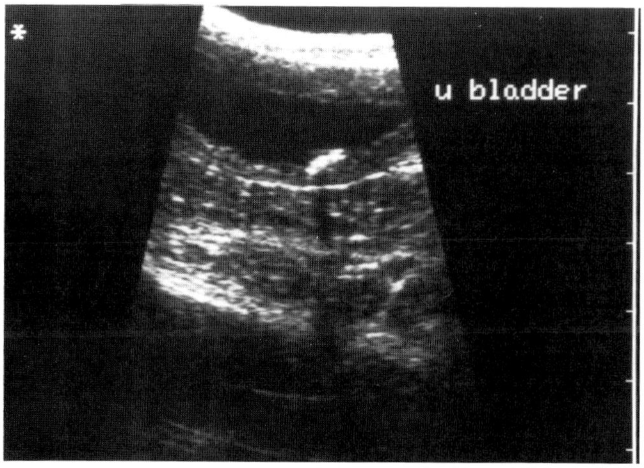

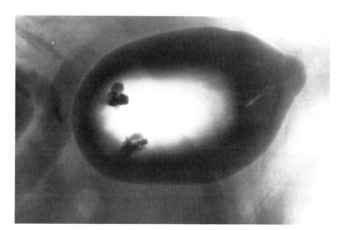

FIG. 6–38. Inflammatory bladder polyps on a double-contrast cystogram cause discrete, sharply marginated filling defects in the positive contrast puddle. (From Brown, S.A., and Barsanti, J.A.: Diseases of the bladder and urethra. *In* Veterinary Internal Medicine. Edited by Ettinger, S.J. Philadelphia, W.B. Saunders, p. 2122, 1989; with permission.)

FIG. 6–36. Ultrasonogram of a dog with a urinary bladder calculus. Urine in the bladder is anechoic. The calculus appears as a bright, echogenic focus that causes acoustic shadowing distally.

teral reflux, which is more common in young than older normal dogs,[49] may occur during cystography, urethrography,[50] or manual expression of the bladder.[51]

The radiographic diagnosis of a flaccid bladder secondary to prolonged urethral obstruction has been reported,[52] but cystography is a poor indicator of urinary bladder tone and detrusor muscle function. The urinary bladder is easily indented by surrounding structures unless intravesical pressure is sufficiently increased to make the bladder taut.[36] In dogs with normal function and large bladder capacity, the bladder may appear large and "flaccid" until completely distended.

Shape

Diverticulum in the cranioventral aspect of the bladder is not uncommon (Fig. 6–39) and may be from traumatic catheterization, urachal remnant, or partial tears of the wall. Urachal remnants may vary in size from small, persistent urachal remnants to a completely patent urachus. Muscular tears with protrusion of the mucosa through the wall may be induced by trauma (Fig. 6–40).

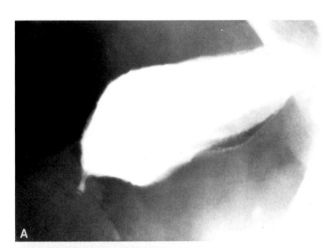

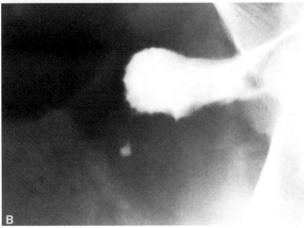

FIG. 6–39. (A) Positive-contrast cystogram in a dog with cystitis and a urachal diverticulum. The mucosa is irregular. (B) When the bladder is less distended, contrast medium is trapped in the diverticulum. The distance between the diverticulum and mucosal surface indicates bladder wall thickening.

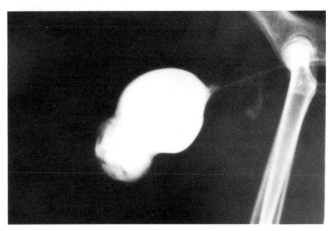

FIG. 6–40. Positive-contrast cystogram of a cat that had been hit by a car and had hematuria. The bladder is abnormally shaped because of an outpouching of the bladder at its vertex. The lesion was thought to be caused by a serosal tear allowing the mucosa to protrude through the wall. Indistinctly margined filling defects were blood clots. The mineral opacity cranial to the pelvis was an avulsion fracture of the pubis. The cat recovered without surgical intervention.

EXAMINATION OF THE URETHRA

The normal urethra is not visible on survey radiographs; therefore, urethrography must be performed to identify urethral tears, mucosal irregularity, strictures, and luminal filling defects.

Urethrography

Technique

As with other contrast procedures, urethrography is always preceded by lateral and VD survey radiographs. Standard abdominal preparation is recommended, but enema administration alone may be satisfactory for rectal evacuation. As with cystography, the animal should be sedated. In male dogs, the femurs should be held perpendicular to the spine on the lateral view. In some instances, the lateral view can be made with the hind legs pulled forward so that the femurs are not superimposed over the distal urethra. Depending on the density of the survey radiograph, the exposure should be increased by about 50% as for positive-contrast cystography.

Two types of positive-contrast urethrography are retrograde and voiding. Retrograde techniques are used most commonly and are technically easier to perform. In male dogs, a Foley balloon-tipped catheter is placed within the urethra at the distal os penis. Sterile lubricant may be used on the catheter tip. The catheter is filled with contrast medium before placement to eliminate air and prevent air bubble artifacts. The balloon is distended enough to prevent catheter withdrawal but not enough to collapse the lumen of the catheter. The balloon-tipped catheter has the advantage of preventing contrast medium leakage and allowing the radiographer to inject the media farther from the primary x-ray beam. A simple straight urethral catheter is not recommended because the urethral lumen must be occluded by digital pressure, making it impossible to keep one's fingers out of the primary beam. Also, it is difficult to prevent contrast medium leakage completely, and the catheter must be inserted further into the urethra, potentially bypassing a lesion. With balloon-tipped catheters, the urethra can be more completely evaluated.

Simple straight rubber urethral catheters may have to be used in smaller dogs because Foley balloon catheters are not available in sizes smaller than 6 Fr gauge. Cardiovascular balloon-tipped catheters are available in small size (Swan-Ganz flow-directed balloon catheter, American Edwards Laboratories, Irvine, CA 92714), but they are expensive and fragile. Balloon-tipped catheters are essential for urethrography in female dogs. A Foley catheter may be used, but because the inflatable bulb is not located at the catheter tip, the tip occupies a relatively large length of the urethra.[53] The cardiovascular catheter has the advantage of having the bulb located at the tip. The catheter should be advanced so that the bulb is approximately 1 cm cranial to the urethral orifice.[54] Although the procedure can be performed with the dog heavily sedated, it is much easier to perform if the dog is anesthetized to prevent straining and movement.

An aqueous, organic, tri-iodinated contrast medium, as for cystography or IU, is used for urethrography. Contrast medium is diluted to 100 to 150 mg I/ml with sterile saline or water to decrease the risk of obscuring filling defects. Mixing contrast medium with aqueous sterile lubricants is not advantageous.[55] Enough contrast medium is used to distend the entire urethra. In male dogs, 10 to 15 ml is usually adequate. Injection is continuous, and the exposure is made during injection of the last few milliliters so that the urethra is still distended. To evaluate the prostatic urethra, the bladder should be fully distended before urethrography. Lateral and slightly obliqued VD views are recommended (Fig. 6–41). The slightly obliqued VD view avoids superimposition of the pelvis and penile portions of the urethra. Injection must be repeated after each repositioning. In female dogs, routine lateral and VD views are made during injection of contrast medium. If urethral stricture is suspected on initial radiographs, the study is repeated after bladder distention because the normal diameter of the proximal urethra is larger with bladder distention.[55]

Positive-contrast vaginourethrography is another radiographic technique for evaluation of the urethra of female dogs.[33,34,47,56,57] With this technique, the entire urethra can be identified on the lateral view (Fig. 6–42). On the VD view, however, the urethra is superimposed over the vagina, which is filled with contrast medium. This technique is relatively easy to perform because urethral catheterization is unnecessary. A Foley catheter is filled with contrast medium to prevent introduction of air into the vagina, which could cause artifactual filling defects. After the dog is anesthetized, the Foley balloon-tipped catheter is placed into the vestibule, and the balloon is inflated to prevent contrast medium leakage

from the vulva. Positive-contrast medium (as used for positive-contrast cystography) is injected (approximately 1 ml/kg). Contrast medium should enter the vagina, urethra, and bladder (Fig. 6–42). For detection of ectopic ureters, lateral views are made in right and left lateral recumbency.[33] If urethral strictures are suspected, enough contrast medium is injected to fill the bladder and produce back pressure to distend the urethra (Fig. 6–42). As with other urethrographic techniques, radiographic exposure is made during injection of contrast medium.

In cats, urethrography is best performed with the cat under general anesthesia. Balloon-tipped cardiovascular catheters (4-gauge) are recommended. Straight, stiff urethral catheters (3.5-gauge) may be used in male cats, but contrast medium leakage is likely, making urethral distention difficult. In male cats, the catheter tip should be inserted about 1.5 cm past the urethral orifice so that the balloon is not distended within the penile urethra. The diameter of the penile urethra is too small to allow sufficient inflation of the cuff.[58,59] Balloon-tipped catheters are essential for urethrography in female cats. As with female dogs, the diameter of the proximal urethra in female cats is greater during bladder distention.[55] Therefore, the study should be repeated after bladder distention if stricture is suspected on initial radiographs.

Voiding urethrography is rarely used in animals because of the difficulty in inducing sustained urination during radiographic exposure. The procedure is usually performed with the animal under light general anesthesia. The bladder is filled with positive-contrast medium, and urination is induced by compressing the bladder with a wooden spoon placed on the abdomen. The bladder can be filled with contrast medium by catheterization or IU in animals in which catheterization is not possible. The main reason to perform voiding urethrography is to evaluate the distal urethra that might be obscured by or distal to the catheter balloon during retrograde urethrography.

Potential Complications

A minor complication of urethrography using balloon-tipped catheters is transient submucosal hemorrhage caused by inflation of the balloon.[60] Severe cystitis and bladder rupture may occur when urethrography is performed with a distended bladder to obtain maximal urethral distention.[44,45] Forceful injection into an obstructed urethra may cause urethral rupture. Absorption of contrast medium into the venous system may cause similar adverse reactions as described for IU.

Interpretation of Normal Findings

The urethra of the male dog is divided into prostatic, membranous, and penile portions. The mucosal margin is smooth throughout. A focal filling defect caused by the urethral crest in the prostatic urethra may be seen on the VD view.[25,54] Longitudinal mucosal folds may be seen as linear filling defects when the prostatic ure-

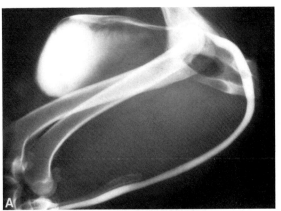
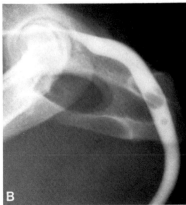
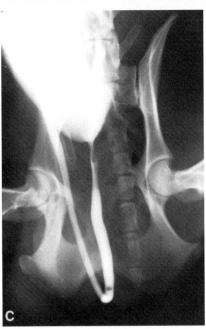

FIG. 6—41. Lateral (A), close-up lateral (B), and oblique VD (C) views of a urethrogram in a normal male dog. Mucosal margins are smooth. (A) The narrowed prostatic urethra is normal because the bladder is not fully distended. (B) Smoothly marginated, lucent filling defects are air bubbles. The largest air bubble is slightly elongated, conforming to the urethral diameter. (C) The linear filling defect in the prostatic urethra seen on the VD view is caused by the urethral crest.

thra is incompletely distended.[61] The diameter of the urethra varies with injection pressure, bladder distention, and urethral spasm. The membranous urethra is frequently narrowed at the ischial arch. Nonpathologic narrowing can be identified by gradual tapering and smooth mucosal margins (Fig. 6–43A) as opposed to abrupt narrowing that occurs more frequently with strictures.[54] If necessary, the study should be repeated to help differentiate between spasm and stricture. A spasm may persist, however, making if difficult to differentiate from a stricture. Infusion of lidocaine before urethrography has been recommended to decrease the likelihood of urethral spasm in unanesthetized dogs.[26,52–54,62] The prostatic urethra may be narrow on retrograde urethrography (see Fig. 6–41A) and wide on voiding urethrography.[61] On maximum distention retrograde urethrography, in which the urinary bladder is fully distended

before urethrography, and during micturition, the prostatic urethra is wider than the membranous urethra (Fig. 6–44),[63,64] but there is no difference in the diameters of the membranous and penile urethra before and after bladder distention.[55] Urethroprostatic reflux of contrast medium may occur during urethrography, especially when the bladder is maximally distended. The amount of reflux expected in dogs with normal prostates is minimal and may appear as small, focal, contrast "blushes" (Fig. 6–44).[64]

The normal female canine urethra has smooth longitudinal folds when the urethra is incompletely distended. The diameter of the distal urethra before and after bladder distention is unchanged, but the proximal urethral diameter is significantly larger after bladder distention.[55]

The male feline urethra is divided into intrapelvic

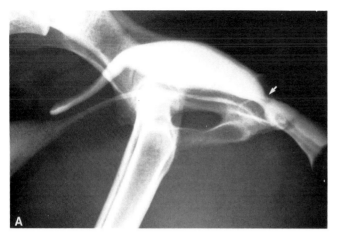

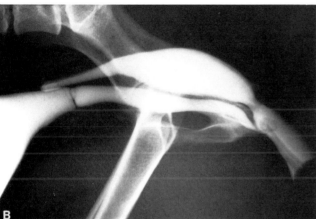

FIG. 6–42. Positive-contrast vaginourethrography in a 5-year-old bitch with a dysuria. (A) On the initial film, the bladder and urethra are incompletely distended, and no abnormalities are identified. The Foley catheter bulb and tip are visible in the vestibule. A rounded filling defect caused by an air bubble overlies the catheter tip. Contrast medium outlines the vagina. The slightly narrowed area (arrow) is the vestibulovaginal junction. (B) A stricture at the bladder-urethral junction is found when the bladder and urethra are more completely distended.

(preprostatic, prostatic, and postprostatic) and penile portions.[59] As in the dog, urethral diameter varies with injection pressure, resistance, bladder distention, and urethral spasm. When the bladder is distended, the intrapelvic urethral diameter is uniform.[66] The diameter of the penile urethra is greatest at the ischiatic arch and becomes progressively smaller toward the distal tip.[59] The female feline urethra is similar to that of the bitch.[52,62,66]

Interpretation of Abnormal Findings

Luminal Filling Defects

Calculi, air bubbles, clots, and cellular debris appear as lucent filling defects in the contrast column. Opaque calculi are readily identified on survey radiographs as mineral opacities lying over the plane of the urethra, but urethrography must be performed to identify radiolu-

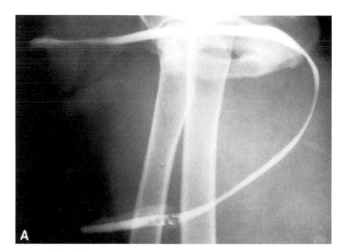

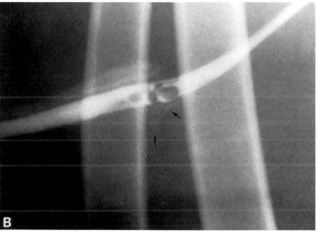

FIG. 6–43. Retrograde urethrogram in a male dog with dysuria. (A) Irregularly shaped filling defects within the urethra at the caudal aspect of the os penis are calculi. Gradual narrowing of the urethra at the ischial arch is caused by urethral spasm. (B) The irregular shape of the filling defects and slight expansion of the urethra around them are indicative of calculi rather than air bubbles. Slight increase in density (arrows) within the soft tissues ventral to the calculi is caused by contrast medium extravasation from the urethra.

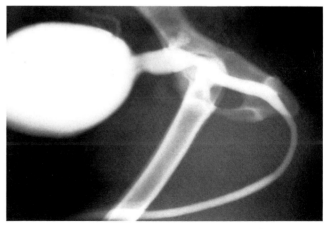

FIG. 6–44. Maximum-distention urethrography in a normal male dog. The prostatic urethra is wider than the membranous urethra. Urethroprostatic and vesicoureteral reflux are present.

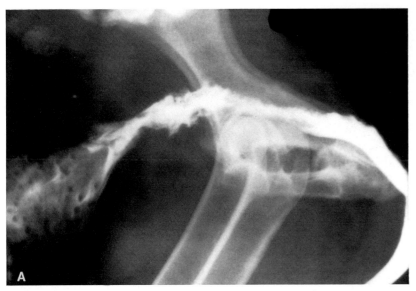
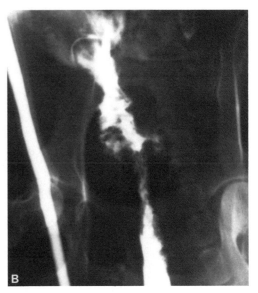

FIG. 6–45. Urethrography ([A] lateral, [B] VD) in a male dog with dysuria caused by transitional cell carcinoma of the urethra. The mucosal margination of the intrapelvic urethra is very irregular, and the luminal diameter is varied. Focal filling defects in the bladder were "islands" of tumor.

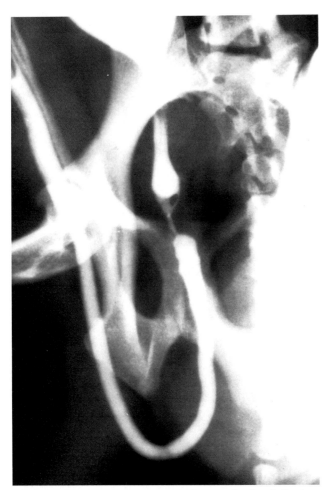

FIG. 6–46. Urethral stricture in a male dog following a traumatic incident. The pelvic urethra is abruptly narrowed, indicating stricture rather than spasm in which urethral narrowing is gradual (see Fig. 6-43[A]).

cent calculi. Calculi often have irregular shapes and indistinct margins and, if large enough, distend the urethral lumen (see Fig. 6–43). In contrast, air bubbles appear as round, smoothly marginated lucent filling defects. Large bubbles conform to the urethral lumen forming elongated lucent filling defects with rounded ends (see Fig. 6–41). Blood clots are uncommon, are variable in shape, and have indistinct margins. Abnormal enlargement of the colliculus seminalis was reported as a cause of urethral filling defects in dogs with Sertoli cell tumors.[67] The colliculus seminalis appeared as a smoothly marginated filling defect originating from the dorsal wall of the prostatic urethra.

Mucosal Margination

Irregular mucosal margination may be caused by neoplasia[68] or urethritis.[69] With severe mucosal irregularity and luminal narrowing, neoplasia should be the primary differential diagnosis (Fig. 6–45).

Shape

Luminal narrowing with smooth mucosal margins may be caused by urethral spasm or stricture. As noted previously, spasms tend to result in gradual urethral narrowing, whereas strictures tend to narrow the urethral lumen abruptly (see Fig. 6–42B; Fig. 6–46). Prostatic disease may cause urethral narrowing. Maximum distention retrograde urethrography is performed to confirm urethral narrowing caused by prostatic disease. Diverticulae appear as outpouchings of the urethral lumen and may result from catheter trauma or urethral surgery (Fig. 6–47).

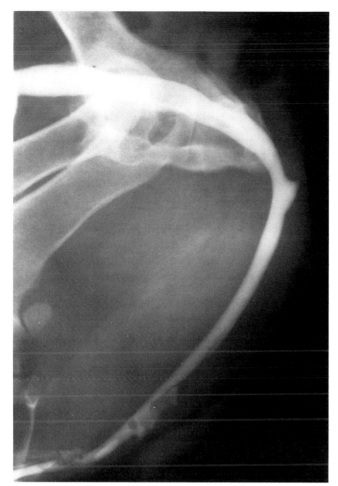

FIG. 6–47. Urethrogram in a male dog with urethral diverticula. The diverticulum at the ischial arch was caused by catheter trauma. The large diverticulum proximal to the os penis occurred secondary to urethrotomy. An air bubble causes a round filling defect within the urethra.

Contrast Medium Extravasation

Contrast medium extravasation from urethral rupture may extend into the retroperitoneal and pelvic canal space or into the peritoneal space, depending on the location of the rupture (see Fig. 6–18). Urethral fistulae (urethrovaginal, urethrorectal) are uncommon, but are readily diagnosed with positive-contrast urethrography.[52,70,71]

EXAMINATION OF THE PROSTATE GLAND

When visible radiographically, the prostate is seen as a rounded, soft tissue dense structure located just caudal to the bladder. Commonly, a triangular shaped, fat, dense area can be seen ventrally between the bladder, prostate, and abdominal wall. The prostate is usually located within the pelvic canal but moves cranially with bladder distention. In immature or castrated dogs, the prostate is small and may be difficult to identify radiographically. On the lateral view, the normal prostatic

diameter should be no greater than 70% of the distance between the pubis and sacral promontory,[72] and on the VD view, the normal prostatic width should be no more than 50% of the width of the pelvic canal.[73]

On ultrasound examination, the normal dog prostate has a diffuse, hypoechoic, granular appearance that has been described as "uniformly inhomogeneous" (Fig. 6–48).[75] It is less echogenic than the surrounding abdominal and pelvic musculature.[75] The capsular surface should be smooth, but it is often indistinct. The prostatic urethra appears on the sagittal view as a tubular hypoechoic structure that is continuous with the bladder and on the transverse scan as a round hypoechoic structure in the center of the prostate. A centrally located hilar echo may be the confluence of prostatic ducts in the urethral area.[74–76] The parenchymal echogenicity of the prostate should be less than that of the hilar echo, but the hilar echo is inconsistently identified.[76] It is helpful to have the urinary bladder full, so that the prostate is pulled cranially and is easier to scan transabdominally.

Interpretation of Abdominal Findings

Size

Enlargement of the prostate commonly occurs in dogs with prostatic abnormalities. Enlargement on the lateral view greater than 90% of the pubic-promontory distance is suggestive of neoplasia, abscess, or paraprostatic cysts.[72]

Shape

Asymmetrical enlargement of the prostate (Fig. 6–49) around the urethra is more common with neoplasia, abscess, or cysts than diffuse conditions such as benign hyperplasia without cysts or prostatitis (Fig. 6–50).[72] Thus, severe prostatic enlargement is an indication for

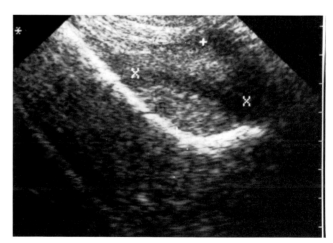

FIG. 6–48. Sagittal sonogram of the prostate of a normal dog. The prostate is outlined by cursors and has a coarsely granular appearance. The prostatic urethra is the hypoechoic line extending between the "x" cursors in a craniocaudal direction. Cranial is to the left, and ventral is at the top.

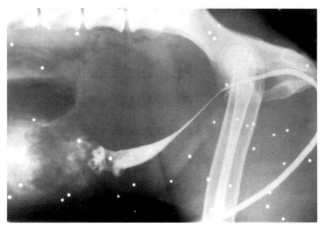

FIG. 6–49. Urethrogram of a dog with asymmetrical periurethral prostatic enlargement caused by a cyst. The urethra is displaced ventrally, and there is a greater amount of prostatic tissue dorsal to the urethra than ventral. The bladder is displaced cranially by the enlarged prostate. Mottled density within the bladder is caused by incomplete mixing of contrast medium with unopacified urine. Gunshot pellets scattered throughout the soft tissues were an incidental finding.

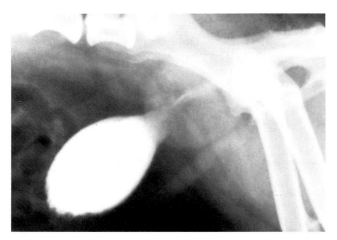

FIG. 6–50. Urethrocystogram in a dog with symmetrical periurethral prostatic enlargement and cystitis. Symmetrical prostatic enlargement is commonly associated with benign hyperplasia or prostatitis.

thorough diagnostic evaluation. Irregular periosteal bone reaction along the ventral aspects of the caudal lumbar vertebrae or on the pelvis (Fig. 6–51) is compatible with metastasis of prostatic or urethral neoplasia. Iliac lymph node enlargement may also be seen with metastasis from prostatic neoplasia or, less commonly, with prostatic abscessation.[25,72,73]

Paraprostatic cysts may become very large and can be located dorsal, ventral, lateral, cranial, or caudal to the prostate (Fig. 6–52).

Density

Mineralization of the prostate may be seen in dogs with chronic prostatitis[77] or prostatic calculi,[78] but prostatic carcinoma should be the primary consideration.[72] The

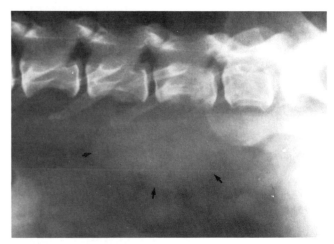

FIG. 6–51. Close-up lateral view of the caudal lumbar region of a dog with irregular periosteal bone reaction on the ventral aspects of the L5–L7 vertebral bodies. The iliac lymph nodes (arrows) are enlarged. These lesions are typical of metastasis from prostatic or urethral neoplasms.

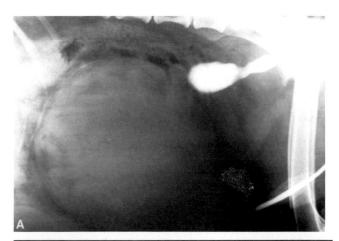

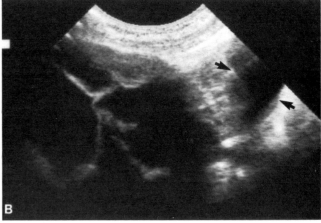

FIG. 6–52. Urethrocystogram (A) and sagittal sonogram (B) of a dog with a large paraprostatic cyst. The cyst was connected to the prostate by a stalk and appears as a large, round soft tissue mass in the midabdomen displacing the bladder dorsally. A portion of the cyst wall is mineralized. (B) On ultrasound examination, the cyst is seen as a large anechoic mass containing hypoechoic septae. The urinary bladder (arrows) is located caudal to the cyst. Cranial is to the left, and ventral is at the top.

walls of paraprostatic cysts may also become mineralized and have an "eggshell" appearance (Fig. 6–52).

Prostatic Reflux

Urethroprostatic reflux during urethrography has been reported in dogs with prostatitis, prostatic hyperplasia, and neoplasia.[79] Because small amounts of contrast medium reflux can be seen in normal dogs during urethrography (see Fig. 6–44),[65,79] mild urethroprostatic reflux does not differentiate normal from abnormal. Massive coalescent urethroprostatic reflux is abnormal, however, and suggestive of neoplasia or abscessation.[72]

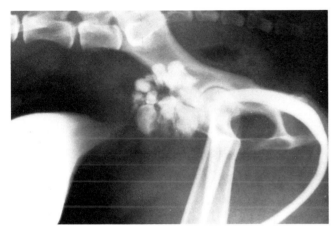

FIG. 6–53. Massive reflux of contrast medium into prostatic cavities during urethrography. Extensive urethroprostatic reflux such as this is abnormal and suggestive of neoplasia or abscessation. The histologic diagnosis was adenocarcinoma.

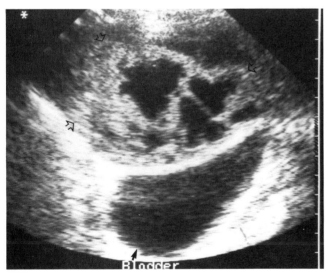

FIG. 6–54. Sagittal sonogram of a dog with prostatomegaly. The prostate is located ventral to the bladder (solid arrow), displacing it dorsally. Prostatic margins are indistinct (open arrows), and the parenchyma is more echogenic than normal. Several thick-walled, anechoic cavities seen within the prostate could be caused by cyst, abscess, or hematoma formation. Cranial is to the left, and ventral is at the top.

Occasionally, cavitary lesions are outlined by contrast medium (Fig. 6–53).

Ultrasonography is used to evaluate prostatic size, shape, and margination but is most useful for differentiating solid from cystic conditions and paraprostatic cysts from parenchymal cystic lesions. Cystic lesions such as prostatic abscessation, prostatic cysts, and hematomas have a hypoechoic to anechoic appearance with distant enhancement (see Fig. 6–52; Fig. 6–54).[76]

Noncavitating prostatic diseases are difficult to differentiate ultrasonographically. Homogeneous increased echogenicity may be caused by hyperplasia,[80] fibrosis, or glandular aging.[76] Focal to multifocal areas of increased echogenicity have been seen with prostatitis and neoplasia.[76] In general, ultrasonography is sensitive for detecting abnormalities and for differentiating solid from cystic lesions but is not specific for type of disease. Therefore, it should be used in conjunction with other diagnostic tests for prostatic evaluation.

REFERENCES

1. Herring, D.S., and Bjornton, G.: Physics, facts, and artifacts of diagnostic ultrasound. Vet. Clin. North Am. [Sm. Anim. Pract.], 15:1107, 1985.
2. Nyland, T.G., Park, R.D., Lattimer, J.C., et al.: Gray-scale ultrasonography of the canine abdomen. Vet. Radiol., 22:220, 1981.
3. Park, R.D., Nyland, T.G., Lattimer, J.C., et al.: B-Mode gray-scale ultrasound: Imaging artifacts and interpretation principles. Vet. Radiol., 22:204, 1981.
4. Rantanen, N.W., and Ewing, R.L.: Principles of ultrasound application in animals. Vet. Radiol., 22:196, 1981.
5. Grandage, J.: Some effects of posture on the radiographic appearance of the kidneys of the dog. J. Am. Vet. Med. Assoc., 166:165, 1975.
6. Finco, D.R., Stiles, N.S., Kneller, S.K., et al.: Radiologic estimation of kidney size of the dog. J. Am. Vet. Med. Assoc., 159:995, 1971.
7. Barrett, R.B., and Kneller, S.K.: Feline kidney mensuration. Acta Radiol., 319(suppl):279, 1972.
8. Walter, P.A., Feeney, D.A., Johnston, G.R., et al.: Ultrasonographic evaluation of renal parenchymal diseases in dogs: 32 cases (1981–1986). J. Am. Vet. Med. Assoc., 191:999, 1987.
9. Walter, P.A., Johnston, G.R., Feeney, D.A., et al.: Applications of ultrasonography in the diagnosis of parenchymal kidney disease in cats: 24 cases (1981–1986). J. Am. Vet. Med. Assoc., 192:92, 1988.
10. Feeney, D.A., Barber, D.L., and Osborne, C.A.: The functional aspects of the nephrogram in excretory urography: A review. Vet. Radiol., 23:42, 1982.
11. Feeney, D.A., Barber, D.L., Johnston, G.R., et al.: The excretory urogram: Part I. Techniques, normal radiographic appearance and misinterpretation. Compend. Contin. Educ. Pract. Vet., 4:233, 1982.
12. Kneller, S.K.: Role of the excretory urogram in the diagnosis of renal and ureteral disease. Vet. Clin. North Am., 4:843, 1974.
13. Thrall, D.E., and Finco, D.R.: Canine excretory urography: Is quality a function of BUN? J. Am. Anim. Hosp. Assoc., 12:446, 1976.
14. Feeney, D.A., Thrall, D.E., Barber, D.L., et al.: The normal canine excretory urogram: Effects of dose, time and individual dog variation. Am. J. Vet. Res., 40:1596, 1979.
15. Feeney, D.A., Barber, D.L., and Osborne, C.A.: Advances in canine excretory urography. In Proceedings 30th Gaines Veteri-

nary Symposium, White Plains, NY, Gaines Dog Research Center, pp. 8–22, 1981.

16. Feeney, D.A., Osborne, C.A., and Jessen, C.R.: Effect of multiple excretory urograms on glomerular filtration of normal dogs: A preliminary report. Am. J. Vet. Res., 41:960, 1980.

17. Talner, L.B.: Urographic contrast media in uremia. Radiol. Clin. North Am., 10:421, 1972.

18. Walter, P.A., Feeney, D.A., and Johnston, G.A.: Diagnosis and treatment of adverse reactions to radiopaque contrast agents. In Current Veterinary Therapy IX. Edited by R.W. Kirk. Philadelphia, W.B. Saunders, pp. 47–52, 1986.

19. Feeney, D.A., Osborne, C.A., and Jessen, C.R.: Effects of radiocontrast agents on the urinalysis with emphasis on specific gravity. J. Am. Vet. Med. Assoc., 176:1378, 1980.

20. Ruby, A.L., Ling, G.V., and Ackerman, N.: Effect of sodium diatrizoate on the in vitro growth of three common canine urinary bacterial species. Vet. Radiol., 24:222, 1983.

21. Yeager, A.E., and Anderson, W.I.: Study of association between histologic features and echogenicity of architecturally normal cat kidneys. Am. J. Vet. Res., 50:860, 1989.

22. Barber, D.L., and Finco, D.R.: Radiographic findings in induced bacterial pyelonephritis in dogs. J. Am. Vet. Med. Assoc., 175:1183, 1979.

23. Barber, D.L., and Rowland, G.N.:Radiographically detectable soft tissue calcification in chronic renal failure. Vet. Radiol., 20:117, 1979.

24. Miller, J.B., and Sande, R.D.: Osseous metaplasia in the renal pelvis of a dog with hydronephrosis. Vet. Radiol., 21:146, 1980.

25. Burk, R.L., and Ackerman, N.: Small Animal Radiology: A Diagnostic Atlas and Text. New York, Churchill Livingstone, pp. 133–233, 1986.

26. Ackerman, N.: Radiology of Urogenital Diseases in Dogs and Cats. Davis, Calif., Venture Press, 1983.

27. Chambers, J.N., Selcer, B.A., and Barsanti, J.A.: Recovery from severe hydroureter and hydronephrosis after ureteral anastomosis in a dog. J. Am. Vet. Med. Assoc., 191:1589, 1987.

28. Barber, D.L.: Postoperative radiography of the urinary system. Vet. Clin. North Am. [Sm. Anim. Pract.], 14:31, 1984.

29. Bjorling, D.E., Mahaffey, M.B., and Crowell, W.A.: Bilateral ureteroileostomy and perineal urinary diversion in dogs. Vet. Surg., 14:204, 1985.

30. Caine, M., and Hermann, G.: The return of peristalsis in the anastomosed ureter, a cine-radiographic study. Br. J. Urol., 42:164, 1970.

31. Greene, R.W., and Griener, T.P.: The ureter: Repair of longitudinal defects and reimplantation. In Current Techniques in Veterinary Surgery. Edited by M.J. Bojrab. Philadelphia, Lea & Febiger, p. 217, 1975.

32. Mason, L.K., Stone, E.A., Biery, D.N., et al.: Surgery of ectopic ureters: Pre and postoperative radiographic morphology. J. Am. Anim. Hosp. Assoc., 26:73, 1990.

33. Holt, P.E., Gibbs, C., and Pearson, H.: Canine ectopic ureter—a review of twenty-nine cases. J. Sm. Am. Anim. Pract., 23:195, 1982.

34. Holt, P.E., Gibbs, C., and Latham, J.: An evaluation of positive contrast vagino-urethrography as a diagnostic aid in the bitch. J. Sm. Anim. Pract., 25:531, 1984.

35. Mahaffey, M.B., Barsanti, J.A., Barber, D.L., et al.: Pelvic bladder in dogs without urinary incontinence. J. Am. Vet. Med. Assoc., 184:1477, 1984.

36. Mahaffey, M.B., Barber, D.L., Barsanti, J.A., et al.: Simultaneous double-contrast cystography and cystometry in dogs. Vet. Radiol., 25:254, 1984.

37. Mahaffey, M.B., Barsanti, J.A., Crowell, W.A., et al.: Cystography: Effect of technique on diagnosis of cystitis in dogs. Vet. Radiol., 30:261, 1989.

38. Ackerman, N., and Nyland, T.G.: Cystography. Calif. Vet., 32:13, 1978.

39. Schwensen, K., Mahaffey, M.B., Barsanti, J.A., et al.: The effect of intravesical lidocaine on urinary bladder distension during cystography in cats. American College of Veterinary Radiology Scientific Program, Incline Village, Nevada, August 11, 1986.

40. Ackerman, N., Wingfield, W.E., and Corley, E.A.: Fatal air embolism associated with pneumourethrography and pneumocystography in a dog. J. Am. Vet. Med. Assoc., 160:1616, 1972.

41. Johnston, G.R., and Feeney, D.A.: Comparative organ imaging, lower urinary tract. Vet. Radiol., 25:146, 1984.

42. Johnston, G.R., Feeney, D.A., and Osborne, C.A.: Urethrography and cystography in cats. Part II. Abnormal radiographic anatomy and complications. Compend. Contin. Educ. Pract. Vet., 4:931, 1982.

43. Zontine, W.J., and Andrews, L.K.: Fatal air embolization as a complication of pneumocystography. J. Am. Vet. Radiol. Soc., 19:8, 1978.

44. Barsanti, J.A., Crowell, W., Losonsky, J., et al.: Complications of bladder distension during retrograde urethrography. Am. J. Vet. Res., 42:819, 1981.

45. Johnston, G.R., Stevens, J.B., Jessen, C.R., et al.: Complications of retrograde contrast urethrography in dogs and cats. Am. J. Vet. Res., 44:1248, 1983.

46. Johnston, G.R., Osborne, C.A., Jessen, C.R., et al.: Effects of urinary bladder distention on location of the urinary bladder and urethra of healthy dogs and cats. Am. J. Vet. Res., 47:404, 1986.

47. Holt, P.E.: Importance of urethral length, bladder neck position and vestibulovaginal stenosis in sphincter mechanism incompetence in the incontinent bitch. Res. Vet. Sci., 39:364, 1985.

48. Root, C.R., and Scott, R.C.: Emphysematous cystitis and other radiographic manifestations of diabetes mellitus in dogs and cats. J. Am. Vet. Med. Assoc., 158:721, 1971.

49. Christie, B.A.: Incidence and etiology of vesicoureteral reflux in apparently normal dogs. Invest. Urol., 9:184, 1971.

50. Klausner, J.S., and Feeney, D.A.: Vesicoureteral reflux. In Current Veterinary Therapy VIII. Edited by R.W. Kirk. Philadelphia, W.B. Saunders, pp. 1041–1043, 1983.

51. Feeney, D.A., Osborne, C.A., and Johnston, G.R.: Vesicoureteral reflux induced by manual compression of the urinary bladder of dogs and cats. J. Am. Vet. Med. Assoc., 182:79, 1983.

52. Park, R.: Radiology of the urinary bladder and urethra. In Radiographic Diagnosis of Abdominal Disorders in the Dog and Cat: Radiographic Interpretation, Clinical Signs, Pathophysiology. Edited by T.R. O'Brien. Philadelphia, W.B. Saunders, pp. 543–614, 1978.

53. Ackerman, N.: Urethrography—technique. Calif. Vet., 33:6, 1979.

54. Ticer, J.W., Spencer, C.P., and Ackerman, N.: Positive contrast retrograde urethrography. A useful procedure for evaluating urethral disorders in the dog. Vet. Radiol., 21:2, 1980.

55. Johnston, G.R., Jessen, C.R., and Osborne, C.A.: Effects of bladder distention on canine and feline retrograde urethrography. Vet. Radiol., 24:271, 1983.

56. Holt, P.E.: Urinary incontinence in the bitch due to sphincter mechanism incompetence: Surgical treatment. J. Sm. Anim. Pract., 26:237, 1985.

57. Osborne, C.A., Low, D.G., and Finco, D.R.: Canine and Feline Urology. Philadelphia, W.B. Saunders, p. 336, 1972.

58. Johnston, G.R., and Feeney, D.A.: Localization of feline urethral obstruction. Vet. Clin. North Am. [Sm. Anim. Pract.], 14:555, 1984.

59. Johnston, G.R., Feeney, D.A., and Osborne, C.A.: Urethrography and cystography in cats. Part I. Techniques, normal radiographic anatomy, and artifacts. Compend. Contin. Educ. Pract. Vet., 4:823, 1982.

60. Johnston, G.R., Stevens, J.B., Jessen, C.R., et al.: Effects of prolonged distention of retention catheters on the urethra of dogs and cats. Am. J. Vet. Res., 44:223, 1983.

61. Poogird, W., and Wood, A.K.W.: Radiologic study of the canine urethra. Am. J. Vet. Res., 47:2491, 1986.
62. Johnston, G.R., Jessen, C.R., and Osborne, C.A.: Retrograde contrast urethrography. In Current Veterinary Therapy VI. Edited by R.W. Kirk. Philadelphia, W.B. Saunders, pp. 1189–1192, 1977.
63. Mygind, T., and Tage, H.: Radiological analysis of urethral morphology and function in male dogs. Invest. Radiol., 1:301, 1966.
64. Feeney, D.A., Johnston, G.R., Osborne, C.A., et al.: Dimensions of the prostatic and membranous urethra in normal male dogs during maximum distension retrograde urethrocystography. Vet. Radiol., 25:249, 1984.
65. Feeney, D.A., Johnston, G.R., Osborne, C.A., et al.: Maximum distension retrograde urethrography in healthy male dogs: Occurrence and radiographic appearance of urethroprostatic reflux. Am. J. Vet. Res., 45:948,1984.
66. Johnston, G.R., and Feeney, D.A.: Radiographic evaluation of the urinary tract in dogs and cats. In Nephrology and Urology. Edited by E.B. Breitschwerdt. New York, Churchill Livingstone, p. 203, 1986.
67. Jacobs, G., Barsanti, J., Prasse, K., et al.: Colliculus seminalis as a cause of a urethral filling defect in two dogs with Sertoli cell testicular neoplasms. J. Am. Vet. Med. Assoc., 192:1748, 1988.
68. Ticer, J.W., Spencer, C.P., and Ackerman, N.: Transitional cell carcinoma of the urethra in four female dogs: Its urethrographic appearance. Vet. Radiol., 21:12, 1980.
69. Burk, R.L., and Schaubhut, C.W., Jr.; Obstructive urethritis in the female dog. Vet. Med. Sm. Anim. Clin., 71:898, 1976.
70. Osuna, D.J., Stone, E.A., and Metcalf, M.: Urethrorectal fistula in a dog. J. Am. Anim. Hosp. Assoc., 25:35, 1989.
71. Whitney, W.O., and Schrader, L.A.: Urethrorectal fistulectomy in a dog using a perineal approach. J. Am. Vet. Med. Assoc., 193:568, 1988.
72. Feeney, D.A., Johnston, G.R., Klausner, J.S., et al.: Canine prostatic disease—comparison of radiographic appearance with morphologic and microbiologic findings: 30 cases (1981–1985). J. Am. Vet. Med. Assoc., 190:1018, 1987.
73. Lattimer, J.C.: The prostate. In Textbook of Veterinary Diagnostic Radiology. Edited by D.E. Thrall. Philadelphia, W.B. Saunders, p. 444, 1986.
74. Johnston, G.R., Feeney, D.A., Osborne, C.A., et al.: Effects of intravesical hydrostatic pressure and volume on the distensibility of the canine prostatic portion of the urethra. Am. J. Vet. Res., 46:748, 1985.
75. Feeney, D.A., Johnston, G.R., and Klausner, J.S.: Two-dimensional, gray-scale ultrasonography, applications in canine prostatic disease. Vet. Clin. North Am. [Sm. Anim. Pract.], 15:1159, 1985.
76. Feeney, D.A., Johnston, G.R., Klausner, J.S., et al.: Canine prostatic disease-comparison of ultrasonographic appearance with morphologic and microbiologic findings: 30 cases (1981–1985). J. Am. Vet. Med. Assoc., 190:1027, 1987.
77. Hornbuckle, W.E., MacCoy, D.M., Allan, G.S., et al.: Prostatic disease in the dog. Cornell Vet., 68(suppl):284, 1978.
78. Knecht, C.D.: Disease of the canine prostate gland. Compend. Contin. Educ. Pract. Vet., 1:385, 1979.
79. Ackerman, N.: Prostatic reflux during positive contrast retrograde urethrography in the dog. Vet. Radiol., 24:251, 1983.
80. Cartee, R.E., and Rowles, T.: Transabdominal sonographic evaluation of the canine prostate. Vet. Radiol., 24:156, 1983.

Section Three

General Principles of
Urologic Surgery

7

Surgical Materials, Instruments, and Urinary Catheters

A successful outcome after a surgical procedure is not only dependent on the surgeon's knowledge and skill, but also on the materials and instruments used before, during, and after the surgery. Suture materials can incite calculi or granuloma formation. Insertion of urinary catheters can cause iatrogenic injury, precipitate urinary tract infection, or both. Improper instruments can prolong the operative time and damage the delicate tissue of the urinary tract. This chapter focuses on the selection and use of materials and instruments and provides the foundation for the specific surgical techniques discussed in Part Two.

SUTURE MATERIALS

An ideal suture material for the urinary tract should be at least as strong as the tissue through which it is placed and should maintain its strength until the wound regains sufficient strength. The suture should cause minimal tissue reaction and should not incite calculi formation. If the suture is in contact with urine, these characteristics should be maintained, even if urine is infected.

When placed entirely within tissue, any of the synthetic absorbable suture materials (Table 7-1) maintain their strength for more than the 14 to 21 days the bladder needs to regain initial strength.[1,2] Infected urine may diminish the strength of some synthetic absorbable suture materials, particularly polyglycolic acid (Dexon) and polyglactin 910 (Vicryl).[3-6] Our in vitro studies demonstrated that Vicryl and Dexon lost strength faster in *E. coli*–infected urine than in sterile urine, but PDS II and chromic gut retained their strength.[5] When sutures were incubated with *Proteus*-infected urine, Vicryl and Dexon lost all strength within 24-hours of immersion.[5] Maxon and PDS retained strength for three to seven days.[5] Chromic gut retained most of its original strength for more than 10 days in either *E. coli*–infected or *Proteus*-infected urine.[4-6] In an in vivo study, PDS II re-

tained 60% and chromic gut 25% of its strength after 7 days in *Proteus*-infected urine. In vitro phagocytosis may accelerate the breakdown of gut suture material. Urine infected with a urea-splitting microorganism (e.g., *Proteus*) is alkaline because of the breakdown of urea to ammonia. The change in pH may alter the hydrolytic degradation of some synthetic absorbable suture materials.[7] Multiple, transverse microfractures were seen with scanning electron microscopy of Dexon suture after incubation in urine infected with *Proteus*.[8]

Placement of nonabsorbable sutures or staples into the lumen of the urinary bladder should be avoided because they predictably promote urolithiasis. Polypropylene, nylon, and silk sutures have been associated

---

TABLE 7–1. SUTURE MATERIAL FOR UROLOGIC SURGERY

Material	Ethicon, Inc* Trade Name	Davis & Geckt Trade Name
Synthetic Nonabsorbable Monofilament		
Monofilament nylon	Ethilon	Dermalon
Polypropylene	Prolene	Surgilene
Synthetic Absorbable Braided		
Coated polyglactin 910 (PG-910)	Vicryl	
Uncoated polyglycolic acid		Dexon "S"
Coated polyglycolic acid		Dexon Plus
Synthetic Absorbable Monofilament		
Polyglyconate		Maxon
Polydioxanone	PDS II	
Natural Fiber		
Chromic gut	Chromic gut	Chromic gut

* Sommerville, NJ 08876
† Wayne, NJ 07470

with calculi formation after clinical surgery in dogs and humans.[9,10] Chromic gut and Dexon within the lumen of the urinary bladder also cause deposition of crystaline substances, but because the sutures slough within 4 to 8 weeks, calculi formation is less likely.[11,12] Braided, nonabsorbable suture, e.g., silk or plastic sheathed twisted nylon (Vetafil, S. Jackson, Inc. Alexandria, VA 22303), should not be used in the urinary tract because it can induce granuloma formation (Fig. 7-1).[13]

Current recommendations for choice of suture material are:

1. If the suture can be placed beneath the mucosa, chromic gut, monofilament synthetic nonabsorbable suture, or synthetic absorbable suture material can be used. For example, for closure of the urinary bladder following a cystotomy, a simple interrupted, Cushing, or Lembert pattern, which does not penetrate the mucosa, is used.
2. If the suture will be in contact with sterile urine, any absorbable suture can be used. A synthetic absorbable suture is preferred for small diameter ureters or urethras, in which the exaggerated inflammatory response of chromic gut is undesirable.
3. If the suture will be in contact with infected urine, especially *Proteus* or other urea-splitting organisms, PDS II or Maxon sutures are recommended (e.g., with ureteral or urethral anastomosis). In animals with diseases associated with delayed wound healing, a nonabsorbable monofilament suture (e.g., nylon or polypropylene) may be required even though the suture can potentially induce encrustation and calculi formation.
4. In the kidney, a monofilament absorbable suture material (PDS II, Maxon) is desirable because it has minimal tissue drag and causes minimal inflammatory reaction in the renal parenchyma.

SURGICAL INSTRUMENTS

General surgical instruments are used to incise the abdomen and the urinary bladder. A vascular clamp or bulldog clamp is used to occlude the renal artery during nephrotomy (Fig. 7-2). Temporary vascular occlusion should never be done with a hemostat because a hemostat damages the vessel wall and can cause clotting and thrombi. A delicate instrument pack can be assembled for surgery on the urethra and ureter. For suturing the ureter and urethra, needle holders must have fine jaws to grasp delicate swedged needles, maximize effective needle length, and minimize straightening stress as the needle holder is applied. Small iris scissors and No. 11 and 15 scalpel blades are helpful for incising the urethra or ureter. Delicate tissue forceps aid in gentle tissue handling. Identification of tissue layers and small lumina is facilitated by the use of magnification loupes (4×).

A suction apparatus allows removal of urine within the abdomen and provides a means of removing large volumes of lavage fluid. It is also useful for quickly draining a full bladder during surgery or evacuating prostatic abscesses. To create a very small hole and to minimize contamination, a hypodermic needle can be attached to the suction tubing and then inserted into the bladder or prostate (Fig. 7-3). The contaminated needle or suction tip should be exchanged before proceeding.

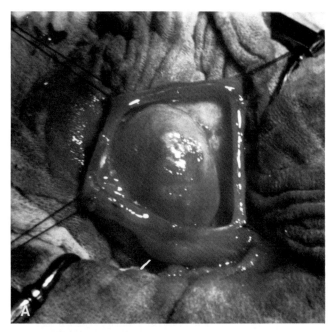

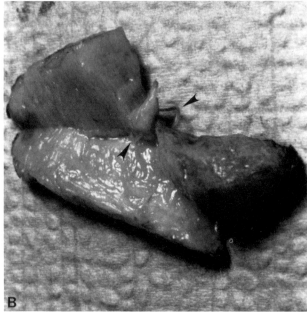

FIG. 7—1. (A) Interior surface of a dog's urinary bladder showing a submucosal mass. The dog had a cystotomy 6 months previously. The incision had been closed with plastic-sheathed, twisted nylon suture material. (B) After excision of the bladder mass, a piece of suture material was found within the mass (arrows). The histologic diagnosis was granuloma.

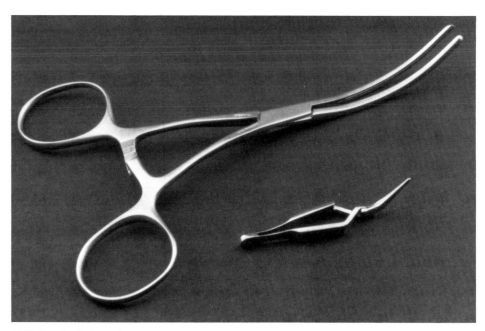

FIG. 7–2. Adjustable pressure bulldog clamp (bottom); angled Diethrich bulldog vascular clamp (top); used for temporary occlusion of vessels.

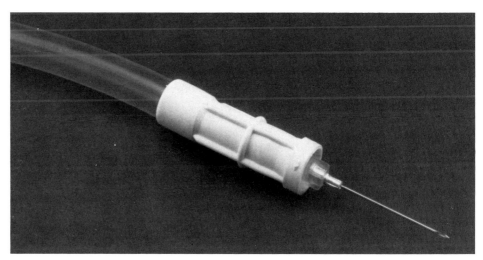

FIG. 7–3. To drain the bladder or a prostatic abscess, a needle can be placed in the end of the suction tubing and then inserted into the area to be drained.

CATHETERS

Urinary catheters are inserted to diagnose problems, drain urine, or maintain anatomic continuity. Catheters can be either self-retaining or non–self-retaining (Fig. 7-4). Sources for self-retaining catheters include Bard Urological Division, Covington, GA 30209; Kendall Co, Boston, MA 02101; and Argyle Catheters, Sherwood Medical Industries Inc., St. Louis, MO 63103. The Foley catheter is the most commonly used self-retaining catheter. It has an inflatable balloon just behind the distal openings, similar to an endotracheal tube. After the catheter is inserted, the balloon is inflated with sterile saline through an inflation channel incorporated into the catheter wall. The distended balloon prevents removal of the catheter. To deflate the balloon, a syringe is reattached to the inflation valve, and the saline is aspirated. A Foley or de Pezzer catheter can be placed surgically as a cytostomy (prepubic) catheter (See Fig. 16-6). The most commonly used catheters that are not self-retaining are simple, straight urethral catheters. These are used for single urine collections or diagnostic procedures or may be secured in place by use of tape or sutures.

Most catheters are sized according to their outer diameter, using the French (Fr scale) system or in millimeters. Each number of the Fr scale equals 0.33 mm, so the French size can be converted to millimeters by

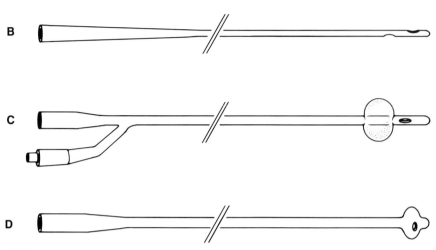

FIG. 7—4. Types of commonly used urinary catheters: (A) Short feline urethral catheter; (B) simple urethral or ureteral catheter; (C) Foley catheter with inflated retention bulb; (D) mushroom or de Pezzer catheter.

dividing by 3 (e.g., size 12 Fr = 4 mm in diameter). The internal diameter is affected by the design of the catheter and the material from which it is made. For example, the inside of an inflatable Foley catheter contains the main drainage lumen and a separate channel for balloon inflation. Consequently, this catheter type has a smaller drainage channel than a nonballoon catheter of the same Fr size.

The catheter material influences a variety of catheter characteristics, including biocompatibility and longevity. Materials used in the urinary tract are subject to special conditions, including deterioration and precipitation of urinary mucoids and crystalloids (encrustation), which can cause irritation, infection, and occlusion of the catheters.[14]

Catheters are constructed of polymeric biomaterials, either naturally occurring (e.g., latex, a rubber plant byproduct) or synthetic (e.g., polypropylene, polyvinyl chloride, polyethylene, silicone, or polyurethane). Foley catheters are composed either of latex with a Teflon coating or of 100% silicone. The soft and flexible properties of these materials allow fashioning of the inflatable bulb. Teflon coating makes the latex catheter more inert and easier to insert than natural latex alone. Silicone is more inert than latex and is much less likely to become encrusted with urinary salts than latex. Silicone Foley catheters have a larger drainage lumen than latex Foley catheters of the same Fr size because of differences in the manufacturing process.[15] Silicone and silicone-coated catheters are considerably more expensive than latex catheters, however, and are probably not sufficiently advantageous to justify the expense for catheters placed for only a few days. They may be useful in very small animals in which the larger internal diameter is beneficial or in animals that need indwelling catheters for prolonged periods. De Pezzer catheters are made of latex, silicone, or polyethylene.

Polyvinyl chloride is stiffer and stronger than latex and silicone. These qualities make a polyvinyl catheter easy to pass and enable use of small external to internal diameter ratios for optimal drainage. Polyvinyl catheters are more rigid when chilled; at body temperature, they soften and become more flexible. Polyvinyl catheters were found to be much less irritating to the urethra in cats than were polypropylene catheters.[16] Polyvinyl catheters are not self-retaining and are commonly used in catheterization of male dogs and cats. (Sovereign Sterile Feeding Tube and Urethral Catheter, Sherwood Medical Industries Inc., St. Louis, MO 63103). The short stiff catheters, sometimes used for unblocking male cats, are made of polypropylene.

USE OF URINARY CATHETERS

Catheterization of the urethra can either be *single* (catheter inserted into the bladder for short period of time), *intermittent* (repeated single catheterizations), or *indwelling* (catheter remains in bladder, urethra, or both).

Complications

The risks of catheterization are iatrogenic injury and induction of infection. The distal urethra, prepuce, and vagina have a normal bacterial flora (including *Staphylococcus aureus* and *epidermitis*, *Mycoplasma*, *Streptococcus canis*, and *E. coli* most commonly in dogs; coagulase-negative *Staphylococcus*, *Streptococcus canis*, and *E. coli* most commonly in cats),[17–19] which can be introduced into the bladder by catheterization.

In general, single catheterization has a much lower frequency of infection than indwelling catheterization, but a risk of infection still exists, particularly in females.[20,21] (See Chapter 2 for interpretation of urinalysis obtained by catheterization.)

When using an indwelling catheter, a closed urine collection system delays the occurrence of urinary tract infection (UTI). With this system, the urinary catheter is connected to sterile tubing and then to a collection bag. Even with closed drainage systems, bacterial UTI developed in about 50% of dogs and cats after 4 days of catheterization.[22] More than 30% of all nosocomial infections in humans are related to catheter-associated UTI, which is the most common predisposing factor in fatal gram-negative sepsis.[23]

Systemic antimicrobial therapy is ineffective in preventing or eradicating catheter-associated infections.[22,24] Instead, antibiotic usage leads to emergence of resistant microbes that may be spread to other animals through contaminated urine.[25] Coating the catheter with antibiotic reduced the incidence of ascending UTI in some humans,[26] but efficacy in dogs and cats has not been studied.

In addition to inducing infection, catheterization can cause direct mechanical trauma to the urethra and bladder. Careless insertion of the catheter can tear the urethra, causing subsequent urine leakage. Long, stiff polypropylene catheters that protrude into the bladder lumen injure the bladder wall and produce gross hematuria.[16] Indwelling polypropylene catheters also produce urethritis, which appears to be a foreign body reaction and is worsened by bacteriuria.[16]

Indications for Urethral Catheterization

Because of the associated complications, urethral catheterization should be avoided as a routine procedure to collect urine samples.

Indications for Single or Intermittent Urethral Catheterization

Indications include:

1. To diagnose or relieve urethral obstruction
2. To obtain urine when cystocentesis is not possible
3. To determine residual volume
4. To permit radiographic study of the urethra and bladder
5. To remove urine in animals unable to void

Indications for Indwelling Urethral Catheterization

Indications include:

1. Persistently poor urine stream because of partial urethral obstruction from tissue swelling or obstructing material
2. Repeated recurrent obstruction during current episode

3. Hypotonic urinary bladder that is not easily expressed
4. Measurement of urine output
5. Collection of urine from paralyzed or immobilized animal with incontinence to keep incisions dry and lessen contamination
6. Selected cases of urethral and prostatic surgery
7. Animal that is medically suited for intermittent catheterization but is uncooperative. Injury to the urethra may be less with an indwelling catheter than with multiple catheterizations. This is often true in female dogs and in male and female cats.

Alternatives to urethral catheterization should be considered before an indwelling catheter is placed. In animals with voiding dysfunction because of pain or housebreaking, allowing an animal access to outside lawn may encourage voiding. In animals with neurogenic voiding dysfunction, emptying of the bladder by gentle compression on the caudal abdomen may be possible. Appropriate pharmacologic agents to stimulate the detrusor muscle and relax the urethral sphincter should be tried. Absorbable diapers can be used to prevent urine soiling in an incontinent animal. An indwelling urethral catheter is chosen when the risks of damage to the bladder from prolonged distention outweigh the risks of UTI, and intermittent catheterization is not feasible.

Selection and Insertion of Urethral Catheters

Polyvinyl, latex, or silicone catheters should be used when continuous drainage of the bladder lumen is necessary. Stiff polyethylene catheters should not be left indwelling. In a female, a self-retaining Foley catheter is useful. The catheter is inserted just far enough to aspirate a small volume of fluid injected with a syringe. Overinsertion may make the catheter double back on itself (Fig. 7-5). As small a catheter as possible to maintain drainage is used.

Before insertion of a catheter in a female dog or cat, the vulvar lips and perineum are washed and the catheter is generously lubricated. Gloves and instruments should be sterile. Use of an anoscope, as shown in Figures 2-2 and 2-3, or a laryngoscope facilitates insertion of the catheter in females dogs. In female cats, the urethral orifice is often visible when the vulvar lips are parted. A catheter can usually be inserted by slowly advancing the catheter in the ventral midline of the vagina. In a male dog or cat, an assistant should gently retract the prepuce and cleanse the end of the penis before the catheter is inserted.

Management of Urinary Catheters

Indwelling catheters are used for as short a time as possible and always connected to a closed drainage system. Personnel should wash their hands whenever handling the catheter or drainage bag. Sterile, closed drainage systems are designed to maintain the sterility of the urinary tract, to avoid cross-contamination among patients, and to reduce spills of urine. Commercial drain-

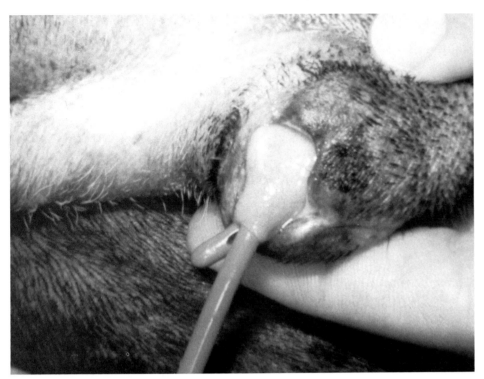

FIG. 7–5. Urethral catheter has been inserted too far, and the end has doubled back on itself.

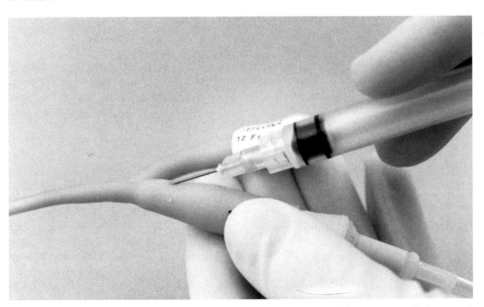

FIG. 7–6. Aspiration of urine from urinary catheter using a 25-gauge needle inserted obliquely through the catheter wall.

age bags are available with ports for evacuating the bag. Veterinary practices commonly use a sterile, empty intravenous fluid bag and administration set, which can be difficult to drain aseptically. A closed drainage system is economically advantageous for the client because the cost of antibiotics to treat UTI is usually greater than that of a drainage bag, which is left in place during the animal's hospitalization.

Aseptic, closed drainage systems prevent colonization of the drainage bag and subsequent ascending infection through the catheter lumen for at least a few days after the catheter is inserted. Bacteria colonize the intraurethral sheath around the catheter and ascend around the catheter to enter the bladder. Persistent infection is aided by the continued presence of the catheter, which acts as a foreign body and reservoir for bacteria.[27,29]

To prevent contamination of the drainage bag or the

catheter lumen, the junction of the catheter with the drainage tube must not be broken once attached, unless it becomes obstructed. Catheters are irrigated only when there is obstruction, and a sterile syringe should be used. The catheter is not replaced, unless it becomes obstructed. The bags should never be inverted or raised above the level of the animal's bladder. If it is necessary to transport the animal, the tubing is clamped first. The bag is not allowed to touch the floor and should not be held upside down while emptying. The bag is emptied every 8 hours or more frequently if it fills rapidly. The only reasons to change the bag are poor flow, leakage, odor, or obstruction. The addition of povidone iodine or hydrogen peroxide to drainage bags does not prevent catheter-associated bladder bacteriuria.[30,32] There may be some value in adding an effective antimicrobial compound to the bag to prevent cross-infection from contaminated drainage bag urine to other animals.

Antibiotic therapy and bacterial cultures are not routinely performed while the catheter is in place, unless the animal shows signs of bacteremia (fever, leukocytosis). Just before the catheter is removed, a urine sample for bacteriologic culture is collected from the proximal lumen of the catheter. Samples for urine cultures should be taken from the catheter, not the bag, because the bag may become contaminated and the catheter remain sterile. The catheter is first cleaned with an alcohol sponge, a 25-gauge needle is inserted through the catheter wall, and then urine is aspirated into a syringe (Fig. 7-6). The tip of the catheter is not cultured because culture of the tip primarily detects contaminants that adhere to the catheter as it is removed through the urethra.[33] Once the catheter is removed, antibiotic administration is based on urine bacteriologic culture and sensitivity results. Such infections should be treated for at least 10 days. Approximately 1 week after therapy is finished, a urine culture should be performed to ensure that the infection has been eliminated.

REFERENCES

1. Rodeheaver, G.T., Thacker, J.G., Owen, J., et al.: Knotting and handling characteristics of coated synthetic absorbable sutures. J. Surg. Res., 35:525, 1983.
2. Rodeheaver, G.T., Powell, T.A., Thacker, J.G., et al.: Mechanical performance of monofilament synthetic absorbable sutures. Am. J. Surg., 154:544, 1987.
3. Crocker, R.H., Lage, A.L., Parsonnet, J., et al.: The physical properties of polyglactin 910 (Vicryl), chromic gut and polydioxanone (PDS) in sterile and infected canine urine. (abst) J. Urol., 139:337A, 1988.
4. El-Mahrouky, A., McElhaney, J., Barone, F.F., et al.: In vitro comparison of the properties of polydioxanone, polyglycolic acid and catgut sutures in sterile and infected urine. J. Urol., 138:913, 1987.
5. Schiller, T.S., Stone, E.A., and Gupta, B.S.: Tensile strength of five absorbable suture materials in sterile and infected canine urine. (abst) Vet. Surg. 20:346, 1991.
6. Sebeseri, O., Keller, U., Spreng, P., et al.: The physical properties of polyglycolic acid sutures (Dexon) in sterile and infected urine. Invest. Urol., 12:490, 1979.
7. Chu, C.C.: A comparison of the effect of pH on the biodegradation of two synthetic absorbable sutures. Ann. Surg., 195:55, 1982.
8. Holbrook, M.C.: The resistance of polyglycolic acid sutures to attack by infected human urine. Br. J. Urol., 54:313, 1982.
9. Brodey, R.S.: Canine urolithiasis: A survey and discussion of fifty-two clinical cases. J. Am. Vet. Med. Assoc., 126:1, 1955.
10. Sherman, J.S., and Thornbury, J.: The fate of non-absorbable intraureteral suture. J. Urol., 110:40, 1973.
11. Kronborg, O., Ostergaard, A., Steven, K., et al.: Polyglycolic acid versus chromic catgut in bladder surgery. Br. J. Urol., 50:324, 1978.
12. Morrow, F.A., Kogan, S.J., Freed, S.Z., et al.: In vivo comparison of polyglycolic acid, chromic catgut and silk in tissue of the genitourinary tract: An experimental study of tissue retrieval and calculogenesis. J. Urol., 112:655, 1974.
13. Pearl, G.S., and Someren, A.: Suture granuloma simulating bladder neoplasm. Urology, 15:304, 1980.
14. Kunin, C.M.: Detection, Prevention and Management of Urinary Tract Infection. Philadelphia, Lea & Febiger, pp. 245–297, 1987.
15. Lange, P.H.: Diagnostic and therapeutic urologic instrumentation. In Campbell's Urology. Edited by P.C. Walsh, A.D. Perlmutter, and T.A. Stamey. Philadelphia, W.B. Saunders, pp. 510–540, 1986.
16. Lees, G.E., Osborne, C.A., Stevens, J.B., et al.: Adverse effects caused by polypropylene and polyvinyl feline urinary catheters. Am. J. Vet. Res., 41:1836, 1980.
17. Ling, G.V., and Ruby, A.L.: Aerobic bacterial flora of the prepuce urethra, and vagina of normal adult dogs. Am. J. Vet. Res., 39:695, 1978.
18. Allen, W.E., and Dagnall, G.J.R.: Some observations on the aerobic bacterial flora of the genital tract of the dog and bitch. J. Sm. Anim. Pract., 23:325, 1982.
19. Clemetson, L.L., and Ward, A.C.S.: Bacterial flora of the vagina and uterus of cats. J. Am. Vet. Med. Assoc., 196:902, 1990.
20. Thomas, J.E.: Urinary tract infection induced by intermittent urethral catheterization in dogs. J. Am. Vet. Med. Assoc., 174:705, 1979.
21. Biertuempfel, P.H., Ling, G.V., and Ling, G.A.: Urinary tract infection resulting from catheterization in healthy adult dogs. J. Am. Vet. Med. Assoc., 178:989, 1981.
22. Barsanti, J.A., Blue, J., and Edmunds, J.: Urinary tract infection due to indwelling bladder catheters in dogs and cats. J. Am. Vet. Med. Assoc., 187:384, 1985.
23. Kreiger, J.N., Kaiser, D.L., and Wenzel, R.P.: Nosocomial urinary tract infections: Secular trends, treatment and economics in a university hospital. J. Urol., 130:102, 1983.
24. Lees, G.E., Osborne, C.A., Stevens, J.B., et al.: Adverse effects of open indwelling catheterization in normal male cats. Am. J. Vet. Res., 42:825, 1981.
25. Garibaldi, R.A., Burke, J.P., Dickman, M.L., et al.: Factors predisposing to bacteriuria during indwelling urethral catheterization. N. Engl. J. Med., 291:215, 1974.
26. Schaeffer, A.J., Story, K.O., and Johnson, S.M.: Effect of silver oxide/trichloroisocyanuric acid antimicrobial urinary drainage system on catheter-associated bacteriuria. J. Urol., 139:69, 1988.
27. Kass, E.H., and Schneiderman, L.J.: Entry of bacteria into the urinary tracts of patients with inlying catheters. N. Engl. J. Med., 256:556, 1957.
28. Garibaldi, R.A., Burke, J.P., Britt, M.R., et al.: Meatal colonization and catheter-associated bacteriuria. N. Engl. J. Med., 303:216, 1980.
29. Daifuku, R., and Stamm, W.E.: Bacterial adherence to bladder urothelial cells in catheter-associated urinary tract infection. N. Engl. J. Med., 314:1208, 1986.
30. Thompson, R.L., Haley, C.E., Searcy, M.A., et al.: Catheter-associated bacteriuria. Failure to reduce attack rates using peri-

odic instillations of a disinfectant into urinary drainage systems. J.A.M.A., *251:*747, 1984.

31. Gillespie, W.A., Jones, J.E., Teasdale, C., et al.: Does the addition of disinfectant prevent infection in catheterized patients? Lancet, *1:*1037, 1983.

32. Sweet, D.E., Goodpasture, H.C., Holl, K., et al.: Evaluation of H_2O_2 prophylaxis of bacteriuria in patients with long-term indwelling Foley catheters: A randomized controlled study. Infect. Control., *6:*263, 1985.

33. Gross, P.A., Harkavy, L.M., Barden, G.E., et al.: Positive Foley catheter tip cultures—fact or fancy. J.A.M.A., *228:*72, 1974.

8

Anesthesia for Urologic Surgery

STEVE C. HASKINS

Acute renal failure may be associated with an otherwise uneventful operative experience in patients with marginal renal function. Renal function should, therefore, be assessed in all middle-aged or older patients and in all patients with diseases or who are receiving drugs that are likely to precipitate renal dysfunction. Owners should be questioned about problems that could be related to poor renal function in any aged pet such as polyuria/polydipsia, intermittent anorexia, depression, vomiting, fetid breath, or oral erosions. A mild abnormality in a renal function test may be indicative of severe renal pathology and should not be disregarded because it is "just a little abnormal." Elective surgery should be postponed in those patients with abnormal renal function tests until the abnormality can be fully characterized and, if possible, corrected.

Anesthesia and surgery are associated with increased sympathetic and renin-angiotensin activity, both of which decrease total renal blood flow and redistribute intrarenal blood flow away from the renal cortex.[1-5] The decreased renal blood flow may cause renal ischemia and hypoxemia, and if a critical number of nephrons are damaged, renal failure will result.[6]

Antidiuretic hormone (ADH) and aldosterone blood levels are both increased during general anesthesia.[7] ADH release, which may be directly stimulated by morphine, decreases free water clearance, urine output, and plasma sodium concentration during and for periods of time after anesthesia. Aldosterone release is responsible for the tendency of surgical patients to retain sodium and water during and after operation. Although neither contributes directly to decreased renal blood flow and nephron hypoxia, both decrease urine output, which is the indirect measure used clinically to evaluate renal blood flow.

Many anesthetic drugs, operative techniques, and perioperative events induce hypotension, which re-duces visceral organ perfusion. Hypovolemic compensatory mechanisms (sympathetic and angiotensin vasoconstriction), although supporting blood pressure, do so at the expense of a further decrement in visceral perfusion.

Renal cortical blood flow is significantly depressed in the hemorrhaged dog when the mean arterial blood pressure decreases to 70 mm Hg.[8] A reduction of renal blood flow of 50 to 75% causes a sustained afferent arteriolar constriction, leading to cortical ischemia, decreased glomerular permeability, tubular backleak, and tubular obstruction.[1,6] Once established, renal cortical blood flow and glomerular filtration may remain low despite cardiovascular stabilization because of acute tubular necrosis or vasomotor nephropathy.[1,6]

EFFECT OF ANESTHETICS ON RENAL FUNCTION

A phenothiazine tranquilizer may increase renal blood flow[9,10] and should be used if induction hypotension is not expected to be a problem. Phenothiazines do impair dopaminergic receptiveness to dopamine,[11] and the intended use of dopamine constitutes a relative contraindication to phenothiazine administration. Sedative doses of narcotics and barbiturates induce little, if any, decrease in glomerular filtration rate (GFR).[9]

Barbiturates generally increase renal vascular resistance and decrease renal blood flow and glomerular filtration;[12,13] however, they may transiently increase renal blood flow and decrease resistance in normovolemic dogs.[14] Thiopental caused a significant increase in renal blood flow and decrease in renal vascular resistance in hypovolemic dogs.[15]

Ketamine causes an increase,[14] no change,[16] or a decrease[17] in renal cortical blood flow in normal dogs.

It causes increased renal vascular resistance,[14,15] and therefore, the enhanced blood flow is attributed to the increased systemic blood pressure. It was associated with a small increase in renal cortical blood flow in hypovolemic dogs.[15] Diazepam decreased renal blood flow and increased renal vascular resistance in normovolemic conscious dogs[14] and children;[18] however, it caused a small increase in renal blood flow and a decrease in vascular resistance in hypovolemic dogs.[15]

We have proposed for years that ketamine is not metabolized in the cat, and that recovery from anesthesia is dependent on renal elimination of the active drug. Several studies have shown that this is not true.[19–21] Ketamine is not metabolized as completely in the cat as it is in other species. It is metabolized only to the level of norketamine, which has 10% of the activity of the parent compound. Norketamine is eliminated mostly in the bile. Ninety minutes after the administration of 25 mg/kg of ketamine IM, only 2.6% of ketamine or norketamine had been recovered in the urine.[20] It appears that recovery is attributable to redistribution and metabolism.

Morphine, meperidine, and fentanyl decrease renal plasma flow, glomerular filtration, and urine output.[22,23] The antidiuresis effect is attributed to ADH release,[24] to a histamine-mediated decrease in arterial blood pressure and renal perfusion (except fentanyl), or to hypercapnia-induced renal vasoconstriction.[25] Innovar causes either no change[10,26] or an increase in renal blood flow[17] in normal dogs and is considered a safe anesthetic drug for patients with renal disease.

Regional anesthesia, presuming adequate fluid therapy to eliminate systemic hypotension, has minimal or no effect on renal blood flow and GFR.[27]

Either halothane or isoflurane is suitable for maintenance of general anesthesia in patients with compensated renal failure. Both agents produce minimal to moderate decreases in renal blood flow and GFR and increases in filtration fraction.[28–33] Halothane does not redistribute intrarenal blood flow away from the cortex[34] and even reduces the renal sympathetic vasoconstriction that occurs in hypovolemia[29,30] and, therefore, may be somewhat protective of renal function from this baseline. A 4-hour hypotensive anesthesia with halothane in a canine remnant kidney model was not associated with renal failure; however, three of eight dogs developed a significant increase in azotemia and signs of uremia (vomiting, dehydration) on the day following anesthesia.[35] The condition was responsive to fluid.

Methoxyflurane has been associated with a polyuric, hypernatremic, low-urine osmolality, azotemic, renal failure syndrome in humans.[36] The nephrotoxicity of methoxyflurane is associated with the fluoride metabolite.[36] Although methoxyflurane-associated renal failure has been reported to occur in the dog,[37–39] given the widespread use of this agent in dogs and cats and the low reported incidence of nephrotoxicity, it would appear that the syndrome is much less a problem in these species compared with humans. Experimental efforts to reproduce the disease in dogs have failed to do so, even though blood fluoride concentrations have risen to lev-els comparable to humans.[40–42] Hepatic microsomal enzyme induction enhances methoxyflurane metabolism[39] and predisposes to the nephrotoxicity of this agent.[37,38]

Although it is generally recommended to avoid the use of methoxyflurane in patients with end-stage renal disease, if for some reason its use is unavoidable, several steps may be taken to attempt to reduce its toxicity:

1. Maintain the patient with the lowest vaporizer settings compatible with the completion of the surgery
2. Keep the anesthetic exposure as brief as possible
3. Maintain active diuresis during the operative period and for several days following, which may or may not[43] help by diluting the tubular fluoride concentration and by accelerating its passage through the nephrons
4. Avoid additive nephrotoxic events (hypotension, vasoconstriction, aminoglycoside antibiotics).
5. Avoid other enzyme-inducing drugs such as phenobarbital or repeated doses of methoxyflurane or halothane. Obesity increases the body storage of methoxyflurane, which increases the amount that is metabolized. This would presumably increase the nephrotoxicity
6. Alkalinization of the urine may increase fluoride elimination[44]

Nitrous oxide has minimal effect on renal function[12] but will potentiate the antidiuresis produced by halothane[45] and morphine.[25]

Many nondepolarizing muscle relaxants depend on renal excretion for the termination of their clinical effects and are, therefore, prolonged in the patient with renal failure (gallamine,[46] metocurine, pancuronium, and d-tubocurarine).[47] The duration of action of vecuronium and atracurium is not significantly prolonged by renal failure.[47] Muscle relaxants have no direct effects on renal function but may indirectly influence renal perfusion as they affect hemodynamics. Succinylcholine should be avoided in hyperkalemic patients because of its potential for releasing excessive amounts of potassium from the muscles.

The decrease in renal blood flow and cortical perfusion induced by most anesthetics is, most likely, an indirect effect (sympathetic/renin-angiotensin-mediated) because in isolated perfused kidneys most anesthetics are vasodilators.[48]

COMPENSATED END-STAGE RENAL DISEASE

The major emphasis of anesthetic protocols for patients with compensated end-stage renal disease, in which there is only a mild abnormality of renal function tests, is to protect the kidney from further damage. Anesthetic procedures that are well tolerated by normal kidneys may not be by diseased kidneys.

The renal ischemia induced by uneventful anesthesia and surgery is enhanced by common anesthetic complications such as hypovolemia,[49,50] hypotension,[51] hypoxemia,[49] or peripheral vasoconstriction,[6] and these events must be minimized as much as possible. A sustained afferent arteriolar constriction and renal cortical ischemia (vasomotor nephropathy) may result if the decrease in renal blood flow is excessive or prolonged and may prevent re-establishment of renal blood flow after restoration of the initial cause.[1,6] Drugs that cause or potentiate renal failure (aminoglycoside and cephalosporin antibiotics, radiocontrast media, prostaglandin inhibitors[52,53]) should also be avoided in these patients. Preinduction fluid loading, to eliminate prerenal ischemia and to minimize intraoperative sympathoadrenal and renin-angiotensin secretion,[13] may help reduce the incidence of acute renal failure.

The choice of drugs to use in the patient with compensated end-stage renal disease is relatively wide, with the possible exception of methoxyflurane, and subsidiary to the physiologic support of the patient in the perioperative period. Regional anesthesia or Innovar may be the preferred induction agents followed by either an ultrashort-acting barbiturate (thiamylal, thiopental), ketamine, or a narcotic (not in any specific order of preference). A mask induction and maintenance with isoflurane or halothane appear also to be quite acceptable. Methoxyflurane should be avoided if possible.

More important than the choices of drug is the physiologic support of the patient during the anesthetic experience. Urine output should be evaluated regularly during the course of the operation as an indirect indication of the adequacy of renal blood flow. A urinary catheter is the preferred method of monitoring. The urinary catheter must be placed in a strict aseptic manner because bladder infections are common with urinary catheterization. The catheter should be soft; introduction of excessive lengths should be avoided; and it must be connected to a closed, sterile collection system. See Chapter 7 for a discussion of catheters. If the patient is or becomes oliguric or anuric, fluids such as lactated Ringer's solution should first be administered in sufficient quantity to eliminate any prerenal component. Ten to 40 ml/kg, administered as a bolus, is an approximate guideline. Physical signs, such as color and capillary refill time, and measurements, such as toe-web temperature and central venous and arterial blood pressure, however, may provide a more finite end point.

If fluid administration does not result in an increased urine output, a diuretic should be administered. Early diuretic therapy may help prevent acute renal failure. The following three diuretics are suggested: furosemide, glucose or mannitol, and dopamine. They may be given in any order or in any combination.

Furosemide (5 mg/kg IV) should produce a brisk diuresis within 10 minutes. Furosemide has a renal vasodilating effect in addition to its potent natriuretic effect.[54] If urine output does not commence within 10 minutes, either readminister one additional dose of furosemide or proceed to the next diuretic. Furosemide may enhance the nephrotoxicity of some antibiotics[55] such as the aminoglycosides and should not be used in concert.

Glucose or mannitol (0.25 to 0.5 g/kg IV) osmotically increases blood volume and renal perfusion and has an osmotic natriuretic effect. The diuretic should be administered over 20 to 30 minutes. If mannitol is administered too rapidly, it may cause circulatory overload and precipitate heart failure and pulmonary edema.[56] Urine should start to flow within 10 minutes of the end of the infusion. If it has not, proceed to the next diuretic.

Dopamine (1 to 5 μg/kg/min IV) stimulates dopaminergic receptors, which cause renal vasodilation and improved renal perfusion and urine output. Dopamine probably also has a tubular effect, which promotes diuresis.[57] Begin the dopamine infusion at 1 μg/kg/min and continue for 15 minutes; if there is no urine output, increase the dopamine infusion rate (in 1 μg/kg/min increments) until urine starts to flow, or until there is evidence of cardiovascular stimulation. Increasing heart rate, increasing arterial blood pressure, or occurrence of premature ventricular contractions indicates cardiovascular stimulation and possible alpha-receptor–mediated renal vasoconstriction, which will override the dopaminergic diuretic effect and cause decreased renal blood flow and oliguria/anuria. The dopamine infusion rate should be decreased.

If none of these diuretics alone have induced urine flow, it may be beneficial to attempt combinations of fluids and diuretics. Early, intraoperative, aggressive fluid and diuresis therapy is a high priority because it may forestall acute renal failure and the necessity for dialysis.

UNCOMPENSATED RENAL FAILURE

Uncompensated renal failure is associated with the excessive accumulation of metabolic waste products, fluid, and electrolyte imbalances and secondary deterioration of other organ systems. These systemic consequences of overt renal failure alter a patient's response to general anesthesia or may have direct detrimental effects on homeostasis. All abnormalities should be characterized as completely as possible and stabilized prior to the induction of general anesthesia.

The systemic consequences of uncompensated renal failure include:

1. Polyuric renal disease may be associated with dehydration, hypernatremia, and hypokalemia. Fluid therapy (with a crystalloid extracellular fluid–replacement solution, such as lactated Ringer's solution) should be generous.
2. Oliguric/anuric renal disease may be associated with edema, hyponatremia, hyperkalemia, and acidosis. Fluid therapy should be conservative. Fluid therapy needs to be tailored to the specific needs of the patient, not necessarily to the presenting condition. A patient may be anuric on presentation, secondary to polyuric-induced dehydration.[58,59] Fluid therapy should be initially generous to eliminate signs of dehydration and any prerenal oliguric component. If oliguria/anuria persists following adequate rehydration, further therapy should be conservative.

3. Hyperkalemia may cause severe electrocardiographic/myocardial abnormalities.
4. Uremic "toxemia" causes central nervous system depression and myocardial depression[60] and potentiates the effect of general anesthetics; anesthetic dosages should be decreased.
5. Metabolic acidosis, secondary to retention of protein metabolites ($PO_4^=$, $SO_4^=$), may directly interfere with cellular enzymatic function if severe. Acidosis decreases protein binding,[61] and ionized fraction of the barbiturates and induction dosages should be appropriately conservative.
6. Anemia, secondary to decreased erythropoietin production and bone marrow depression, may interfere with oxygen delivery to the tissues. Phenothiazine tranquilizers and barbiturates cause significant decreases in hemoglobin concentration and should be avoided in the anemic patient.
7. Uremic patients are highly prone to infection and sepsis,[62] and all invasive techniques should be accomplished in a strictly aseptic fashion. Prophylactic antibiotics were not found to be beneficial.[63]
8. A platelet dysfunction occurs in uremic humans,[64,65] and hemorrhagic tendencies should be treated with fresh plasma or whole blood.
9. Nausea, vomiting, and a delayed gastric emptying time[66] may predispose to induction or early recovery vomition and aspiration. Induction and intubation should be rapid. The endotracheal tube should remain in place during recovery, and patients should be carefully observed for vomition after the tube is removed until recovery is complete. Antacids or H_2-receptor blockers may be advantageous in this regard.[67]
10. Uremic pericarditis leading to cardiac tamponade is reported to occur in 10 to 20% and 3 to 7% of uremic humans, respectively.[66] The existence of pericarditis and cardiac tamponade should be evaluated preoperatively, and an emergency pericardiocentesis should be done when necessary.
11. Severe uremia may impair the ability of the liver to metabolize some drugs.[68]
12. Hypertension caused by high angiotensin blood levels and, perhaps, hypervolemia is more of a problem in humans, who are subject to aneurysmal rupture and arteriosclerotic emboli, than dogs. Hypertension, however, may predispose to heart failure or pulmonary or cerebral edema if worsened by the anesthetic experience.
13. Hypocalcemia owing to decreased intestinal absorption and hyperphosphatemia owing to decreased phosphate excretion may cause calcium phosphate metastatic calcification, osteomalacia, parasthesias, and tetany, if severe.

Severely uremic patients are systemically debilitated, are more susceptible to the direct and indirect effects of general anesthetics, and are candidates for induction and intraoperative hypotension and hypoventilation. Their anesthetic management, therefore, more closely resembles that of a cardiovascularly compromised patient than it does a compensated end-stage renal disease patient. These patients often do not require a preanesthetic sedative. If they do, a small dose of a narcotic would be preferable to a hypotension-prone phenothiazine. An anticholinergic drug should be administered. Uremic unatropinized humans have been reported to succumb to a vagal-mediated cardiac arrest.[69,70] Preoperative antacids and H_2-receptor blockers help decrease the acidity and volume of gastric fluid. Intraoperative alkaline gavage, if preoperative antacids were not given, could be beneficial.

Barbiturates are more potent in uremic patients by an effect independent of the potentiating effects of hypoproteinemia and acidemia previously discussed.[71] Nitrogenous end products may competitively bind to albumin,[72] or there may be an increased blood-brain barrier permeability.[73] Ketamine should be avoided in hypertensive patients. A narcotic-diazepam induction (oxymorphone, fentanyl) may be a primary choice; mask induction and maintenance with halothane or isoflurane may also work well but may be excessively hypotensive. Fluid overloading should be avoided, and drugs that depend on renal excretion to a significant extent for the termination of their clinical effects (gallamine, d-tubocurarine, pancuronium, metocurine, neostigmine, phenobarbital) should not be administered.

ANESTHESIA FOR FELINE URETHRAL OBSTRUCTION

The cat sustaining a urethral obstruction is often presented with many of the systemic consequences common to the uncompensated renal failure patient: dehydration, hyperkalemia, uremia, and metabolic acidosis. An isoelectrolyte crystalloid, such as lactated Ringer's, should be administered (10 to 40 ml/kg) to restore an effective circulating blood volume prior to induction of anesthesia. If bradycardia or electrocardiographic evidence of hyperkalemia persists, calcium (1 to 2 ml of 10% calcium chloride), glucose (0.5 g/kg) and insulin (0.3 units/kg), or bicarbonate (1 to 3 mEq/kg) may be administered. Anesthesia is often helpful in the urethral catheterization procedure. If used, anesthesia should be induced with the least hypotensive agent available, e.g., ketamine (administered IV in 1 to 2 mg/kg dosages at 1-minute intervals) and diazepam (0.2 mg/kg administered IV after the first dose of ketamine), to help with muscle relaxation.

If the cat is uremic, an indwelling urethral catheter should be placed and the cat stabilized with regard to its fluid and electrolyte disturbances and uremic condition. Urethral surgery, if desirable, can then be accomplished with routine anesthetic protocols. If surgery is deemed necessary before adequate stabilization, anesthesia should be induced with ketamine and diazepam and maintained with halothane or isoflurane as long as blood pressure can be monitored and supported. If not, a ketamine (1 to 2 mg/kg IV every 20 to 30 minutes) and diazepam (0.2 mg/kg IV every 30 minutes) maintenance technique may be preferable.

REFERENCES

1. Sladen, R.: Can we prevent postoperative renal failure intraoperatively? Refresher Course No. 129, American Society of Anesthesiologists, 1981.
2. Rosen, S.M.: Effects of anaesthesia and surgery on renal hemodynamics. Br. J. Anaesth., 44:252, 1972.
3. Cousins, M.J., and Mazze, R.I.: Anaesthesia, surgery, and renal function; immediate and delayed effects. Anaesth. Intens. Care., 1:355, 1973.
4. Utting, J.E.: Anaesthesia and the kidney. In General Anaesthesia. Edited by T.C. Gray, et al. London, Butterworths, pp. 763–777 1980.
5. Berne, R.M.: Hemodynamics and sodium excretion of denervated kidney in anesthetized and unanesthetized dog. Am. J. Physiol., 171:148, 1952.
6. Myers, B.D., and Moran, S.M.: Hemodynamically mediated acute renal failure. N. Engl. J. Med., 314:97, 1986.
7. Mazze, R.I.: Renal physiology and the effects of anesthesia. In Anesthesia. 2nd Ed. Edited by R.D. Miller. New York, Churchill Livingstone, pp. 1223–1248, 1986.
8. Rosen, S.M., Traniger, B.P., Kreik, H.R., et al.: Intrarenal distribution of blood flow in the transplanted dog kidney: Effect of denervation rejection. J. Clin. Invest., 46:1239, 1967.
9. Papper, S., and Papper, E.M.: The effects of preanesthetic, anesthetic, and postoperative drugs on renal function. Clin. Pharmacol. Ther., 5:205, 1964.
10. Gorman, H.M., and Craythorne, M.W.B.: The effects of a new neuroleptanalgesic agent (Innovar) on renal function in man. Acta Anaesthesiol. Scand., 24(Suppl):111, 1966.
11. Bradshaw, E.G., Pleuvry, B.J., and Sharma, H.L.: Effect of droperidol on dopamine-induced increase in effective renal plasma flow in dogs. Br. J. Anaesth., 52:879, 1980.
12. Deutsch, S., Bastron, R.D., Pierce, E.C. Jr., et al.: The effects of anesthesia with thiopentone, nitrous oxide, narcotics and neuromuscular blocking drugs on renal fucntion in normal man. Br. J. Anaesth., 41:807, 1969.
13. Burger, B.M., Hopkins, T., Tulloch, A., et al.: The role of angiotensin in the canine renal vascular response to barbiturate anesthesia. Circ. Res., 38:196, 1976.
14. Priano, L.L.: Alteration of renal hemodynamics by thiopental, diazepam, and ketamine in conscious dogs. Anesth. Analg., 61:853, 1982.
15. Priano, L.L.: Renal hemodynamic alterations following administration of thiopental, diazepam, or ketamine to conscious hypovolemic dogs. Adv. Shock Res., 9:173, 1983.
16. Bevan, D.R., and Bhudu, R.: The effect of ketamine on renal blood flow in greyhounds. Br. J. Anaesth., 47:634, 1975.
17. Hirasawa, H., and Yonezawa, T.: The effects of ketamine and Innovar on the renal cortical and medullary blood flow of the dog. Anaesthetist, 24:349, 1975.
18. Guignard, J.P., Felloux, B., Lavoie, J., et al.: Effect of intravenous diazepam on renal function. Clin. Pharmacol. Ther., 18:401, 1975.
19. Baggot, J.D., and Blake, J.W.: Disposition kinetics of ketamine in the domestic cat. Arch. Int. Pharmacodyn. Ther., 220:115, 1976.
20. Waterman, A.E.: Influence of premedication with xylazine on the distribution and metabolism of intramuscularly administered ketamine in cats. Res. Vet. Sci., 35:285, 1983.
21. Heavner, J.R., and Bloedow, D.C.: Ketamine pharmacokinetics in domestic cats. Vet. Anesth., 6:16, 1979.
22. Handley, C.A., and Keller, A.D.: Changes in renal function produced by morphine in normal dogs and dogs with diabetes insipidus. J. Pharmacol. Exp. Ther., 99:33, 1950.
23. Bidwai, A.V., Liu, W.S., Stanley, L.H., et al.: The effects of large doses of fentanyl and fentanyl with nitrous oxide in the dog. Can. Anaesth. Soc. J., 23:296, 1976.
24. Duke, H.N., Pickford, M., and Watt, J.A.: The antidiuretic action of morphine; its site and mode of action in the hypothalamus of the dog. Q. J. Exp. Physiol., 36:149, 1951.
25. Bidwai, A.V., Stanley, T.H., Bloomer, H.A., et al.: Effects of anesthetic doses of morphine on renal fucntion in the dog. Anesth. Analg., 54:357, 1975.
26. Järnberg, P.O., Santesson, J., and Eklund, J.: Renal function during neurolept anaesthesia. Acta Anaesthesiol. Scand., 22:167, 1978.
27. Kennedy, W.F., Sawyer, T.K., Gerbershagen, H.V., et al.: Simultaneous systemic cardiovascular and renal hemodynamic measurements during high spinal anaesthesia in normal man. Acta Anaesthesiol. Scand. 37(Suppl):163, 1970.
28. Eger, E.I.: Isoflurane, A Compendium and Reference. Ohio Medical Products, Cleveland, Ohio 1981.
29. MacDonald, A.G.: The effect of halothane on renal cortical blood flow in normotensive and hypotensive dogs. Br. J. Anaesth., 41:644, 1969.
30. Priano, L.L.: Effect of halothane on renal hemodynamics during normovolemia and acute hemorrhagic hypovolemia. Anesthesiology, 63:357, 1985.
31. Barry, K.G., Mazze, R.I., and Schwartz, F.S.: Prevention of surgical oliguria and renal haemodynamics suppression by sustained hydration. N. Engl. J. Med., 270:1371, 1964.
32. Mazze, R.I., Cousins, M.J., and Barr, G.A.: Renal effects and metabolim of isoflurane in man. Anesthesiology, 40:536, 1974.
33. Gelman, S., Fowler, K.C., and Smith, L.R.: Regional blood flow during isoflurane and halothane anesthesia. Anesth. Analg., 63:557, 1984.
34. Leighton, K., and Bruce, C.: Distribution of kidney blood flow: A comparison of methoxyflurane and halothane effects as measured by heated thermocouple. Can. Anaesth. Soc. J., 22:125, 1975.
35. Stone, E.A., Rawlings, C.A., Finco, D.R., et al.: Renal function after prolonged hypotensive anesthesia and surgery in dogs with reduced renal mass. Am. J. Vet. Res., 42:1675, 1981.
36. Mazze, R.I., and Cousins, M.J.: Renal toxicity of anaesthetics: With specific reference to nephrotoxicity of methoxyflurane. Can. Anaesth. Soc. J., 20:64, 1973.
37. Ndiritu, C.G., and Weigel, J.: Hepatorenal injury in a dog associated with methoxyflurane. Vet. Med. Sm. Anim. Clin., 72:545, 1977.
38. Trim, C.: Anesthesia and the kidney. Compend. Contin. Educ. Pract. Vet., 1:843 1979.
39. Stubbs, S., Fuerg, H., Wade, J.G.: High output renal failure following methoxyflurane anesthesia in the dog. Anesthesia and the Kidney Conference, Winnepag, Manatoba, Canada 1971.
40. Pedersoli, W.M.: Serum fluoride concentration, renal, and hepatic function test results in dogs with methoxyflurane anesthesia. Am. J. Vet. Res., 38:949, 1977.
41. Brunson, D.B., Stowe, S.M., and McGrath, C.J.: Serum and urine inorganic fluoride concentrations and urine oxalate concentrations following methoxyflurane anesthesia in the dog. Am. J. Vet. Res., 40:197, 1979.
42. Messick, J.M., Wilson, D.M., and Theye, R.A.: Canine renal function and V̇O₂ during methoxyflurane anesthesia. Anesth. Analg., 51:933, 1972.
43. Oikkonen, M., Rosenberg, P.H., and Collan, R.: Effects of mannitol and furosemide on urinary fluoride excretion of surgical patients anesthetized with enflurane and halothane. Acta Anaesthesiol. Scand., 26:82, 1982.
44. Jainberg, P.O., Ekstrand, J., and Irestedt, L.: Renal fluoride excretion during and after endlurane anesthesia. Dependency on spontaneous urinary pH variations. Acta Anaesthesiol. Scand., 24:129, 1980.
45. Hill, G.E., Lunn, J.K., Hodges, M.R., et al.: N₂O modification of halothane-altered renal function in the dog. Anesth. Analg., 56:690, 1977.

46. Feldman, S.A., Cohen, E.N., and Golling, R.C.: The excretion of gallamine in the dog. Anesthesiology, *30:*593, 1969.
47. Mazze, R.I.: Anesthesia for patients with abnormal renal function and genitourinary operations. *In* Anesthesia. 2nd Ed. Edited by R.D. Miller. New York, Churchill Livingstone, 1986.
48. Bastron, R.D., Pyne, J.L., and Inagaki, M.: Halothane-induced renal vasodilation. Anesthesiology, *50:*126, 1979.
49. Bastron, R.D., and Deutsch, S.: Anesthesia and the Kidney. New York, Grune & Stratton, 1976.
50. Selkurt, E.E.: Current status of renal circulation and related nephron function in hemorrhage and experimental shock. Circ. Shock, *1:*3, 1974.
51. Guthrie, R.H., and Cucin, R.L.: Renal circulation curing hypotension. Am. J. Surg. *125:*280, 1973.
52. Henrich, W.L., Pettinger, W.A., and Cronin, R.E.: The influence of circulating catecholamines and prostaglandins on canine renal hemodynamics during hemorrhage. Circ. Res., *48:*424, 1981.
53. Clive, D.M., and Stoff, J.S.: Renal syndromes associated with nonsteroidal anti-inflammatory drugs. N. Engl. J. Med., *310:*563, 1984.
54. Gerber, J.G., and Nies, A.S.: Furosemide-induced vasodilation: Importance of the state of hydration and filtration. Kidney Int., *18:*454, 1980.
55. Lawson, D.H., Macadam, R.F., Singh, H., et al.: Effect of furosemide on antibiotic-induced renal damage in rats. *J. Infect. Dis.*, *126:*593, 1972.
56. Warren, S.E., and Blantz, R.C.: Mannitol. Arch. Intern. Med., *141:*493, 1981.
57. D'Orio, V., Elallaf, D., Juchmés, J., et al.: The use of low doses of dopamine in intensive care medicine. Arch. Int. Physical Biochem., *92:*S11, 1984.
58. Finco, D.R., Osborne, C.A., and Low, D.G.: Physiology and pathophysiology of renal failure. *In* Textbook of Veterinary Internal Medicine. Edited by S.J. Ettinger. Philadelphia, W.B. Saunders, pp. 1453–1464, 1975.
59. Low, D.G., and Cowgill, L.D.: Emergency management of the acute uremic crisis. *In* Current Veterinary Therapy VIII. Edited by R.W. Kirk. Philadelphia, W.B. Saunders, pp. 981–989, 1983.
60. Scheuer, J., and Stezoski, S.W.: The effects of uremic compounds on cardiac function and metabolism. J. Molec. Cell Cardiol., *5:*287, 1973.
61. Ghoneim, M.M., and Pandya, H.: Plasma protein binding of thiopental in patients with impaired renal or hepatic function. Anesthesiology, *42:*545, 1975.
62. Montgomerie, J.Z., Kalmanson, G.M., and Guze, L.B.: Renal failure and infection. Medicine, *47:*1, 1968.
63. Linton, A.L.: Diagnostic criteria and clinical course of acute renal failure. *In* Acute Renal Failure. Edited by A. Chapman. New York, Churchill Livingstone, pp. 14–28, 1980.
64. Eknoyan, G., Wacksman, S.J., Glueck, H.I., et al.: Platelet function in renal failure. N. Engl. J. Med., *280:*677, 1969.
65. Dodds, A., and Nicholls, M.: Haematological aspects of renal disease. Anaesth. Intens. Care, *11:*361, 1983.
66. Müller, M.C.: Anesthesia for the patient with renal dysfunction. *In* The Kidney in Anesthesia, International Anesthesia Clinics. Edited by H.J. Priebe. Boston, Little, Brown, *22:*169, 1984.
67. Maddern, P.J.: Anaesthesia for the patient with impaired renal function. Anaesth. Intens. Care, *11:*321, 1983.
68. Reidenberg, M.M.: Renal Function and Drug Action. Philadelphia, W.B. Saunders, 1971. pp. 19–31.
69. Lunding, M.: The anaesthetist and acute renal failure. Acta Anaesthesiol. Scand., *15*(Suppl):139, 1965.
70. Deutsch, S.: Anesthetic management in acute and chronic renal failure. Vet. Clin. North Am., *3:*57, 1973.
71. Dundee, J.W., and Richards, R.K.: Effect of azotemia upon the action of intravenous barbiturate anesthesia. Anesthesiology, *15:*333, 1954.
72. Ghoneim, M.M., and Pandya, H.: Plasma protein binding of thiopental in patients with impaired renal or hepatic function. Anesthesiology, *42:*545, 1975.
73. Freeman, R.B., Sheff, M.F., Maher, J.F., et al.: The blood cerebrospinal fluid barrier in uremia. Ann. Intern. Med., *56:*233, 1962.

9

Preoperative Management

The purpose of preoperative management is to improve the animal's condition for anesthesia and surgery, maximize the benefits of surgery, prevent deterioration of renal function, prevent infectious complications, and provide prognostic information to the owner. Formulation of a preoperative management plan requires review of the animal's history, physical examination, and laboratory and radiographic findings. Refer to Section One to prepare a diagnostic plan for urinary tract problems. Other organ systems should be thoroughly evaluated, particularly in older animals or in animals with suspicious historical or clinical findings. In an animal with renal disease, hydration, electrolyte, acid-base, and cardiovascular status are scrutinized in addition to the animal's renal function.

IMPROVING THE ANIMAL'S CONDITION FOR ANESTHESIA AND SURGERY

The goal of preoperative preparation is to achieve an improved level of urinary tract function for that particular animal but not necessarily to reach a normal level of function. Disease states and medications that may cause problems are identified so that complications can be anticipated and treated before surgery. The anesthetic and fluid management of azotemic and uremic animals is discussed in Chapter 8.

An indwelling intravenous catheter is placed for administration of fluid therapy as outlined in Chapter 8. Urine output is monitored by an indwelling urethral catheter in animals with suspected renal failure. If the uremia is secondary to urine accumulation in the abdomen or urine outflow obstruction, the urine is drained by alternate routes (see Chapters 13, 15, 16 and 21). A decision is made as to whether the surgery is critical or if it can be postponed until the animal is stabilized.

Nausea and Vomiting

Nausea and vomiting associated with uremia may cause volume depletion and decline in blood pressure and renal perfusion. Chlorpromazine (Thorazine, 0.5 mg/kg) or trimethobenzamide (Tigan, 3.0 mg/kg) can be used to suppress vomiting from stimulation of the chemoreceptor trigger zone by circulating uremic toxins. Cimetidine reduces the increased gastrin concentrations in uremic dogs and may be helpful in treating related hemorrhagic gastroenteritis. The recommended dosage is 5 to 10 mg/kg IV bid followed by 5 mg/kg sid to bid.[1] Because cimetidine inhibits the hepatic metabolism of many drugs, anesthetic dosages of barbiturates should be carefully titrated.

Chronic Metabolic Acidosis

The metabolic acidosis of chronic renal failure is often mild. Preoperative treatment is usually not necessary, but the acid-base status should be monitored during and after surgery.

Anemia

The anemia of chronic renal failure is usually well tolerated because it is chronic and compensatory changes have occurred. When the hematocrit (packed cell volume [PCV]) is less than 20%, a blood transfusion is administered before surgery. Crossmatching and administration of DEA-1.1 and DEA-1.2 negative blood are important because future transfusions may be needed. Packed red blood cells are preferable to whole blood to help prevent circulatory overload in the normovolemic animal. The cells can be prepared by controlled centrifugation or gravity sedimentation. The volume needed can be calculated according to the formula:

$$\text{ml of donor blood in anticoagulant needed} = \frac{\text{recipient blood volume} \times (\text{PCV desired} - \text{PCV recipient})}{\text{PCV of donor blood in anticoagulant}}$$

The approximate blood volume of a dog is 90 ml/kg; of a cat, 70 ml/kg. The hematocrit of sedimented cells is usually about 60%.

For example, to calculate the amount of packed red blood cells needed by a 25-kg dog with PCV = 15% (0.15) and a desired PCV = 30% (0.30):

$$\frac{(25 \text{ kg BW} \times 90 \text{ ml}) \times (0.30 - 0.15)}{0.60}$$

= 563 ml packed red blood cells needed

The blood should be infused slowly to minimize circulatory overload. When the hematocrit is above 20% and the animal's physiologic status is stable, preoperative blood transfusions are not required. If severe operative blood loss is anticipated, however, the animal should be crossmatched with the proposed donor in preparation for transfusion of whole blood. Collection, storage, and administration of blood therapy have been reviewed.[2,3]

Coagulopathy

The most common coagulation defect associated with uremia is defective platelet aggregation, with normal platelet numbers.[4] No increased bleeding has been reported in humans with chronic renal failure.[5] Congenital clotting abnormalities, e.g., von Willebrand's disease in Doberman pinschers, and previous therapy with drugs that interfere with coagulation, e.g., aspirin and phenylbutazone, are diagnosed from the history, physical examination, and laboratory tests. A platelet count, bleeding time, and activated coagulation time may help detect abnormalities in animals with suspicious findings during the routine preoperative evaluation. Further diagnosis may require evaluation of prothrombin time, partial thromboplastin time, thrombin time, and coagulation factor assays. Disseminated intravascular coagulation (DIC) can occur in animals with ruptured prostatic abscesses, peritonitis, and gram-negative sepsis. Treatment of DIC is discussed in Chapter 11.

Nutritional Status

The total body fat and protein content may be reduced in the uremic animal because of anorexia, vomiting, nausea, and diarrhea. In addition, the animal may be on a low-protein diet for management of renal failure or dissolution of calculi. Maintaining an adequate nutritional regimen may be of critical importance in managing seriously ill surgical patients with pre-existing weight loss and depleted energy reserves. The surgical procedure, perioperative management (e.g., Elizabethan collars, feeding restrictions), and postoperative complications may interfere with food intake and increase the animal's energy output. In these situations, the severely undernourished animal is unable to maintain the high-priority protein pools for wound healing and immunocompetence. The most common complications of protein-calorie malnutrition are wound infection and sepsis because of impaired immunologic activity involving both the T- and B-cell systems. Undernutrition is also associated with impaired wound healing and decreased mechanical wound strength causing abdominal and skin wound dehiscences.

Most animals can easily withstand the brief period of catabolism and starvation associated with the stress of surgery because energy losses and impaired nutrient intake are not critical in the previously well-nourished animal. In simple early starvation, the protein is lost primarily from muscle. High-priority protein pools (for wound healing and immune function) are maintained. Between these two extremes are animals for whom nutritional support is not essential for life but may serve to shorten the postoperative recovery phase and minimize complications.

The following guidelines are used to select animals for nutritional support:

1. An animal that has lost more than 20% of its body weight, is hypoalbuminemic (serum albumin < 2.5 mg/dl), or both
2. Septic or severely traumatized animals that may have a prolonged increase in basal metabolic rate
3. A previously healthy animal that has had or will have delayed feeding, anorexia, or gastrointestinal malfunction for more than 7 to 10 days

Preoperative nutritional therapy may be administered by mouth or nasogastric tube. Force-feeding can be used for animals that are able to ingest adequate amounts of nutrients by mouth, but the procedure is time-consuming and stressful for an uncooperative animal. A nasogastric tube (small-bore feeding tube) can be passed through the nose and into the stomach for administration of a liquid diet.[6,7] If the animal requires prolonged nutritional therapy, placement of a gastrostomy tube in an animal that is not vomiting or a jejunostomy catheter may be the most efficacious method.[8,9]

MAXIMIZING THE BENEFITS OF THE SURGERY

Careful planning minimizes the operative time and maximizes the benefits of the surgery. The proposed surgery should be reviewed and all possible equipment and supplies assembled, including specimen bottles for biopsy specimens, culture tubes, syringe and needle for urine culture, catheters, and drains. Warm sterile isotonic lavage fluids are used to keep the tissues moist and for diluting any contamination during the procedure from urine or purulent material. Plans can be made to place a gastrostomy or jejunostomy catheter during the laparotomy for postoperative enteral feeding. A warm water blanket may help prevent a critical loss of body heat in smaller animals. Azotemic and uremic animals may be predisposed to hypothermia because of a reduction in basal heat production.[10]

PRESERVING RENAL FUNCTION

With compensated renal disease, the animal already has reduced nephron capability, and the occurrence of acute renal failure (ARF) following an anesthetic and surgical procedure could lead to decompensation and death.

Prerenal azotemia and pre-existing renal failure complicate the diagnosis and treatment of ARF. An animal with polyuric chronic renal failure manages its inability to concentrate by increasing fluid intake. After hospitalization, water restriction, either planned (e.g., preoperative orders) or inadvertent (e.g., empty water bowl), may contribute to dehydration and further compromise of renal function.

The factors most commonly associated with operative ARF in humans are iatrogenic problems, surgical complications, and alterations related to the primary disease. Iatrogenic factors may be the use of nephrotoxic antibiotics, failure to adjust drug dosages in animals with chronic renal disease, and technical mishaps during surgery. The development of ARF during surgery can best be prevented by careful attention to hydration status and avoidance of nephrotoxic anesthetics and drugs. Neomycin and bacitracin should not be added to the lavage fluids because metabolism of neuromuscular blocking agents is altered by renal failure. Careful intraoperative hemostasis may help prevent hemorrhagic hypotension with subsequent reduction of renal blood flow. Monitoring urine output may allow early detection of oliguria during surgery and subsequent adjustment of anesthetics, fluid therapy, and diuretics (see Chapter 8).

PREVENTING INFECTIOUS COMPLICATIONS

Infectious processes in animals with end-stage renal disease require aggressive management in view of the depressed immunologic response in uremia. Many urinary tract problems are associated with urinary tract infection in addition to renal failure, e.g., calculi, neoplasia, or any cause of decreased voiding. In all of these instances, it is best to have the results of a urine culture before surgery if time allows. The animal is then started on appropriate antibiotics so that there are adequate blood and tissue levels at the time of surgery. Leakage of infected urine or purulent material from renal or prostatic abscesses into the abdomen may cause peritonitis and subsequent sepsis. In the event of intraoperative spillage, the abdomen should be lavaged with warm sterile saline (100 to 150 ml/kg BW) and suctioned dry. (For management of sepsis, see Chapter 11.)

INFORMING OWNER OF PLAN

The proposed surgery is discussed with the owner, realizing that the plan may be changed during surgery depending on surgical findings. The owner is told why the surgery is needed, what may happen if no surgery is performed, and what alternative modes of therapy are available. Postoperative management and risks (such as the need for catheters and the risk of incontinence) are also described. The owner should be aware of the expected benefits and end results as well as projected expenses.

REFERENCES

1. Chew, D.J., and DiBartola, S.P. Manual of Small Animal Nephrology and Urology. New York, Churchill Livingstone, 1986.
2. Greene, C.D.: Blood transfusion therapy: An updated overview. *In* Proceedings 49th Annual Meeting American Animal Hospital Association, pp. 187–189, 1982.
3. Tangner, C.H.: Transfusion therapy for the dog and cat. Comp. Cont. Educ. Pract. Vet., *4*:521, 1982.
4. Eknoyan, G., Wacksman, S.J., Glueck, H.I., et al: Platelet function in renal failure. N. Engl. J. Med., *280*:677, 1969.
5. Brenowitz, J.B., Williams, C.D., and Edwards, W.E.: Major surgery in patients with chronic renal failure. Am. J. Surg., *134*:765, 1977.
6. Crowe, D.T.: Clinical use of an indwelling nasogastric tube for enteral nutrition and fluid therapy in the dog and cat. J. Am. Anim. Hosp. Assoc., *22*:675, 1986.
7. Crowe, D.T.: Enteral nutrition for critically ill or injured patients—Part I. Comp. Cont. Educ. Sm. Anim., *8*:603, 1986.
8. Crowe, D.T.: Enteral nutrition for critically ill or injured patients—Part II. Comp. Cont. Educ. Sm. Anim., *8*:719, 1986.
9. Mathews, K.A., and Binnington, A.G.: Percutaneous incisionless placement of a gastrostomy tube utilizing a gastroscope: Preliminary observations. J. Am. Anim. Hosp. Assoc., *22*:601, 1986.
10. Eaton, A.G., Cordell, S.G., and Couaux, J.L.: Metabolism of nephrectomized dogs. Am. J. Med. Sci., *194*:214, 1937.

10

General Surgical Approaches

CHOOSING THE APPROACH

The appropriate surgical approach provides adequate exposure with the least amount of tissue trauma. The choice of surgical approach is based on the preoperative evaluation and the intended surgical procedure. If the problem has been localized to the abdomen, but the extent or scope of the disease is unknown, a complete abdominal exploratory procedure is indicated. Examples include abdominal trauma, suspected abdominal neoplasia, and renal and cystic uroliths. The best surgical approach for a complete abdominal exploratory procedure is through a midline abdominal incision extending from the xiphoid to the pubis, with a parapreputial skin incision in male dogs. For a biopsy of the prostate or a simple cystotomy, a caudal abdominal incision is used. In a female dog and in cats, a midline skin incision is made, but a parapreputial incision is required in male dogs.

For kidney biopsy, nephrotomy, or nephrectomy, either kidney can be reached through a cranial midline incision extending from the xiphoid to 1 to 2 cm caudal to the umbilicus. If the clinician has concluded from the preoperative evaluation that only one kidney requires scrutiny, a paracostal incision can be used. Emergency examination of the renal pedicle for bleeding is best done through a midline approach because the renal vessels are not as obvious through a paracostal approach.

To gain access to an intrapelvic prostate, the prostatic urethra or the membranous urethra in males, and the intrapelvic urethra in females, a midline incision is extended caudally and the pubis (pubic osteotomy) or pubis and ischium (pubic and ischial osteotomy) are removed. This approach is used for a complete prostatectomy or for urethrectomy prior to urinary diversion.

For correction of defects of the terminal urethra in a female, an episiotomy is performed because it exposes the vaginal vault and urethral papilla.

The penile urethra in the perineal and prescrotal regions in male dogs is approached through a midline skin incision directly over the urethra and body of the penis. The scrotal portion of the penile urethra can be accessed only after a castration and scrotal ablation. (See Chapter 19 for approach to penile urethra in the scrotal and prescrotal regions; Chapter 31 for penile urethra in perineal region.)

For access to the distal portion of the penile urethra in male dogs, the penis is extruded. To hold it in extension, the preputial orifice is partially occluded around the penis just caudal to the bulbus glandis, using a towel clamp through the edges of the prepuce.

APPROACH FOR THE KIDNEYS

After a routine abdominal incision, the left kidney is exposed by using the descending colon and mesocolon as a retractor for the jejunum. The colon is gently grasped between thumb and forefinger and pulled toward the midline (Fig. 10–1A). After the jejunum and spleen are tucked medially, the left kidney and paravertebral space are visible (Fig. 10–1B). The viscera are covered with moist laparotomy sponges.

To expose the right kidney, the duodenum and mesoduodenum are used as a retractor. The duodenum is elevated, taking care not to damage the pancreas (Fig. 10–2A). After the jejunum is placed medial to the duodenum, the caudal pole of the right kidney is seen in close proximity to the caudal vena cava (Fig. 10–2B). The right lobes of the liver cover the cranial pole. To expose the entire kidney, the right liver lobe is retracted cranially, and the hepatorenal ligament is severed, avoiding the caudal vena cava and the renal vessels (Fig. 10–2C).

PARAPREPUTIAL ABDOMINAL INCISION

The prepuce is draped out of the surgical field. After the last surgical scrub, the prepuce is positioned to one side using a sterile towel clamp (Fig. 10–3A). If the prepuce must remain in the surgical field to allow access to the urethral opening, a urethral catheter is placed and connected to a sterile collection system to prevent urine contamination of the abdomen. The midline skin incision begins at the umbilicus or as far cranially as necessary for a particular procedure. At a point 1 cm cranial to the prepuce, it curves laterally and courses lateral to the prepuce (Fig. 10–3B). Incision of the prepuce increases the risk of postoperative edema and seroma. The preputial muscle and fat are incised. The preputial vessels are isolated, ligated, and severed (Fig. 10–3C). The prepuce is retracted toward the opposite side, and a stab incision is made on the midline through the linea alba (Fig. 10–3D). In the caudal abdomen, the linea alba is often indistinct. In these instances, the incision is made between the rectus abdominis muscle. The incision is extended with a scalpel, using a tissue forceps to protect the internal organs (Fig. 10–3E). For closure, the linea alba is closed first. The preputial muscle and fat are closed separately from the subcutaneous fascia to lessen the risk of postoperative seroma (Fig. 10–3F). Skin closure is routine.

PUBIC AND ISCHIAL OSTEOTOMY

A pubic *osteotomy*, sometimes referred to as a cranial *pubic osteotomy*, is used to remove the ventral pubis and expose the prostate and cranial pelvic urethra. A *pubic and ischial osteotomy*, sometimes referred to as a complete pubic osteotomy, is used to remove the ventral pubis and ischium and expose the entire pelvic urethra, rectum, and vagina in females.

The skin incision begins as a parapreputial abdominal incision (Fig. 10–3) and extends to the cranial edge of the scrotum in a male dog (Fig. 10–4A). The prepuce is retracted laterally and the scrotum retracted caudally to expose the pelvic symphysis. In a cat or female dog, a ventral midline incision extends two-thirds the length of the pelvic symphysis for pubic osteotomy and to the caudal edge of the pelvic symphysis for pubic and ischial osteotomy. After fat is dissected from the pelvic symphysis, the attachments of the rectus abdominis, adductor, and gracilis muscles are severed with a scalpel blade (Fig. 10–4B). Using a periosteal elevator, the adductor and gracilis muscles are elevated from the pubis and ischium (Fig. 10–4C). Holes for closure wire are predrilled (Fig. 10–4D). For a pubic osteotomy, the bone is cut bilaterally from the cranial edge of the pubis into the obturator foramen and transversely across the symphysis (Fig. 10–4D, upper insert). The cranial osteotomies are made into the medial side of the obturator foramen to avoid the obturator nerve located laterally. For pubic and ischial osteotomy, the transverse cut is not made, and the ischium is osteotomized from the obturator foramina to the caudal edge of the ischium (Fig. 10–4D, lower insert). An osteotome and mallet or a power saw are used for the osteotomy (Fig. 10–4E). The bone segment is elevated caudally (Fig. 10–4F) and wrapped in a moist sponge. After a pubic and ischiatic osteotomy, the bone segment can be removed, wrapped in a moist sponge, and placed in the abdominal cavity for safe-keeping. To close the osteotomy, 20-gauge orthopedic wire is preplaced through the drilled holes, the bone segment is repositioned, and the wires tightened (Fig. 10–4G). In a cat or small dog, the bone segment can be discarded. The adductor and gracilis muscles are apposed using 0 or 2–0 absorbable suture material in a mattress pattern. The rectus abdominis muscle is sutured to the adductor muscle and the periosteum of the pubis. After skin closure, hobbles are placed on the rear legs to prevent abduction for 2 weeks.

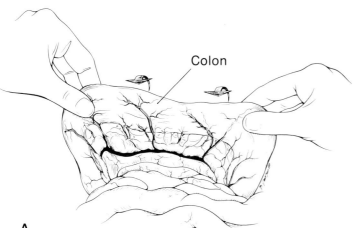

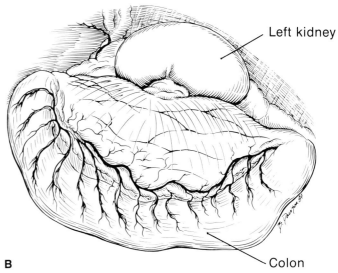

FIG. 10–1. (A) Approach for left kidney. The colon is gently grasped and pulled toward midline. (B) After the jejunum is placed medial to mesocolon, the left kidney is visible.

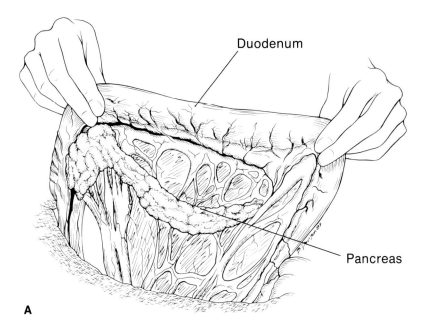

Duodenum

Pancreas

FIG. 10–2. (A) Approach for right kidney. The duodenum is elevated and moved toward the midline. The pancreas is identified and protected.

A

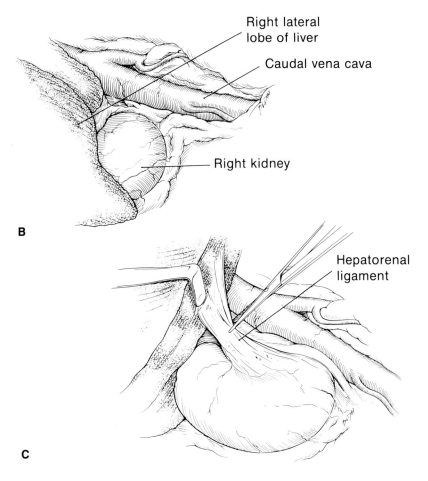

Right lateral
lobe of liver

Caudal vena cava

Right kidney

FIG. 10–2. (*Cont.*). (B) With jejunum medial to mesoduodenum, the caudal pole of the right kidney is visible next to the caudal vena cava. (C) For access to the cranial pole and hilus of the right kidney, the right lateral liver lobe is retracted and the hepatorenal ligament is severed.

B

Hepatorenal
ligament

C

FIG. 10—3. (A) Parapreputial abdominal incision. The prepuce is secured laterally using a sterile towel clamp after last surgical scrub. (B) Skin incision starts on midline and extends caudally. At about 1 cm from the prepuce, the incision curves and continues lateral to the prepuce. (C) Preputial vessels are ligated and severed.

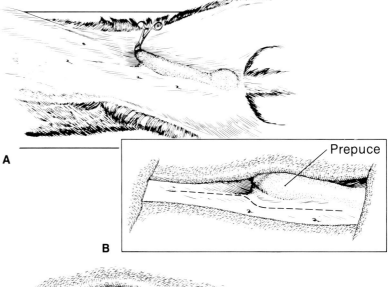

A

B

Prepuce

Preputial vessels

C

FIG. 10—3. (*Cont.*). (D) After preputial muscle and fat are incised, the prepuce is retracted toward the opposite side, and a stab incision is made through the linea alba. (E) the incision is extended with a scalpel, using tissue forceps as a guide. (F) After the linea alba is closed, preputial muscle and fat are closed as a separate layer, followed by subcutaneous fascia and skin.

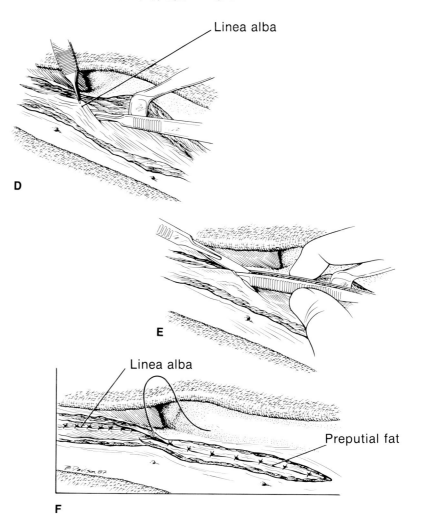

Linea alba

D

E

Linea alba

Preputial fat

F

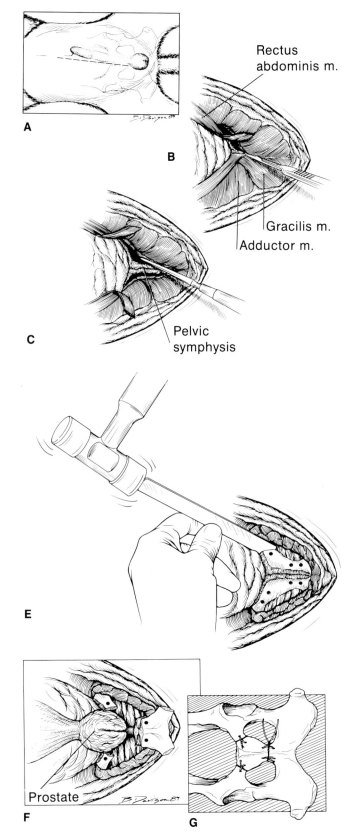

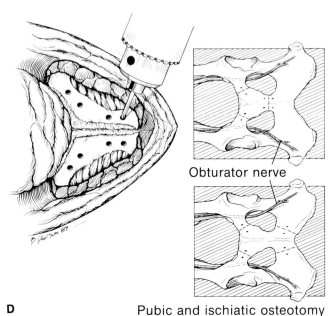

A

B

Rectus
abdominis m.

Gracilis m.

Adductor m.

C

Pelvic
symphysis

D

Obturator nerve

Pubic and ischiatic osteotomy

E

F

Prostate

G

FIG. 10—4. (A) Pubic and ischial osteotomy. Skin incision extends to the cranial edge of the scrotum in a male dog. In a cat or female dog, the incision may extend to the caudal edge of the ischium. (B) Rectus abdominis, adductor, and gracilis muscles are severed at their attachments to the pelvic symphysis. (C) Adductor and gracilis muscles are elevated from the pubis and ischium.

FIG. 10—4. (*Cont.*). (D) Holes for reattaching the bone segment are drilled. For a pubic osteotomy, the bone is cut bilaterally from the cranial edge of pubis into the obturator foramina and transversely across the symphysis (upper insert). For a pubic and ischial osteotomy, the ischium is osteotomized from the obturator foramina to the caudal edge of the ischium (lower insert). Note the location of the obturator nerve.

FIG. 10—4. (*Cont.*). (E) The osteotomy is performed with a hammer and mallet or with a power saw. (F) The bone segment is elevated caudally. A pubic osteotomy is illustrated. (G) To close the osteotomy, 20-gauge orthopedic wire is preplaced through the drilled holes. The bone segment is repositioned, and the wires are tightened.

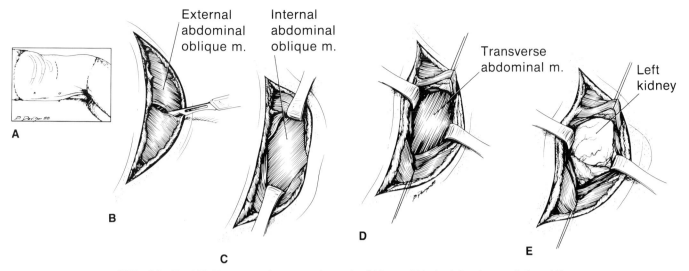

External abdominal oblique m.
Internal abdominal oblique m.
Transverse abdominal m.
Left kidney

A

B

C

D

E

FIG. 10—5. (A) Paracostal approach to the kidney. Skin incision is parallel and 2 cm caudal to last rib. (B) The external abdominal oblique muscle is divided between muscle fibers. (C) Retraction of the external abdominal oblique muscle reveals internal abdominal oblique muscle. (D) Division and retraction of the internal abdominal oblique muscle reveals the transverse abdominal muscle. (E) After the transverse abdominal muscle is separated, the kidney is located.

PARACOSTAL APPROACH TO THE KIDNEY

For a paracostal approach, the dog is placed in lateral recumbency. The skin incision is made parallel and 2 cm caudal to the last rib (Fig. 10–5A). The external abdominal oblique muscle is divided between muscle fibers (Fig. 10–5B). Retraction of this muscle reveals the internal abdominal oblique muscle (Fig. 10–5C). Division and retraction of the internal abdominal oblique muscle reveals the transverse abdominal muscle (Fig. 10–5D). Once the transverse abdominal muscle is separated, the kidney is located (Fig. 10–5E). If the kidney is enlarged, it may be necessary to cut some of the muscle layers to provide a larger opening than is possible with muscle separation. Umbilical tape can be placed around the cranial and caudal poles to help elevate the kidney from the incision (Fig. 10–6). For closure, the muscles are reapposed with absorbable suture material in a continuous pattern. Skin closure is routine. The major disadvantages of this approach are (1) no access to the opposite kidney and abdomen and (2) difficult exposure of the kidney in an obese dog. It is used most frequently for kidney biopsy in animals with generalized renal disease and for unilateral nephrotomy. A limited paracostal approach is used for the "fingerhole" method of needle biopsy of the kidney.

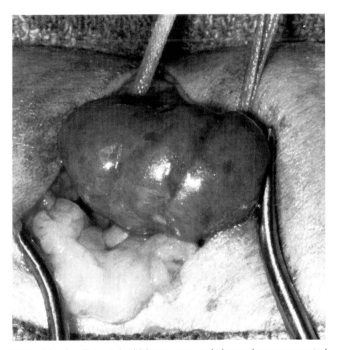

FIG. 10—6. The right kidney exposed through a paracostal incision. Umbilical tape is used to help elevate the kidney from the incision.

EPISIOTOMY

The animal is positioned in a perineal position (Fig. 10–7A). The table should be padded, and care is taken not to overextend the hind legs. A pursestring suture is placed around the anus. The skin incision extends from

1 to 2 cm distal to the anus to the edge of the vulvar lips (Fig. 10–7B,C). Straight, blunt scissors are inserted into the vagina to use as a guide for the incision into the vestibule. A scalpel is used to incise through the vestibular muscle and mucosa (Fig. 10–7D). The incision extends dorsally to provide exposure of the vestibule and cranial vagina without entering the external anal

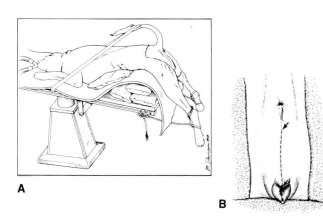

A

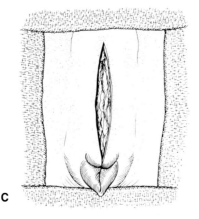

B

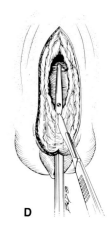

C

D

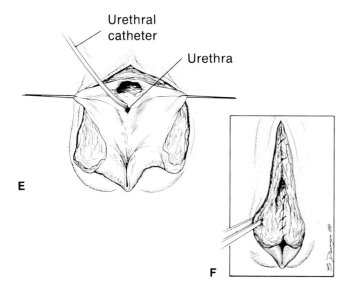

Urethral
catheter

Urethra

E

F

FIG. 10–7. (A) Episiotomy. The animal is positioned in a perineal position.

FIG. 10–7. (*Cont.*). (B and C) After a pursestring suture is placed, the skin incision extends from 1 to 2 cm distal to the anus to the edge of vulvar lips. (D) Scissors are placed into the vagina to guide the incision through vestibular muscle and mucosa.

FIG. 10–7. (*Cont.*). (E) Retention sutures are used to retract cut edges. A catheter is positioned in the urethra. (F) Vestibular mucosa is closed as a separate layer, followed by muscle and subcutaneous layers.

sphincter. Hemorrhage can be controlled with ligatures, pressure, or electrocoagulation. If excessive hemorrhage occurs, straight Doyen intestinal forceps can be clamped along the edges of the incision. Retention sutures are used to retract the cut edges (Fig. 10–7E). A catheter is placed to identify the urethral opening. The episiotomy is closed in three or four layers using a simple interrupted pattern (Fig. 10–7F). In a large dog, the mucosa, muscle, and subcutaneous layers are closed separately. In small dogs and cats, the muscle and subcutaneous layers can be closed together. Skin closure is routine.

11

General Postoperative Wound Healing, Management, and Complications

WOUND HEALING

After any trauma to the urinary tract, including surgery, return to function is dependent on the mode and extent of wound healing. An understanding of wound healing in the different organs of the urinary tract helps the surgeon to minimize postoperative complications.

Kidney

The kidney is composed of nephrons and interstitial tissue with an extensive and intricate blood supply and is covered by a well-developed fibrous capsule. Surgical incision destroys nephron units, which do not regenerate, along the line of the incision. Healing occurs primarily by fibrous protein synthesis. Wound contraction secondarily damages other functioning nephrons, but, fortunately, contraction does not predominate during the healing process of the renal parenchyma.[1] The extent of scar formation is largely dependent on the degree of vascular injury. If interlobar vessels are transected, a wedge-shaped infarct may result.[2,3]

Ureter

Healing of a wound in the area of the ureteropelvic junction (i.e., where the ureter joins the renal pelvis) is associated with more contraction than in a wound to the renal parenchyma. Contracture of the ureteropelvic junction can cause stenosis and urine outflow obstruction.

The urothelium of the ureter has enormous proliferative potential. The epithelium and submucosal tissue, particularly with urine contact, may have an inductive effect on mesenchymal stem cells, causing osteogenesis of fibrous and muscle tissue. After injury to the ureter, there is a rapid proliferation of urothelium by mitosis and migration of dedifferentiated cells. When at least 50% of the circumference of the ureter remains, the ep-

ithelium can seal a leak within 48 hours if the urine is diverted from the healing wound. The defect is closed by epithelialization, fibrous protein synthesis, and longitudinal, not circumferential, wound contraction. In a severed ureter, primary wound healing, with regular alignment of all layers of the ureteric wall, occurs after a tension-free, watertight anastomosis.[4]

Bladder

The bladder has great reparative capability, even though it is one of the weakest organs, with wall strength similar to the colon. If the entire bladder is denuded of mucosa, regeneration from ureteral epithelium, and possibly urethral sources, occurs within 30 days. Regeneration of mucosa, which is accelerated by urine contact, depends on mitotic division and migration of cells.[1] Removal of all epithelium by cautery or laser may cause enough inflammatory response and fibrous tissue formation to diminish bladder capacity greatly.[5]

After an incision through the bladder wall, collagen content is temporarily diminished. Collagen synthesis is measurable by the fifth day and returns to the level of surrounding healthy tissue by 70 days. A scar is formed as the collagen is deposited and remodeled without regeneration of smooth muscle in the wound. The wounded tissue gains almost 100% of its original strength within 14 to 21 days.[6] Enlargement of the bladder after partial cystectomy is a combination of epithelial regeneration, synthesis and remodeling of scar tissue, hypertrophy and proliferation of smooth muscle, and stretching of the bladder remnant.[1] In humans, it is reported that more than 75% of the bladder can be excised, with the trigone left intact, and the remnant closed around a 5-ml Foley catheter bulb. In a few weeks, the bladder develops a 30-ml capacity. Within 3 months, the capacity of the bladder may be as much as 300 ml. Similar figures are not available for animals, but our clinical impression is that after partial cystectomy with preservation of only enough bladder to ensure closure, animals initially urinate very frequently, but after a few months appear to regain normal voiding volume.

Urethra

The urethra heals by epithelialization, fibrous protein synthesis, and scar contraction. As long as one third to one half of the urethral circumference remains intact, the urethra can regenerate a defect of 4 to 5 cm in length within 3 to 4 weeks. Suture apposition is not necessary, but urine flow must be diverted by cystostomy catheter or indwelling catheter.[7] The urethra does not bridge a complete gap even with splinting because scar tissue causes complete occlusion after removal of the splint.[7] After a primary urethral anastomosis, fibrous tissue production can also be excessive if there is urine leakage, excessive tissue trauma, or both.[1] Urinary diversion by cystostomy catheter may help prevent urine leakage. (See Chapter 16.)

GENERAL POSTOPERATIVE MANAGEMENT AND COMPLICATIONS

Any operation carries with it a risk of complications, which can involve the surgical site or affect other systems (e.g., respiratory, cardiovascular). Immediate complications occur within the first 24 hours, early complications during the first 2 to 3 weeks after surgery, and late complications during any subsequent period, often long after the animal has left the hospital.

General complications associated with surgery may result from improper operative technique, unfamiliarity with pertinent anatomy, poor surgical judgment, intraoperative contamination and bleeding, inappropriate use of instruments and suture material, and concurrent disease.

Hemorrhage

Postoperative hemorrhage may be caused by iatrogenic operative injury to vessels or organs such as the spleen or liver, by faulty ligation of a major vessel such as the renal artery, or by coagulation abnormalities. Bleeding from a vessel or organ must first be differentiated from bleeding caused by abnormal coagulation. If microscopic examination of a peripheral blood smear reveals 3 to 5 platelets per high-power field ($400\times$) and if the blood in a test tube clots within 1 minute, it is initially assumed that the bleeding is from an unligated vessel. If there is bleeding into the abdomen, an abdominocentesis, using a syringe and needle, should retrieve blood. The hematocrit of the abdominal fluid will be similar to the peripheral blood hematocrit. Radiographs are usually not helpful in diagnosing abdominal bleeding but may be suggestive of retroperitoneal hemorrhage.

The decision for reoperation depends on the rate and duration of bleeding as well as cardiovascular status. Bleeding from cutaneous sites, such as a urethrostomy, may be controlled by cold packs, pressure, and tranquilization. Persistent bleeding mandates re-examina-

tion in the operating room. To correct vessel bleeding, proper exposure with adequate light and suction is necessary. The most common error in control of hemorrhage is a hasty attempt to apply clamps in a field obscured by accumulating blood. Manual or finger compression may slow the bleeding enough to identify the source. It may be helpful to occlude temporarily major arterial supply to an area while the vessel is located. The aorta can be compressed against the spine, the iliac vessels against the pelvic brim.

If disseminated intravascular coagulation (DIC) is suspected because of fewer than 3 to 5 platelets per high-power field, poor clotting, or other signs suggestive of DIC, a platelet count and an activated coagulation time test (ACT) are performed. In acute DIC, platelet counts are fewer than 100,000/ul, and ACT is 120 to 200 seconds for dogs and 75 to 120 seconds for cats. With end-stage DIC, platelet counts are fewer than 75,000/ul and ACT is more than 200 seconds (dog) or more than 120 seconds (cat).[8]

The most important aspect of treatment for DIC is effective therapy of the underlying disease so that the coagulatory stimulus is removed. As long as the initiating cause remains, treatment of DIC is, at best, only temporarily effective. Suppression of DIC itself is beneficial only in that it allows sufficient time for diagnosis and initiation of effective therapy of the underlying condition.

Two common causes of DIC in humans with urologic problems are bacterial sepsis, with endotoxin release, and prostatic cancer, with thromboplastin release.[9] When septicemia is the triggering mechanism, administration of appropriate antibiotics and surgical drainage of the source of infection should help prevent further release of endotoxin. In addition to treatment of the underlying cause of DIC, all conditions that promote DIC should be evaluated and reversed if present. These include hypovolemia, dehydration, acid-base imbalance, and electrolyte disorders.

These supportive measures may be sufficient in some cases. If DIC continues or is severe, however, further therapy with anticoagulants and replacement of clotting factors may be required. In DIC arising after surgery for urinary tract disorders, heparin is generally the anticoagulant of choice, although efficacy is controversial. The dose of heparin recommended varies with the stage of DIC.

If DIC is in an early stage, as indicated by only mild to moderate reductions in platelet count with other coagulation tests being normal, a low dose of heparin is used. This dose is 75 to 150 IU/kg in dogs and 75 to 100 IU/kg in cats. The heparin is given subcutaneously, using a 25-gauge needle, every 8 hours. Such a dosage does not significantly prolong coagulation time, so monitoring of activated partial thromboplastin time (APPT) or ACT is performed primarily to determine whether DIC is worsening. These tests should be performed just before the next scheduled heparin dose. Risk of inducing bleeding with these dosages is small.[8,10]

If DIC is of known recent onset and is rapidly progressive, with a platelet count that drops markedly and

ACTs that first shorten and then begin to prolong, higher dosages of heparin are recommended. These dosages are 375 to 500 IU/kg SQ every 8 hours in dogs and 250 IU/kg SQ every 8 hours in cats, which increase the APTT 1.5 to 2 times normal and carry a potential risk of hemorrhage. The APTT is a more accurate monitor of changes in coagulation than the ACT in this situation. If the APTT or the ACT is prolonged more than twice its normal value, either the dosage of heparin is too high or DIC is becoming end stage. Only careful evaluation of the patient's status, the platelet count, and other coagulation tests can separate these two possibilities. In either case, the dosage of heparin should be reduced.[10]

If DIC is in an end stage with low platelet counts and markedly long APTT or ACTs (> 4 minutes), low-dose heparin should be begun (75 to 150 IU/kg SQ every 8 hours in dogs and 75 to 100 IU/kg SQ every 8 hours in cats), and clotting factors should be immediately replaced with fresh whole blood or plasma.[8,10]

Once started, administration of heparin should be continued without interruption at regular intervals until DIC is no longer evident (normalization of patient status, platelet count, and clotting times). If DIC is not resolved, heparin withdrawal may result in rebound hypercoagulability. To avoid rebound hypercoagulability, heparin therapy should always be withdrawn gradually while monitoring clotting time.[8,10]

Postoperative Shock

The major causes of shock after urologic surgery are (1) significant systemic hypotension from hypovolemia and (2) sepsis. The signs of postoperative shock are decreased arterial pressure, weak or thready pulse, rapid heart rate, decreased capillary refill, pale mucous membranes, and decreased or absent urine output. The persistent effects of preoperative sedation, anesthesia, and postoperative analgesia may confuse the diagnosis. A septic animal might also display signs of peritonitis (e.g., abdominal pain, vomiting, fever).

Systemic Hypotension

Uncorrected volume deficit before surgery, insufficient intraoperative fluid therapy, and continuing postoperative hemorrhage can all contribute to postoperative hypovolemia. A balanced electrolyte solution is administered as the initial treatment of hypotensive shock. The fluid rate can be as high as 80 ml/kg/hr for a dog, 60 ml/kg/hr for a cat. Hematocrit and plasma protein concentrations are monitored. If the hematocrit falls rapidly to below 20%, compatible whole blood is given. Total amount of fluids and blood is determined by return to normal physiologic status, e.g., by arterial blood pressure and urine output (2 to 3 ml/kg/hr). Corticosteroids are probably beneficial if administered relatively early in hypotensive shock (methylprednisolone sodium succinate, 30 mg/kg IV, once, or dexamethasone sodium phosphate, 3 mg/kg IV, once).[11] If the animal does not improve or initially responds and then slowly regresses,

there is probably continuing bleeding or sepsis, and further evaluation is necessary.

Sepsis

Sepsis after urologic surgery is not commonly reported, but it can occur after surgery on a pyelonephritic kidney or an abscessed prostate. Leakage of infected urine into the peritoneal cavity from the kidney, ureter, or bladder could also cause peritonitis and sepsis.

An abdominocentesis may reveal toxic degenerative neutrophils with intracellular and extracellular bacteria. An increase in neutrophil numbers is commonly seen in abdominal fluid after surgery, but neutrophils should not be degenerate or contain bacteria.[12] Abnormal laboratory tests in sepsis include hypoglycemia, hypoalbuminemia, increased alkaline phosphatase, neutrophilia, thrombocytopenia, and metabolic acidosis.[11] DIC can be a complicating factor.

Preliminary treatment includes administration of lactated Ringer's solution or replacement electrolyte solution at 20 to 40 ml/kg with maintenance at 10 ml/kg because of continued losses into the peritoneal space. If total solids decrease below 4 g/dl, plasma, dextran, or albumin should be started.[11]

Intravenous broad-spectrum systemic antibiotics (e.g., cephazoline or cefoxitin) are administered after samples for culture have been collected. In an animal with normal renal function, a combination of aminoglycoside and metronidazole or clindamycin could be used when bacteria are resistant or when there is poor response to initial treatment. Development of nephrotoxicity from aminoglycosides should be monitored by microscopic examination of the urine for casts. The use of steroids and nonsteroidal anti-inflammatory drugs for septic shock is controversial and has been reviewed elsewhere.[11]

Determining and correcting the cause of the sepsis is the primary treatment. The source of the infection should be removed or drained surgically. If there is generalized peritonitis, the abdomen is lavaged with 100 ml/kg warm lactated Ringer's solution. The abdomen is suctioned, removing all fluid and blood.

Hypokalemia

In the postoperative period, hypokalemia occurs in animals on prolonged fluid therapy without potassium supplementation. Diuresis accelerates excretion of potassium, and withholding food precludes adequate intake of potassium. Signs can include muscle weakness, anorexia, and gastrointestinal ileus. Hypokalemia can be prevented by adding potassium to the balanced electrolyte solution. As a rough guideline, for a normokalemic animal, 20 mEq potassium is added to 1 L of lactated Ringer's solution. Larger amounts are required for hypokalemic animals (Table 11-1). If the animal is able to tolerate oral medications without vomiting, potassium can be supplemented orally at 1 to 3 mEq/kg/day. The oral route is the safest way to supplement potassium.

TABLE 11–1. RECOMMENDED AMOUNTS OF POTASSIUM CHLORIDE SUPPLEMENTATION IN HYPOKALEMIC DOGS AND CATS REQUIRING INTRAVENOUS OR SUBCUTANEOUS FLUID THERAPY

Serum Potassium (mEq/l)	IV Supplementation (mEq/250 ml LRS)	SC Supplementation (mEq/250 ml LRS)
3.0–3.5	5	10
2.5–3.0	7	14
2.0–2.5	10	20
<2.0	12	24

Note: Intravenous administration of solutions containing potassium chloride should never exceed 0.5 mEq potassium/kg/hr. If serum potassium returns to normal and the animal is eating, potassium therapy can be discontinued. If serum potassium returns to normal, but anorexia continues, potassium therapy should be continued at a level determined by consideration of continuing losses of potassium and by daily monitoring of serum potassium. If the serum potassium does not return to normal, level of supplementation should be increased.

LRS = lactated Ringer's solution.

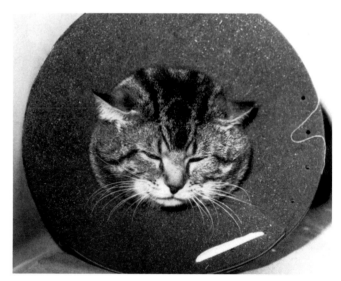

FIG. 11–1. An Elizabethan collar should extend beyond a cat or dog's muzzle.

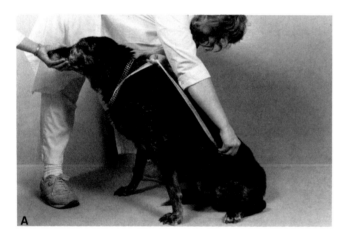

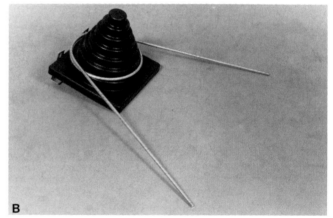

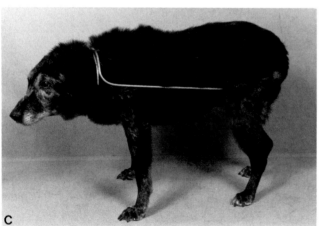

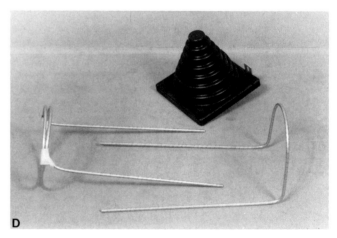

(*Legend appears on facing page*)

Postoperative Azotemia and Oliguria

The first cause of postoperative oliguria to consider is blockage or incorrect positioning of a urethral catheter. If the catheter is in place and patent, consider all three potential causes of azotemia: prerenal, renal, and postrenal (see Chapter 3). Elevations in blood urea nitrogen after surgery may have prerenal causes such as hypovolemia or hypotension. The urine specific gravity value helps to ascertain hydration status in an animal with functioning kidneys. If the animal is hypotensive or hypovolemic, appropriate fluid therapy is given. Preoperative findings should be reviewed to determine whether prerenal azotemia is exacerbating underlying renal disease. See Chapter 8 for discussion of fluid therapy in renal failure.

Excoriation and Self-Inflicted Trauma

Damage to the surgical site by the animal can cause hemorrhage, wound dehiscence, and stricture of a urethrostomy. Self-restraint devices are useful in preventing this trauma and also in preventing early removal of indwelling catheters or drains.

Elizabethan Collar

The Elizabethan collar can be purchased or constructed from cardboard, radiographic film, or plastic buckets (Fig. 11-1). The diameter must be great enough to prevent the animal's muzzle from reaching around the edge of the collar. It is secured to the animal's neck with gauze or attached to a buckled collar. Animals with Elizabethan collars sometimes have difficulty eating and drinking. It may be necessary to remove the collar during feeding and replace it afterward.

Sidebrace

The sidebrace allows greater mobility than the Elizabethan collar and does not interfere with eating. Because it is more difficult than a collar for a dog to remove, a sidebrace is used whenever there are indwelling catheters or drains that should not be pulled out prematurely. Cats usually will not tolerate a sidebrace. A sidebrace is easy to make and can be reused on other dogs of similar size. First, the dog's neck and torso length are measured (Fig. 11-2A). The center of an aluminum rod is bent in a circle to fit comfortably around the dog's neck (Fig. 11-2B). The ends of the rod are bent

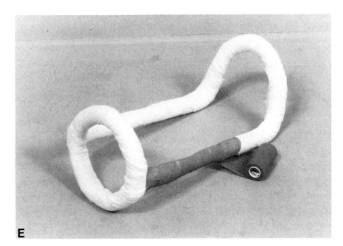

E

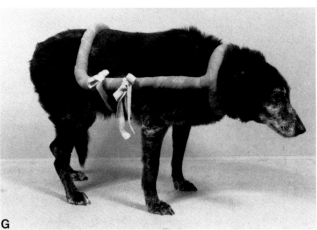

G

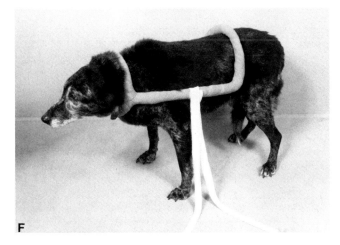

F

FIG. 11-2. (A) Sidebrace. The dog's neck and torso length are measured. (B) Using the measurement of the dog's neck, the center of an aluminum rod is bent in a circle to fit comfortably around the dog's neck. (C) The ends of the rod are bent to fit along the dog's thorax and abdomen. (D) The middle of another aluminum rod is bent to conform to the dog's back, just cranial to the ilium, with the ends extending along the abdomen. (E) The two rods are taped together, padded with cotton, and covered with tape. (F) The sidebrace is placed on the dog. The middle of an elastic tape is taped to the side brace, and each strip is folded longitudinally so that the adhesive surfaces are inward. (G) The tape strips are passed under the dog and tied loosely on the opposite side bar. An additional tape can be placed caudally to secure the sidebrace further.

to fit along the dog's thorax (Fig. 11-2C). The middle of another aluminum rod is bent to conform to the back, just cranial to the ilium, with the ends extending along the abdomen (Fig. 11-2D). The two pieces are taped together, padded with cotton, and covered with tape (Fig. 11-2E). The sidebrace is placed on the dog and secured with a loose piece of tape, which is attached to one of the side bars, passed under the abdomen, and tied to the opposite sidebar (Fig. 11-2F,G).

Wound Dehiscence

Factors associated with wound dehiscence include inadequate technical closure (excessive tension, poor suture placement, unsecured knots, or inadequate suture), poor suture quality, hematoma, wound infection, excessive movement (exercise, coughing, vomiting), previous irradiation, or metabolic disease (Cushing's disease, diabetes mellitus, starvation, or uremia). The first sign of impending dehiscence is a pink fluid discharge from the abdominal incision. This represents a serous effusion present within the abdominal cavity after surgery, which seeps through the separating wound and becomes tinged with blood.

Sometimes the skin sutures hold, but the deeper layers are disrupted (Fig. 11-3). The abdomen is carefully bandaged until surgical repair can be performed. If the animal's condition is critical, the animal should be stabilized before surgery.

An animal with complete abdominal wound dehiscence (Fig. 11-4) requires immediate attention because of the danger of self-mutilation. Exposed viscera are covered with sterile, moistened lap pads, and the abdomen is bandaged to prevent self-mutilation. After the animal is anesthetized and positioned for surgery, the bandage and skin sutures are removed. The wound edges are cleaned. The exposed viscera are lavaged with warm, balanced electrolyte solution and returned to the abdomen. It may be necessary to remove the remaining sutures to enlarge the opening. The body wall sutures are examined to determine the cause of the wound

breakdown. For closure, nonabsorbable sutures (nylon, stainless steel, polypropylene) are passed through all layers of the abdominal scar (dorsal fascia, muscle, and ventral fascia). The sutures are placed at least 1 cm from the wound edge and approximately 0.5 cm apart and tied without tension. If the original sutures have come untied, extra care is taken to tie square knots and leave sufficiently long tags on the knot when the suture is cut.

Wound Infection

Wound infection can occur because of pre-existing infections such as urinary tract infection, peritonitis, or skin infection. Operative sources of infection include lapses in surgical technique, inadequate sterilization of instruments, and contamination from infected urine. After surgery, wound infection can occur from feces or urine contamination from operated or other animals.

Clinical signs of wound infection usually develop a few days after surgery, but they may be delayed if the animal is receiving antibiotics. Initially, there is pain and swelling in the wound. Pyrexia may develop. Treatment requires adequate drainage, which is maintained until the wound cavity heals, beginning with the deepest involved tissue. Otherwise, superficial layers can close and deep-seated infection persist. It may be necessary to remove some of the sutures and allow areas to granulate as open wounds. Antibiotics are ineffective without adequate drainage because they cannot diffuse in sufficient concentrations to sterilize such a wound. Antibiotics are administered for deep-seated infection, for systemic infections, or for spreading cellulitis.

Abdominal Adhesions

Postoperative adhesions may be caused by rough handling of tissues, drying of the tissues, localized or generalized infections, reactive suture material, or foreign bodies such as gauze sponges or laparotomy pads. Particular attention is needed to avoid leaving gauze sponges in very bloody surgeries such as prostatecto-

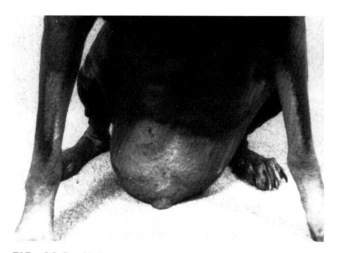

FIG. 11-3. Abdominal wall dehiscence in a dog following prostatic biopsy.

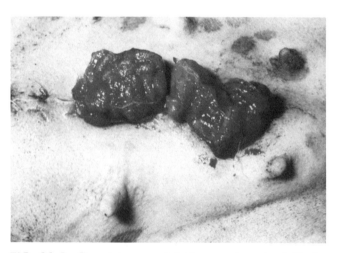

FIG. 11-4. Complete wound dehiscence in a dog following a cystotomy.

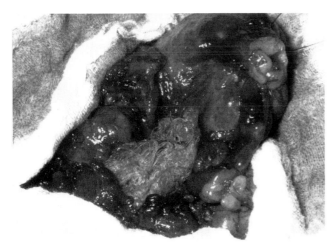

FIG. 11-5. Caudal abdominal exploratory surgery revealed a sponge surrounded by adhesions. The sponge had been left in the abdomen during previous prostate surgery.

mies (Fig. 11-5). A sponge count before surgery and immediately before closure helps prevent inadvertent loss of a sponge in the abdomen. Gauze sponges with radiopaque markers should be used in all abdominal surgeries so that a misplaced sponge can be identified on abdominal radiographs. Symptomatic abdominal adhesions following uncomplicated surgeries in dogs and cats are uncommon, probably because an active fibrinolytic system helps prevent adhesions.

The clinical signs associated with postoperative adhesions depend on location and extent of the adhesions. Adhesions can compress the lumen or blood supply of the ureters or intestines. Obstruction of a single ureter may not initially cause signs. The resultant hydronephrotic kidney may be palpated as an abdominal mass. If both ureters or the urethra is occluded, signs of uremia develop within 48 hours. Involvement of the intestines may produce signs of intestinal obstruction, strangulation, or both. Radiographs may reveal the presence of an abdominal mass. Mechanical ileus is apparent if there is intestinal obstruction and dilation of the proximal segment of the intestine. Radiopaque tabs and markers in sponges and laparotomy pads can also be seen.

An exploratory laparotomy is indicated to determine the cause of the obstruction. Often a ureter obstructed by adhesions cannot be salvaged; thus, a nephroureterectomy is indicated. If the intestine is viable, an attempt is made to excise any bands of adhesions. Intestinal resection is performed if necessary. Following peritonitis or a misplaced sponge, the adhesions may involve the entire intestinal tract, with loops of intestine entering and exiting the tangle of adhesions. Large amounts of intestine may have to be resected to restore continuity to the intestinal tract.

REFERENCES

1. Peacock, E.E.: Wound Repair. Philadelphia, W.B. Saunders, 1984, pp. 472–484.
2. King, W.W.: Renal wound healing: Histologic and histochemical sequences in the repair of intersegmental nephrotomies. Inv. Urol., 4:278, 1974.
3. Stone, E.A., Metcalf, M.R., and Robertson, J.L.: Glomerular filtration rate after nephrotomy: A comparison of intersegmental and bisection nephrotomy. Vet. Surg., 19:76, 1990.
4. Jonas, D., Kramer, W., and Weber, W.: Splintless microsurgical anastomosis of the ureter in the dog. Urol. Res., 9:271, 1981.
5. Osuna, D.J., Stone, E.A., Monteiro-Riviere, N., et al.: Bladder healing after laser treatment in dogs. Vet. Surg., 18:71, 1989.
6. Hastings, J.C., Van Winkle, W., Barker, E., et al.: The effect of suture materials on healing wounds of the bladder. Surg. Gynec. Obstet., 140:933, 1975.
7. Weaver, R.G., and Schulte, J.W.: Experimental and clinical studies of urethral regeneration. Surg. Gynec. Obstet., 115:729, 1962.
8. Greene, C.E.: Management of DIC and thrombosis. In Current Veterinary Therapy VIII. Edited by R.W. Kirk. Philadelphia, W.B. Saunders, 1983, pp. 401–405.
9. Pergament, M.L., Swaim, W.R., and Blackard, C.E.: Disseminated intravascular coagulation in the urologic patient. J. Urol., 116:1, 1976.
10. Slappendel, R.J.: Disseminated intravascular coagulation. In Current Veterinary Therapy X. Edited by R.W. Kirk. Philadelphia, W.B. Saunders, 1989, pp. 451–457.
11. Hardie, E.M., and Rawlings, C.A.: Septic Shock. Part II Prevention, recognition, and treatment. Compend. Contin. Educ. Pract. Vet., 5:483, 1983.
12. Bjorling, D.E., Latimer, K.S., Rawlings, C.A., et al.: Diagnostic peritoneal lavage before and after abdominal surgery in dogs. Am J. Vet. Res., 44:816, 1983.

PART II

SPECIFIC TECHNIQUES OF UROLOGIC SURGERY

Section Four

Feline Urethral Obstruction

12

Diagnosis and Medical Management of Feline Urethral Obstruction

Feline urethral obstruction defines a medical problem rather than a specific disease entity. With urethral obstruction, the cat senses bladder fullness and attempts to void. The obstruction in the urethra, however, prevents bladder emptying, either completely with a total obstruction or partially with an incomplete obstruction. The bladder remains totally to partially distended. The cat repeatedly attempts to urinate. If the cat cannot void any urine, uremia results within 48 to 72 hours. There are several potential causes of urethral obstruction.

CAUSES OF URETHRAL OBSTRUCTION

Obstruction of the feline urethra can occur as a result of a physical obstruction, spasm, or neurologic dysfunction (inability of the urethra to relax) (Table 12-1).[1,2] All causes of obstruction are more common in male cats than females because the male urethra is longer, narrower, and less distensible (Fig. 12-1).

Physical causes of obstruction are most common. Physical causes include urethral plugs, uroliths, neoplasia, strictures (owing to connective tissue, prostatic lesions, or other extraluminal masses), and inflammatory swelling of the urethra. The precise cause of urethral obstruction is often not determined. A prospective study at the University of Minnesota found that approximately 62% of cats with urethral obstruction had urethral plugs, whereas the rest had urolithiasis (10%) or no identifiable cause (28%).[1]

Urethral plugs are disorganized precipitates, which are composed of variable amounts of crystals (primarily struvite) in a colloidal matrix (Figs. 12-2, 12-3, 12-4).[1,3–7] Urethral plugs are contrasted with true uroliths, which are concretions of organized crystalline structure (Fig. 12-5). Most lower urinary tract uroliths in cats are composed of struvite, but other types, including calcium oxalate, calcium phosphate, and urate, have also been found.[1,8]

Neoplasia generally occurs in old cats (average age 10 years),[9] whereas the majority of cats with urethral plugs or uroliths are young (1 to 6 years).[8] Age is used only to decide what is most likely however, and not to make a definitive diagnosis, since the age ranges for neoplasia, urolithiasis, urethral plugs, and idiopathic obstruction overlap. Contrast radiography and biopsy are necessary to identify and diagnose definitively urethral or bladder trigonal neoplasia as a cause of urethral obstruction (see Chapter 30).

Trauma should be ruled out by careful history and physical examination as well as contrast-enhanced radiography. Trauma usually results in urethral tears or stricture.

Urethral spasm is infrequently described as a primary cause of urethral obstruction. Urethral spasm may contribute, however, to continued difficulty with urination after a physical obstruction caused by a urolith or urethral plug having been removed. Urethral spasm in these instances is thought to be caused by urethral irritation and inflammation.

Neurologic dysfunction causing the urethra to fail to relax during attempted micturition (reflex dyssynergia) has been a postulated cause of functional urethral obstruction but has been described rarely.[10]

Because most cases of feline urethral obstruction are caused by urethral plugs, these are discussed further.

ETIOLOGY OF URETHRAL PLUGS

The etiology of urethral plugs is unknown, although several areas have been investigated, including infectious agents, diet, and individual cat characteristics. Each of these is reviewed separately. Because urethral plugs seem to be heterogeneous with variable amounts of matrix and crystals, it is possible that there are different causes for their formation. In some cats, the matrix may be primary with crystals trapped within. In other cats,

TABLE 12–1. CAUSES OF URETHRAL OBSTRUCTION IN CATS		
Intraluminal	**Extraluminal**	**Functional**
Urethral plugs	Neoplasia	Reflex dyssynergia
Uroliths	Strictures	Urethral muscle spasm
Neoplasia	Prostatomegaly (uncommon)	
	Inflammatory swelling	

crystal formation may be dominant, leading to irritation and matrix production.

The proportions of crystalline material to matrix vary, with some plugs being completely matrix and other being more sabulous. Although over 90% of cats have struvite (ammonium magnesium phosphate hexahydrate) as the predominant mineral in the crystals (see Fig. 12-4), crystals with various other minerals such as ammonium acid urate, calcium phosphate, and calcium oxalate have been predominant in a few cats.[1,5,11] In addition to crystals, urethral plugs may contain cells such as red blood cells within the colloidal matrix. The specific chemical composition and tissue of origin of the matrix is unknown.

Infectious Agents

Bacterial infection is uncommon in cats with urethral obstruction. Even nonroutine culture methods to iden-

tify anaerobes, spirochetes, mycoplasma, or fastidious organisms requiring feline urine or tissue to grow have failed to identify potentially causative organisms.[11,12] Bacteria were also not seen on scanning electron microscopy of urinary sediment.[11] Thus, it seems unlikely that bacterial infection is the cause of either matrix formation or mineral precipitation in cats with urethral plugs or idiopathic obstruction.

The relationship of viral infections to urethral plugs remains controversial. One study induced urethral obstruction by injecting urine from a cat with naturally occurring urethral obstruction into the bladders of normal cats.[13,14] Despite efforts in other laboratories, obstruction has not been produced again by urine transfer,[11,15,16] even with the use of glucocorticoids as immunosuppressants.[15] Viruses also have not been recovered from urine of affected cats in any higher proportion than from urine of normal cats.[11,12,15,16] The original investigators have attributed this to their finding that the picornavirus and syncytial virus, originally isolated from urine of affected cats, cannot cause disease alone but can only worsen signs induced by a cell-associated herpesvirus, which cannot be recovered from urine but only from urinary tract tissues.[17]

The cell-associated herpesvirus was initially isolated from kidney tissue from normal kittens.[18] The only isolation from a spontaneous case was from a 4.5-month-old laboratory kitten with urethral obstruction.[19] In this kitten, the virus was isolated from kidney but not lower urinary tract tissue. This herpesvirus alone was found to induce urethral obstruction in specific pathogen free (SPF) cats, as a result of urethral swelling, as well as

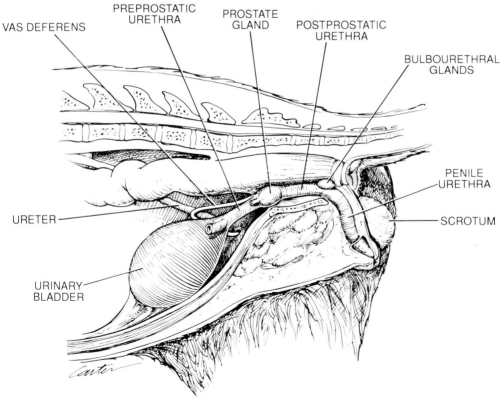

FIG. 12–1. Normal urethra in a male cat.

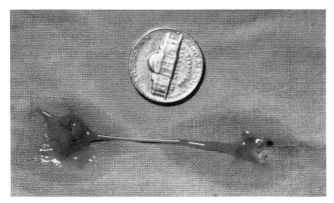

FIG. 12–2. Urethral plug composed primarily of mucus. (From Barsanti, J.A.: Feline hematuria and dysuria: A diagnostic approach. *In* Proceedings, Feline Medicine II, 2nd Annual Kal Kan Symposium, p. 5, 1986; with permission.)

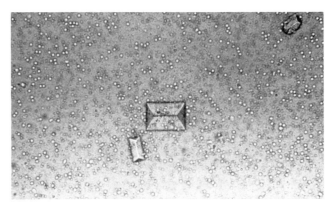

FIG. 12–4. Struvite crystals in urine sediment. (From Barsanti, J.A.: Feline hematuria and dysuria: A diagnostic approach. *In* Proceedings, Feline Medicine II, 2nd Annual Kal Kan Symposium, p. 7, 1986; with permission.)

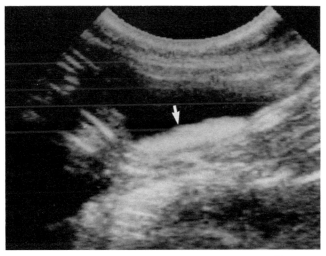

FIG. 12–3. Abdominal ultrasonogram showing disorganized crystalline (arrow) material within the bladder lumen. The cat was presented for hematuria and dysuria without urethral obstruction. Passage of quantities of such crystals into the urethra, however, is one postulated cause of feline urethral obstruction.

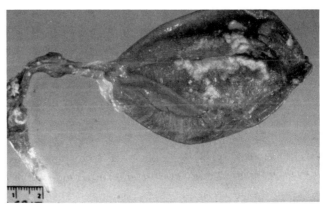

FIG. 12–5. Feline bladder and urethra, showing several urethral calculi and multiple small cystoliths as well as disorganized crystalline material. The urethral calculi caused urethral obstruction, resulting in bladder overdistention and bladder wall injury. The bladder is from a cat on an experimental diet study,[27] rather than a natural case.

inducing hematuria either intermittently or persistently.[20,21] Hemorrhages were found in the bladder and urethra, in addition to crystalline material and calculi. The virus could be reisolated from affected cats.

Despite the experimental induction of cystitis in SPF cats with the cell-associated herpesvirus, only subclinical infection could be induced in conventionally reared laboratory cats.[1] Also, despite laboratory evidence for horizontal and vertical transfer,[20,21] one case control study showed no association of urethral obstruction with multiple cat households and, thus, no evidence for an easily transmitted infectious agent as a cause of feline urethral obstruction.[22]

Thus, although the cell-associated herpes virus may be able to induce lower urinary tract disease in SPF cats, there remains no evidence that this virus is involved in natural cases. Further research in this area is needed.

Diet

As already noted, struvite is the predominant mineral component of crystals in most cats with urethral plugs. Causes of struvite precipitation in urine include increased concentration of ammonium, magnesium, or phosphate; a change in pH to one in which these minerals are less soluble; or a change in other crystallization enhancers or inhibitors in urine. Increased mineral concentration in urine can be caused by an increased quantity of mineral to excrete or a decrease in the amount of water in urine. Ammonium and phosphate are considered abundant in feline urine, so attention has been focused on magnesium as the rate-limiting mineral. Diet may be involved relative to its mineral content, caloric content, caloric density, digestibility, water content, and ability to acidify urine.

Mineral Content

The relationship of mineral content of the diet to urethral obstruction has received the most experimental attention. Various studies from different groups of investigators have produced urethral obstruction in previously normal male cats by increasing the magnesium content of the diet.[23-26] In most of these studies, the cause of obstruction was true uroliths. Renoliths were also noted.[24,26] The mineral components of these induced uroliths were magnesium and phosphate. Urine from cats with uroliths was often alkaline. The relationship of this experimental form of urolithiasis with naturally occurring lower urinary tract disease in cats has been questioned for a number of reasons, including the following (1) Spontaneous urethral obstruction is not often associated with uroliths, especially renoliths that are uncommon in cats[8]; (2) the crystals associated with spontaneous cases are magnesium ammonium phosphate (struvite); and (3) urine from cats with naturally occurring obstruction is usually acidic at the time of obstruction. The use of magnesium oxide in the experimental diets, which alkalinizes the urine and which is not the source of magnesium in cat foods, is now thought to explain the experimental findings.

One study did induce urethral obstruction with dense deposits of struvite crystals in cats fed 0.45% magnesium in a dry diet (six of eight cats) or 0.5 or 1.0% magnesium in a moist diet (six of eight cats in each group).[27] In addition, one of four cats fed 0.15% magnesium in a dry diet developed urethral obstruction. Struvite calculi were also found in cats fed 1.0% magnesium. One difference in this study from those done previously was that the alkalinity induced by the supplemental magnesium oxide was corrected before the experimental moist food was fed. The type of obstruction was still not identical to that seen in natural cases because the urethral plugs consisted only of packed struvite crystals with no matrix.

Commercial cat foods contain less magnesium than has been added to produce calculogenic diets, with the exception of one 0.15% magnesium experimental diet on which one of four experimental cats developed urethral obstruction.[27] This experimental diet induced consistently alkaline urine (pH > 7.0), however. In commercial diets in the United States, the mean magnesium content on a dry weight basis was 0.03 to 0.15% for canned foods, 0.07 to 0.16% for semimoist food, and 0.15 to 0.16% for dry food.[28,29] The amount of minerals in commercial foods was found to be fairly consistent lot to lot.[30] In one study, feeding the 0.16% magnesium found in commercial dry foods did not produce obstruction in normal cats.[23] Examining only the magnesium content on a dry weight basis can be misleading. The amount of other minerals such as calcium and phosphorus affects how calculogenic a diet is.[25]

Cat owners are often confused about the relationship of dietary ash content to urethral obstruction. This confusion has been fostered by some cat food manufacturers. Ash simply refers to all noncombustible components of a diet and, thus, includes most of the mineral content without relationship to any one mineral. In one study, the diet used was 30% ash but only 0.03% magnesium, and no urinary tract signs developed.[31] Thus, ash content is not related to magnesium content.

The amount of magnesium that must be excreted in the urine also depends on how much magnesium is consumed and its intestinal absorption. Thus, caloric density, palatability, and digestibility of a diet may be as important in determining the amount of magnesium that must be excreted as the amount of magnesium on a dry weight basis.[32] Cats eating 0.45 or 0.15% magnesium in a dry diet were found to consume as much magnesium as those eating 1.0 or 0.5% magnesium, respectively, in a canned diet in one study in which food intake was carefully monitored.[27] The cats ate more of the dry diet because of its apparently lower caloric content to maintain body weight and, thus, ingested more magnesium. Despite similar magnesium intake, urine magnesium concentration was less on the experimental dry diet than the moist, probably owing to decreased magnesium absorption associated with the high calcium content of the dry diet. This study points out the necessity of studying magnesium intake and excretion as well as clinical signs when evaluating a diet. The amount of magnesium in urine correlated with magnesium ingested so that the cats stayed in magnesium balance. The greater the quantity of magnesium in the urine, the greater was the likelihood of obstruction with struvite crystals and at higher amounts with urolith formation. The urine magnesium content, however, was not the only factor involved in obstruction because there was no difference in urine magnesium content between cats in each group that developed obstruction and those that did not.[27]

The question that arises from these experimental studies is whether cats with naturally occurring urethral plugs have higher than normal urine magnesium content, because of diet, intestinal hyperabsorption, or renal hyperexcretion. One study has found that cats with naturally occurring lower urinary tract disease had markedly lower urine magnesium content than those fed the high magnesium experimental diets.[27] Thus, most naturally occurring cases are probably not caused by increased absorption or excretion of magnesium.

Water Intake

Water intake on different diets has been studied because of the relationship of urine volume to mineral concentration. Some studies have looked only at water intake or water intake and urine volume, whereas others have examined total water balance, which includes measuring urine and fecal water output and extrapolating to estimate insensible water loss. Studies of water intake alone cannot be extrapolated to conclusions about urine volume since fecal water loss is an important excretory pathway, which varies with factors such as diet.[16,33] The total energy content and fat content of diets are more important than whether a diet is dry or moist in determining urine water loss. A high fat (approximately 30%)/high caloric diet increased urine volume, whereas low fat/lower energy caloric diets caused more water to be excreted in the feces.[33] Total water intake was similar with all diets, whether canned or dry (125 to 230 ml/cat/day).[33] The best conclusion for a clinician is that merely looking at canned versus dry food, in general, is too simplistic. Climatic conditions, specific components of the diets (fat in particular), age of the cat, the means of providing water and food, and the degree of stress may all affect water intake.[34] For the clinician, consideration of the urine specific gravity of cats is more important in measuring degree of urine concentration than determining whether the diet is canned or dry. These considerations become more important in preventing recurrence of urethral plus, rather than identifying cats prone to urethral plug formation. When water balance was compared between male cats with a history of urethral obstruction and normal male cats matched by age and body weight, no significant difference was found.[34]

Urine Acidification

Because struvite crystals are less soluble at a pH greater than 6.8,[7,35,36] the relationship of diet to urine pH has also been studied. Any food induces a shift to alkalinity in urine in the hours immediately after eating. The degree of this postprandial alkaline tide varies with the diet.[37] The frequency of feeding may also affect urine alkalinity. Once a day feeding causes a higher urine pH than ad libitum feeding,[38] but the duration of alkalinity may be less. Urine pH seems to remain fairly constant throughout the day with ad libitum feeding.[38] The relationship of the postprandial alkaline tide to formation of urethral plugs is unknown. Epidemiologic studies have been conducted that considered frequency of feeding to risk of lower urinary tract signs. Results have been inconsistent.[39–41] After naturally occurring urethral obstruction develops, urine pH is usually acidic,[7,35,36,42,43] but urine pH before the obstruction is unknown.

The origin of the crystals found in urethral plugs is not known. Although one study found microcrystals inside renal tubules,[42] this finding was not duplicated in another study.[27]

Despite studies of experimental calculogenic diets, water balance, and effect of feeding on urine pH, the question still remains as to the association of these factors with urethral obstruction in cats. Urethral plugs contain matrix as well as mineral. Whether mineral or matrix came first to form the obstruction is not known. Matrix is suspected because of the unorganized nature of the crystalline material. There is no known relationship between diet and matrix composition, although the biochemical composition of the matrix has received little study to date.

Epidemiologic Studies

Epidemiologic studies have been widely used in the hope that possible etiologic factors of urethral plugs would be suggested. A major drawback has been the definition of the population studied. Most studies have relied only on owners' histories or retrospective studies of case diagnoses and have focused only on clinical signs of hematuria, dysuria, or urethral obstruction. The populations were not defined by any diagnostic criteria, such as urinalysis, urine culture, radiographs, or urine

mineral excretion. Thus, these studies are limited because they considered all lower urinary tract disease rather than any one disease, and the general conclusion that lower urinary tract disease is multifactorial is not unexpected. The incidence rate for all lower urinary tract disease in cats has been found to be about 0.85%.[44,45]

In general, these studies have found an increased risk of lower urinary tract disease in cats that are older than 2 years, neutered, overweight, and "lazy."[5,39,40,41,46–49] Peak age range was 2 to 6 years.[47] The data on obesity may be questioned because one study did not have an unaffected group for comparison[40] and because subjective opinions as to whether the cat was obese were used rather than actual body weight.[47] Determining the activity level of cats was also subjective, based on owner impression[39,40] or on the cat being kept indoors or allowed outdoors.[40,46] Another interpretation of this data would be that outdoor or "active" cats are at "less" risk only because the problem is less likely to be detected with outdoor and unobserved urination. The risk association with neutering was unassociated with age of neutering.[40,49] The risk association with castration could not be associated with decreased urethral size.[5,50,51] Effect of castration on urethral compliance has not been studied, however, and an increase in fibrocyte numbers in the urethra has been found that might cause a decrease in urethral distensibility.[51] Not all studies have confirmed these findings. Some studies have found no association with neutering.[22,52,53]

Congenital Defects

Bladder diverticula (Figs. 12-6, 12-7) associated with a urachal remnant have been identified in cats with lower urinary tract signs.[54–57] Urachal remnants are common in all cats, however. One study of 735 cats used for anatomy dissections indicated that 22% of males and 26.5% of females had identifiable urachal remnants.[54] Comparing this to the incidence of lower urinary tract signs (0.85%) suggests that most cats with urachal rem-

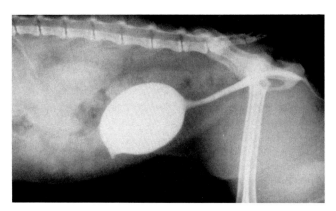

FIG. 12–6. Lateral abdominal radiograph (retrograde urethrocystogram), showing a normal feline urethra and a small urachal diverticulum in a male cat with a history of hematuria and dysuria.

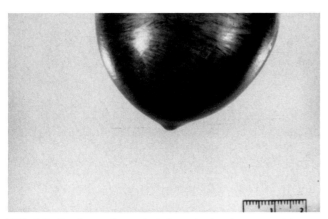

FIG. 12–7. A small urachal diverticulum in a cat with urethral obstruction at necropsy. (Courtesy of Dr. W. Crowell, Department of Pathology, University of Georgia.)

nants do not have signs of lower urinary tract disease. Radiographic evidence of urachal remnants has been shown to resolve spontaneously with resolution of clinical signs.[57] Appearance of urachal remnants in cats with urethral obstruction is considered a consequence of bladder wall injury secondary to obstruction, rather than a possible etiologic factor.

PATHOPHYSIOLOGY

The site of obstruction is usually considered to be the distal penile urethra based on clinical impression. The feline urethra, however, is also narrow just caudal to the bulbourethral glands at the ischial arch[5,58] and between the bladder and the prostate gland (see Fig. 12-1).[59] There are few studies of the site of obstruction in clinical cases, although obstruction in sites other than the penile urethra (intrapelvic, preprostatic) have been reported.[5,58] Determination of the site of obstruction is important in clinical cases since perineal urethrostomy may be recommended for prevention of recurrence. This surgery removes the distal penile urethra and makes a new urethral opening just cranial to the caudal edge of the bulbourethral glands. Thus, it would not prevent recurrence of a more proximal obstruction.

Regardless of the cause, obstruction to urine outflow leads to predictable clinical and biochemical changes, which vary with the duration and degree of obstruction. With complete urethral obstruction, the bladder gradually becomes distended. The rate at which the bladder distends depends on rate of urine flow, bladder capacity, and previous bladder injury. The pressure associated with overdistention results in ischemia, edema, hemorrhage, loss of epithelium, and infiltration of neutrophils around blood vessels (Fig. 12-8).[60–63] The urethra proximal to the obstruction has similar injuries, with desquamation of epithelium, edema, and infiltration of neutrophils around blood vessels and in the lamina propria and muscle layer.[60] The increased pressure is transmitted up the ureters to the kidneys, causing the kidneys to appear somewhat swollen and congested with hemorrhage, particularly in the medulla.[60]

Azotemia results from inability to excrete urine. Obstructive nephropathy is defined as the functional and biochemical alterations that occur in the kidneys as a result of obstruction to urine outflow. Obstruction causes a decrease in renal blood flow (RBF) and glomerular filtration rate (GFR) and changes in reabsorption of solutes and water.[64] The mechanisms for these changes continue to be studied. With increased intraluminal pressure in the bladder and ureters, intratubular pressure increases at a rate dependent on rate of urine flow at the time of obstruction. GFR decreases because of the increased intratubular pressure, which opposes glomerular capillary hydrostatic pressure and leads to decreased effective filtration pressure. Preglomerular vasoconstriction also contributes to the decrease in GFR and RBF. Most nephrons apparently stop filtering completely, whereas others continue but at a markedly reduced rate.[64] In experimental studies, the decrease in GFR was completely reversible over approximately a week, if the period of obstruction was less than 36 hours.

Most *physical findings* in cats with urethral obstruction are related to uremia, resulting from retention of waste products of metabolism, and to hyperkalemia, which results from lack of potassium excretion, acidemia, and possibly reabsorption of potassium through the damaged bladder wall. The severity of these changes is related to the degree and duration of obstruction. Signs associated with uremia (e.g., anorexia, depression, weakness, vomiting, hypothermia, and dehydration) occurred in most experimentally obstructed cats 48 hours after obstruction; longer times were required for signs to develop in some cats.[62]

Signs associated with hyperkalemia include bradycardia and ventricular arrhythmias. Lack of P waves, widened QRS interval, and spiked T waves can be found by electrocardiography.[65] These signs develop when serum potassium concentrations are approximately 10 mEq/L or greater.[65] Bradycardia is not a consistent finding in cats, however, even with marked hyperkalemia.[65] Thus, a normal heart rate does not eliminate the possibility of severe hyperkalemia. Hyperkalemia affects the heart by depressing conduction rate and contractility.[65] The acidemia associated with uremia may exac-

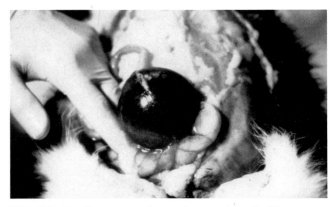

FIG. 12–8. Necropsy of a male cat that died from prolonged urethral obstruction. Note that the bladder is distended and discolored, indicating ischemia.

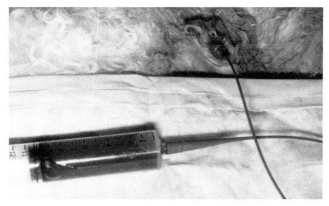

FIG. 12–9. Hemorrhagic urine being removed from a cat's bladder via a flexible urethral catheter after relief of urethral obstruction.

erbate the effects of hyperkalemia on the myocardium.[65] Hyperkalemia also causes generalized muscle weakness. In cats with experimental obstruction, serum potassium increased after the development of uremia.[62] From 48 to 96 hours of complete urethral obstruction were required for severe hyperkalemia (serum potassium > 8 mEq/L) to develop. Acidemia, dehydration, and hyperkalemia are probably responsible for death in untreated cats with urethral obstruction.

Laboratory biochemical changes associated with complete urethral obstruction include azotemia and hyperphosphatemia, both related to decreased GFR and hyperkalemia, as already discussed. Acidemia also occurs as a result of retention of acidic metabolic waste products. Another occasional change is hypocalcemia (serum calcium < 8.0 mg/dl).[65] The hypocalcemia has been attributed to hyperphosphatemia, causing the calcium/phosphorus solubility product to be exceeded, leading to calcium precipitation in tissues. Serum calcium is usually not less than 7 mg/dl. Because acidemia causes a greater percentage of serum calcium to be ionized (active), hypocalcemia usually causes no adverse clinical signs. Mild hyperglycemia also develops in cats with urethral obstruction, secondary to epinephrine or glucocorticoid release from stress, and perhaps caused by peripheral inhibition of insulin by uremic toxins. This hyperglycemia may be associated with glycosuria.[7] A few cats have glycosuria with normoglycemia, and the glycosuria may persist several days after relief of obstruction.[7] This may result from proximal tubular cell injury leading to decreased glucose reabsorption. Nonglucose oxidizing substances (pseudoglycosuria) have also been found in urine from cats with urethral obstruction.[66]

Hematuria is the principal finding on *urinalysis* (Fig. 12-9). The hematuria may be secondary to bladder wall injury from distention or may be primary and related to the cause of the obstruction. In clinical cases, it is usually unknown whether hematuria preceded or followed development of urethral obstruction. Urine is usually acidic and concentrated at the time of obstruction. Pyuria, if present, is usually mild (< 20 white blood cells/high-power field).

DIAGNOSIS

Affected cats try to urinate frequently, often in "unusual" places (such as the sink or bathtub). They may strain during urination but produce little urine. If any urine is expelled, it may appear hemorrhagic. Frequent attempts and straining to urinate may be mistaken by the owner as constipation, since little or no urine is seen with severe obstruction. Frequent licking of the penis, which is discolored and congested, is common. Vomiting, weakness, and depression will be noted if the early signs of obstruction are missed.

The first diagnostic step for a cat with suspected hematuria or dysuria is to determine whether urethral obstruction is present. This can usually be done by physical examination. Finding a distended, tense bladder, which may cause discomfort when palpated, is indicative of urethral obstruction.

When urethral obstruction is suspected on the basis of physical examination, the rest of the cat's history and physical examination should help determine the duration and severity of the obstruction. Signs of uremia indicate that complete obstruction has been present at least 48 hours.[62] Signs of hyperkalemia, such as generalized weakness, cardiac arrhythmias, or bradycardia, indicate a longer duration of complete obstruction.

The combination of uremia and hyperkalemia are potentially life-threatening. Any diagnostic effort other than collecting blood and urine in a cat with such signs should be postponed until treatment is instituted and the cat's condition stabilized. Some data can be collected as treatment is begun. As one tries to remove the obstruction by catheterization, the location and texture of the obstructing material is noted. Any retrieved obstructing material is saved for analysis, either by microscopy for a mucoid plug or by crystallography for a calculus. If a cystocentesis is used to relieve bladder pressure before urethral catheterization, urine is saved for a complete urinalysis. If cystocentesis is not done, urine obtained after catheterization is used for urinalysis.

If the urinalysis indicates pyuria or bacteriuria in addition to hematuria or if the client wishes optimal medical care without regard to cost, urine is cultured for aerobic bacteria. A quantitative culture is performed on urine obtained by catheterization because urethral organisms may contaminate the urine sample. Contamination with urethral organisms has been found to result in counts up to 1000 organisms per milliliter of urine.[67] Very few cats presented for a first episode of urethral obstruction have bacterial urinary tract infection (UTI). If the cat's urinary tract has been catheterized in the past, however, or if the cat has had a perineal urethrostomy, the risk of UTI is increased.

The presence or absence of crystalluria in the urine sediment is noted as well as the type of crystals. One must remember that crystals form as urine cools outside the body. Thus, the presence of crystals in vitro does not necessarily indicate crystalluria in vivo if the urine sample is not fresh. Also, crystalluria can be found in normal cats.

A blood sample is obtained for complete blood count, blood urea nitrogen (BUN) and serum creatinine, and electrolyte concentrations. This blood sample is an additional indicator of the severity of the cat's condition and can help determine type and efficacy of therapy.

If urethral obstruction is suspected but the cat shows no signs of uremia on presentation (obstruction incomplete or of less than 48 hours duration), one must decide whether to perform radiography in addition to the diagnostic tests already discussed. Because obstructing material in cats is often not visible on survey radiographs, a contrast-enhanced procedure, usually a retrograde urethrogram and, occasionally, a cystogram are necessary. Techniques for performing these procedures are discussed in Chapter 6. Contrast-enhanced radiographs are usually not done on most cats during the first episode of obstruction. Such procedures are indicated, however, if the obstruction is difficult to remove or characterize; if the cat has UTI, may have been traumatized, is of an older age (possibility of neoplasia), is a female, has had repeated episodes of obstruction; or if a perineal urethrostomy is planned.[58,68]

The question arises as to whether mineral excretion should be studied in cats with urethral obstruction after the obstruction is removed and the cat stabilized. In an initial study, no increase in mineral excretion was found in cats with lower urinary tract signs, whether obstructed or unobstructed.[27] A few cats did have elevated magnesium excretion, however, comparable to cats on calculogenic diets. Whether these cats might represent a subpopulation of cats that have an abnormality in mineral excretion and might be helped by a low magnesium diet remains unanswered.

TREATMENT

Treatment is directed in two areas. The first is basically symptomatic therapy, i.e., to relieve urethral obstruction and institute fluid therapy to stimulate urine flow. The second is specific therapy for the cause of the obstruction. Symptomatic therapy for the obstructed cat is fairly well defined, although some controversy exists. Knowledge of specific therapy is more limited. Therapy for neoplasia and urolithiasis depends on the type of neoplasia or urolith. Since the cause of urethral plugs remains unknown, no specific therapy is available at this time. To summarize current recommendations, this discussion is divided into three parts: management of cats with urethral obstruction, management of cats with hematuria/dysuria without urethral obstruction, and prevention of recurrent episodes of urethral obstruction.

Management of Urethral Obstruction

Feline Urethral Obstruction

The management of cats with urethral obstruction depends on the severity of the resultant clinical signs, which vary with the degree and duration of the obstruction. If the cat is not yet azotemic, relief of obstruction may be sufficient therapy. In an azotemic but nonuremic cat, relief of obstruction is essential and fluid therapy is beneficial. In a uremic cat, both relief of obstruction and fluid therapy are essential for survival.[62] Whether fluid therapy or relief of obstruction should be attempted first depends on the condition of the cat. If the cat is depressed and weak, we usually start fluid therapy first and may use cystocentesis to relieve bladder distention temporarily. If the cat is alert, we try to relieve obstruction first.

Relief of Obstruction

In all cats with urethral obstruction, the obstruction must be relieved. This is most often accomplished by retrograde flushing of the urethra with a sterile solution such as saline or lactated Ringer's through a lubricated urethral catheter (Fig. 12-10).

Many instruments are available for urethral catheterization. Because the urethra of an obstructed male cat is already damaged as the result of the pressure of the obstructing material, the pressure of the retained urine, and the pressure exerted during the cat's attempts to urinate, gentle technique is necessary to avoid further urethral trauma. Polypropylene catheters such as Tom Cat catheters (Sovereign Open End Tom Cat Catheter, Sherwood Medical Industries Inc., St. Louis, MO 63103) or intravenous catheters may be less traumatic than metal instruments such as a blunted lacrimal cannula or a silver abscess needle. The potential for urethral trauma, however, is related to the care of the operator and the sharpness of the instrument tip more than the instrument's composition.

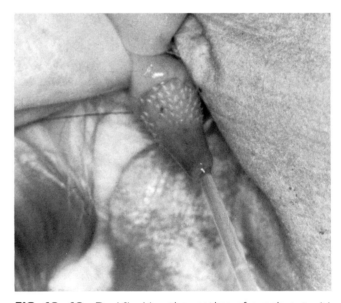

FIG. 12–10. Backflushing the urethra of a male cat with urethral obstruction. A Tom Cat Catheter (Sovereign Open End Tom Cat Catheter, Sherwood Medical Industries, Inc., St. Louis, MO 63103) has been advanced to the site of obstruction. Sterile saline is being injected through the catheter to dislodge the obstructing material, pushing it back into the bladder or flushing it out the urethral orifice.

Sufficient sedation should be used to facilitate catheterization. The degree of sedation required depends on the cat's condition and temperament. All anesthetics should be administered cautiously because of postrenal uremia.[69] Intravenous short-acting barbiturates, inhalant anesthetics, or low doses of ketamine (2 to 6 mg/kg IM or IV) can be used. Use of ketamine may result in prolonged recovery in some cats. (See Chapter 8 for further information on anesthesia.) Avoidance of local anesthetic agents in reverse flushing solutions has been recommended because they may induce systemic toxicity if absorbed in sufficient quantity. Absorption may be enhanced by uroepithelial damage and their toxicity worsened by postrenal uremia.[70]

Once the necessary materials have been gathered and the cat restrained, the penis is cleansed with warm water or dilute povidone-iodine or hexachloradine scrub. As aseptically as possible, a catheter with sterilized lubricant is advanced to the site of obstruction. The location and texture of the obstruction is recorded. The sterile solution is flushed into the urethral lumen and allowed to reflux out the urethral orifice, in the hope of dislodging the obstruction and flushing it out the urethra or into the bladder without greatly increasing intraurethral pressure (see Fig. 12-10). As possible, the catheter is slowly advanced to the bladder. The penis is displaced dorsally until the long axis of the urethra is parallel to the vertebral column to eliminate the natural curvature of the male feline urethra (Fig. 12-11). Occlusion of the distal urethra as fluid is injected may help repulse the obstructing material into the bladder.

If the obstruction is not dislodged by initial retrograde flushing of the urethra, the bladder is emptied by cystocentesis. The technique of cystocentesis is described in Chapter 2. When all urine is to be removed from the bladder, the cystocentesis needle should be placed in the bladder lumen near the bladder neck, so that the needle remains within the lumen as the bladder is emptied. A three-way valve attached to the needle is used to empty the syringe without removing the needle. Use of a 20- or 60-ml syringe reduces the number of times the syringe needs to be emptied. An overdistended feline bladder usually contains 50 to 100 ml of urine. Potential complications of cystocentesis are extravasation of urine into the abdominal cavity and further injury to the bladder wall. These adverse effects are not common if most of the urine is aspirated from the bladder. Gentle manipulation of the bladder is used to avoid bladder rupture, since the bladder wall is distended and injured by increased intravesicular pressure. Once bladder pressure has been relieved, flushing the obstruction out of the urethra via the urethral catheter is often successful.

After the obstruction is relieved, a flexible 3.5 Fr polyvinyl (red rubber) catheter (Sovereign Sterile Feeding Tube and Urethral Catheter, Sherwood Medical Industries, Inc.) is inserted into the bladder, collecting a urine sample for urinalysis if one has not already been obtained by cystocentesis (see Fig. 12-9). This type of catheter is preferred because of its longer length. Ten-centimeter polypropylene catheters (Sovereign Open End

Tom Cat Catheter) often do not reach the bladder lumen.[71] Flexible polyvinyl catheters also produce less bladder and urethral trauma.[71] The catheter should be inserted just into the bladder by determining the point at which urine is first obtained by aspiration. Inserting the catheter too far can result in trauma to the bladder. If large quantities of crystalline material or blood are evident in the urine, the bladder is repeatedly flushed with a sterile isotonic solution.

The decision to remove or retain the catheter is based on the characteristics of each individual case. Leaving the catheter in place prevents immediate reobstruction and facilitates monitoring of urine output but also leads to bacterial UTI and urethral irritation.[72-74] Administration of a broad-spectrum bactericidal antibiotic (ampicillin) while the catheter was in place was shown to reduce the incidence of infection, but infection with antibiotic-resistant bacteria developed in some cats.[72] If the urethral catheter is retained, a closed drainage system is established, by connecting the urethral catheter via extension tubing to a recently emptied sterile fluid bottle or bag (Figs. 12-12, 12-13) or a commercial drainage bag. An Elizabethan collar may be necessary to prevent the cat from removing the urethral catheter or disconnecting the drainage system (Fig. 12-13).

At present, the best recommendation is to retain the catheter only if one of the following four conditions is present: (1) The obstruction was relieved with difficulty, (2) the urine stream is weak and small after relief of obstruction, (3) the cat is uremic, (4) detrusor dysfunction is present secondary to overdistention. In uremic cats, rapid reobstruction should be prevented and urine output monitored. Unless clinical signs of UTI develop, antimicrobial therapy is not used so that infection with resistant organisms is avoided. The catheter is left in place until the uremic signs abate, usually within 24 hours. To avoid catheter-induced complications, the catheter should be removed as soon as possible. A urine sample is collected for urinalysis and culture when the catheter is removed. If bacterial infection is present, antibiotic therapy is instituted for 10 days. A urine culture should be performed again 3 to 5 days after the antibiotic regimen is completed to ensure that the infection was eliminated. In evaluating culture results, any bacteria isolated should be considered significant, as long as the sample was collected using aseptic technique from the catheter (see Fig. 7-6) or by cystocentesis.

If a catheter cannot be inserted into the bladder because of persistent obstruction, emergency surgery may be necessary. Placement of a cystostomy catheter in the bladder (see chapter 16) allows urinary drainage, without repeated cystocentesis, to provide time to reverse uremia and hyperkalemia, stabilize the cat, and allow diagnostic testing to localize further and identify the cause of such a severe obstruction.

Body Temperature Support

Uremic cats are often hypothermic. Support of normal body temperature by blankets or a heating pad is rec-

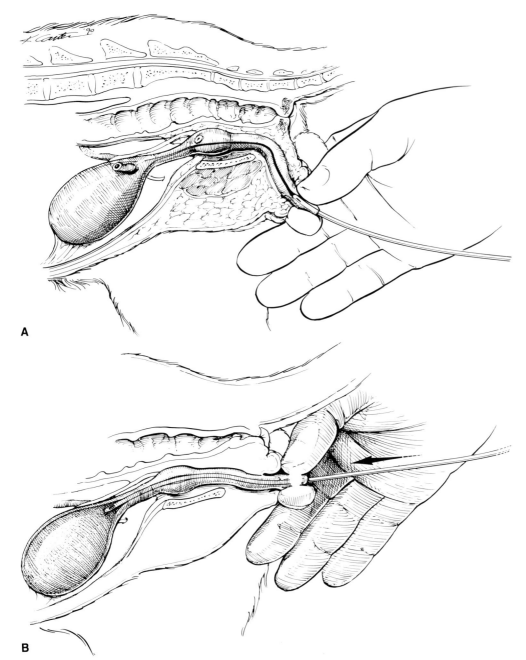

A

B

FIG. 12–11. Catheterization of the male cat urethra. (A) The male cat urethra normally curves ventrally. (B) During catheterization, the penis should be displaced dorsally so that the long axis of the urethra is parallel to the vertebral column.

ommended. Intravenous fluids can be warmed to body temperature before use. A blanket or drape is placed over the metal examining table during urinary and intravenous catheterization. Temperature support should be continued until the cat's temperature reaches the low normal range and the cat's activity increases.

Fluid Therapy

Cats that are uremic at the time of presentation are usually hyperkalemic and acidemic.[75] For survival, these cats require intravenous fluid therapy, in addition to relief of obstruction.[76] The major goals of fluid therapy are to reduce hyperkalemia and azotemia, to improve acid-base balance, and to correct dehydration. Alkalinizing electrolyte solutions such as lactated Ringer's have been shown to reverse acidemia and hyperkalemia in experimentally induced urethral obstruction, even though these fluids do contain a small amount of potassium.[62,76] Solutions containing dextrose and insulin have been recommended[77] as well as combinations of saline and dextrose,[75] but no evidence exists that such therapy is more beneficial than alkalinizing electrolyte solutions alone. Adding sodium bicarbonate to the treatment regimen more rapidly reverses the acidemia of obstructed cats,[75] but no benefit in survival over cats

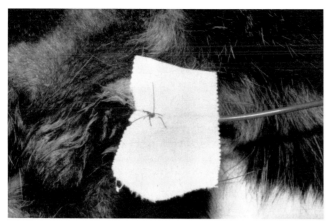

FIG. 12–12. A flexible urethral catheter has been inserted through the urethra to the bladder neck. It is kept in place by putting adhesive tape on the catheter and suturing the adhesive tape to the prepuce.

treated with electrolyte solutions containing the equivalent of 53 mEq/L $NaHCO_3$ (Multisol, Abbott Laboratories, Chicago, IL 60064) has been shown.[62,76] We usually use only a balanced, alkalinizing electrolyte solution such as lactated Ringer's.

The amount of fluids to administer is based on the severity of dehydration, uremic signs, and hyperkalemia. Approximately 5% body weight is given if the signs are mild, 8% if moderate, and 12% if severe (1 pound equals approximately 500 ml and 1 kg 1000 ml). This amount should be administered over approximately 2 hours. These are general guidelines only. Actual volume replacement must be individualized for each cat based on vital signs, changes in hydration status, mental attitude, and urine output. Hyperkalemia, acidemia, and uremia do not rapidly reverse with too slow a rate of fluid administration. Pulmonary edema may result from too rapid fluid replacement. No evidence of pulmonary edema developed when experimentally obstructed cats were given a balanced electrolyte solution at a rate of 50 to 60 ml/kg/hr.[62,76]

In general, after the initial fluid amount is given, the cat's mental attitude improves, urine output is sustained, and severe hyperkalemia is reversed (as shown by biochemical measurement, the cat's improved attitude, or reversal of electrocardiographic abnormalities). When the cat's condition has thus improved, the rate of fluid administration can be reduced. Sufficient volume is given over 24 hours to replace insensible water losses (estimated at 20 ml/kg/day) and urine losses. If urine output is not measured, sufficient fluids should be given to provide maintenance needs (estimated at 66 ml/kg/day) plus correct any dehydration that is detected by changes in skin turgor or moisture of the mucous membranes. Food and water can be offered as soon as vomiting stops, which is usually within the first 24 hours.

Fluid therapy is continued until the azotemia is resolved or minimal. Subcutaneous fluids can be substituted for intravenous fluids, once the uremic signs abate and serum potassium is normal (usually within 4 to 24

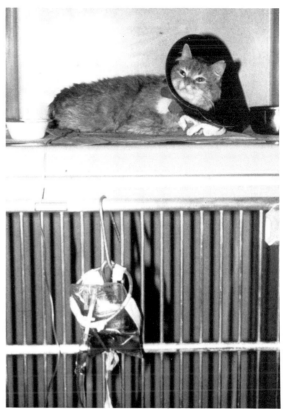

FIG. 12–13. Male cat after relief of urethral obstruction with an indwelling urethral catheter. Note the Elizabethan collar on the cat to prevent his licking at or pulling on the catheter. Also note that the catheter is connected via sterile tubing to a urine collection bag (a "closed" urinary drainage system). (From Barsanti, J.A.: Feline hematuria and dysuria: A diagnostic approach. *In* Proceedings, 2nd Annual Kal Kan Symposium, p. 6, 1986; with permission.)

hours). A postobstructive diuresis that leads to renal water and electrolyte losses makes continued fluid therapy necessary.[62] The cause of this diuresis is unknown, but both decreased renal tubular function and the necessity to excrete solutes retained during obstruction have been postulated. What percentage of cats are affected by a diuretic phase of recovery from obstruction that predisposes them to dehydration is unknown. The daily amount of fluids to be given can be determined by providing for insensible water losses and replacement of urine losses or by providing maintenance needs plus an amount sufficient to correct detectable dehydration. Postobstructive diuresis can persist several days.

Cats with partial or total anorexia and a postobstructive diuresis may become hypokalemic a few days after obstruction is relieved. Recurrent or worsening weakness and lethargy may be the only clinical signs. Hypokalemia was a problem within 24 hours in clinical cases treated with potassium-free fluids and sodium bicarbonate[75] but was not a problem in laboratory cats treated with isotonic, balanced electrolyte solutions.[62,76] If hypokalemia is suspected, it should be confirmed by measurement of serum potassium concentration. If present, potassium supplementation can be given

TABLE 12–2. AMOUNT OF POTASSIUM CHLORIDE TO ADD TO ISOTONIC FLUIDS BASED ON DEGREE OF HYPOKALEMIA

Serum Potassium Concentration (mEq/L)	Intravenous Therapy (mEq Potassium chloride/250 ml)	Subcutaneous Therapy (mEq Potassium chloride/250 ml)
3.0–3.5	5	10
2.5–3.0	7	14
2.0–2.5	10	20
<2.0	12	24

orally if the cat is not vomiting, or 20 mEq potassium chloride can be added to each liter of balanced electrolyte solution. If hypokalemia is severe (< 3.0 mEq/L), additional potassium supplementation may be needed (Table 12-2).

Optimal medical care includes measurement of BUN, serum creatinine, and serum electrolytes daily until the cat is eating and acting normally. We usually continue fluid therapy until BUN and serum creatinine levels are normal.

Experimentally obstructed cats were catabolic after relief of obstruction.[62] Weight loss occurred despite normal hydration, gradual return of food intake, and gradual normalization of laboratory data. Feeding cats highly palatable foods or force feeding after vomiting ceases might help alleviate this catabolic state. In obese cats, such a catabolic state may predispose to hepatic lipidosis.

Prior to use of any drug in cats with urethral obstruction, the necessity, side effects, dose, and frequency of administration of each drug should be reviewed in light of the necessity for renal metabolism or excretion.[70] Urinary acidifiers should not be given to uremic or azotemic cats because they may aggravate existing metabolic acidemia. Nephrotoxic drugs such as aminoglycoside antibiotics are avoided and are administered only for a proven bacterial infection that is sensitive only to these antimicrobials. Although hypocalcemia may be present, treatment with calcium is contraindicated. Treatment with calcium in the presence of hyperphosphatemia may result in metastatic calcification, which could cause permanent renal damage. Treatment with calcium is also unnecessary because sufficient ionized calcium is usually present to prevent adverse clinical signs. Correction of hyperphosphatemia by restoring renal function results in return of eucalcemia.

The use of anti-inflammatory agents is controversial. Some investigators have advocated glucocorticoids to minimize urethral inflammation[60,78]; however, glucocorticoids may aggravate uremia by inducing gluconeogenesis and protein catabolism.[1] We have found that prednisolone in anti-inflammatory dosages increased the risk of bacterial pyelonephritis in experimental cats with indwelling urinary catheters, without reducing lower urinary tract inflammation.[79] Although dimethyl sulfoxide (DMSO) was reported to be beneficial when instilled into the bladder of cats after relief of urethral obstruction,[80] we were unable to document any beneficial effect in laboratory cats with induced cystitis.[79]

Management of Hematuria/Dysuria Without Obstruction

Some cats that have had an episode of urethral obstruction are presented for hematuria and dysuria but have a small bladder on physical examination. Possible causes of hematuria and dysuria without urethral obstruction in cats include bladder uroliths, neoplasia of the bladder, trauma, bacterial infection (secondary to urinary tract manipulation during the bout of obstruction), or idiopathic *feline urologic syndrome*. The diagnostic plan should include a urinalysis and urine culture. Radiographic and ultrasonographic studies should be pursued if the problem is persistent or frequently recurrent or occurs in an aged cat.

Antibiotic therapy is reserved for cats with documented bacteriuria. Antibiotic therapy is no more effective than a placebo in cats without bacteriuria.[81] A prospective study of subcutaneous fluids (100 ml lactated Ringer's) or a smooth muscle relaxant (Pro-Banthine, Searle, San Juan, Puerto Rico 00936) (propantheline bromide, 7.5 mg by mouth) versus 24 hours of hospitalization also indicated no difference in response in cats with these signs.[81] Most cats were normal within 5 days regardless of therapy.[81]

Based on the limited studies discussed here and clinical impression of others,[1] feline urologic syndrome without obstruction seems to be a self-limiting condition in the majority of cats. If the signs do not abate within 5 to 7 days, a diagnostic plan to rule out other causes of hematuria and dysuria should be instituted, including survey and contrast-enhanced radiography (see Chapters 1, 2 and 6).

If no cause is diagnosed but the cat continues to have dysuria and hematuria, symptomatic therapy is recommended, although proof of efficacy is lacking. The most common therapeutic approach is to assume the hematuria and dysuria are related to struvite crystalluria, even though urolithiasis is not evident. Change of diet to a prescription diet that reduces mineral intake and acidifies the urine is often the approach recommended. Alternatively, acidifiers may be used in conjunction with nonprescription cat food. The most effective urinary acidifiers are d,l-methionine and ammonium chloride. Prolonged use of acidifying therapy may be associated with adverse effects. (See next section.)

Other drugs that have been used in cats with idiopathic hematuria and dysuria include diuretics such as furosemide[82] to cause urine dilution and glucocorticoids to reduce any lower urinary tract inflammation.[1] As already noted, these therapeutic methods have not been well evaluated for efficacy.

Urinary products that contain methylene blue or that contain phenazopyridine should not be used in cats because of their potential for causing methemoglobinemia and Heinz body anemia.[83,84]

Prevention of Recurrence of Urethral Obstruction from Urethral Plugs

One of the most frustrating aspects of urethral obstruction is the high rate of recurrence.[40,85] In cats with urethral obstruction, 22% died within 6 months of recurrent obstruction.[40] In another study of cats with urethral obstruction, only 40% were alive without recurrence of obstruction at 6 months.[85] Cats experiencing their first episode of obstruction at less than 4 years of age appeared to have a higher incidence of recurrence than older cats (68 versus 32%).[85] Various recommendations have been made to reduce this recurrence rate, including long-term use of urinary acidifiers, low magnesium diets, increasing water intake and urine output, and perineal urethrostomy. Only one prospective study[2] has been done to evaluate the efficacy of these treatment regimens, and, unfortunately, this prospective study did not have a control group. In this study, cats were treated with a prescription diet (feline s/d, Hill's Pet Products Inc, Topeka, KS 66601), surgery (perineal urethrostomy), or both. No recurrences of urethral obstruction were found in any cat within 1 year, suggesting both surgery and dietary therapy were effective in preventing recurrence. Unfortunately, UTI occurred in about 15% of the cats treated with perineal urethrostomy,[2] and concern has been raised about prolonged use of acidification.[86] Prescription diet s/d is recommended to be fed only for 2 to 3 months.[87] Thus, other treatment regimens are still in use.

Despite concern about prolonged acidification, one such therapy has been the use of urinary acidifiers. Only one acidifier has been evaluated in clinical cases of urethral obstruction. Ertylenediamine dihydrochloride (Chlorethamine, Pitman-Moore, Washington Crossing, NJ 08560), when given for 21 days after obstruction, did not prevent future obstruction.[85] Whether obstruction would have been as likely if the acidifier had been continued was not answered by this study. Ethylenediamine hydrochloride has also been found to be only a weak urinary acidifier in cats.[85,88] In normal cats, ammonium chloride (15 grains/day)[89] and high doses of d,l-methionine (1000 to 1500 mg/day)[90] were the only acidifiers shown to prevent the postprandial alkaline tide. Other than this alkalinity, which occurs a few hours after eating, normal cat urine is acidic.[89] Inclusion of ammonium chloride or a combination of ammonium chloride and d,l-methionine in food fed ad libitum to cats was shown to maintain a much lower urine pH than the same diet without ammonium chloride.[38,91,92] The majority of cats with obstruction have acidic urine. Whether maintenance of a more acidic urine by urinary acidifiers would be beneficial in clinical cases is unknown.

Urinary acidifiers have potential adverse effects. Fatal toxicity, of a common ammonium chloride d,l-methionine combination (Uroeze-FUS, Daniels Pharmaceuticals, St. Petersburg, FL 33713) in kittens receiving the amount in food recommended for adult cats, has been reported.[93] Negative calcium and potassium balance has been found in cats ingesting 1.5% ammonium chloride in their food.[86] Ammonium chloride at 1.5% is at the lower end of amounts often recommended. Hypokalemia with severe muscle weakness has been reported in cats eating acidifying diets, especially cats with underlying renal insufficiency.[94] High doses of acidifiers can produce chronic metabolic acidemia.[92]

Reducing mineral intake and increasing water intake have also been recommended to prevent recurrence of urethral obstruction. Feeding moist cat foods, moistening dry cat foods, salting the food, and giving diuretics are done to increase water turnover. Increasing water intake does not necessarily increase urine output because additional water may be eliminated in the feces. Urine specific gravity should be measured to determine urine dilution. Although one case-controlled study found a higher incidence of an initial episode of urethral obstruction in cats eating greater than 50% dry food,[22] the risk of recurrence of obstruction was not associated with percentage of dry food intake.[39,85] One brief clinical report with few case details indicated prevention of recurrence of urethral obstruction by adding water to a low magnesium diet.[5] Another clinical study, which was not well controlled, suggested a decreased risk of recurrence of urethral obstruction using addition of salt and water to a cat's food for life.[78] D,l-methionine was also administered to affected cats for at least a month. Another poorly controlled study[95] is often cited as proving efficacy of a prescription diet (feline c/d, Hill's Pet Products Inc) even though the study also employed commercially canned cat food, acidifiers, and antimicrobials. As already noted, cats fed prescription diet feline s/d had no recurrence of urethral obstruction in 1 year.[2] This diet, however, is not generally recommended for more than 2 to 3 months.[87] Prospective, controlled studies of the efficacy of other diets, of increasing water consumption, or both are needed.

Limited work has not demonstrated any efficacy of crystallization inhibitors such as tripolyphosphate and of chelators of calcium and magnesium (CureCal, Albion Laboratories Inc, Clearfield, UT).[14] Manufacturer's claim of efficacy is based solely on a limited number of uncontrolled empirical observations.[90]

Surgical techniques to prevent recurrence of urethral obstruction are discussed in Chapter 13.

There is currently no method to prevent recurrence of urethral obstruction from urethral plugs in cats that does not have potential adverse effects. We generally institute use of prescription diet feline c/d after the first episode of obstruction. If obstruction recurs, a perineal urethrostomy is recommended. In all cases, diagnostic efforts should be made to determine the cause and site of obstruction. If the cause is urolithiasis, the urolith should be analyzed and appropriate preventative measures initiated (see Chapter 18).

CONSEQUENCES OF URETHRAL OBSTRUCTION

The consequences of urethral obstruction can be divided into those related to the obstruction itself and those related to treatment of the obstruction.

Consequences of Obstruction

The life-threatening consequences of urethral obstruction are related to the development of postrenal uremia and hyperkalemia, as described under "Pathyphysiology." In experimental urethral obstruction, permanent renal dysfunction did not occur unless obstruction was maintained longer than 96 hours.[64] Normal renal function returned over a week when obstruction was less than 36 hours. Urethral obstruction of 96 hours or longer results in severe uremia, hyperkalemia, and death in cats.[62] Therefore, permanent renal lesions would be considered unlikely in most cats presented for urethral obstruction. One study of renal histology in cats, however, found a high incidence of renal lesions (five of eight cats) in cats more than 7 days after an episode of obstruction, as compared with the incidence of renal lesions in cats of similar age in a necropsy study of over 300 cats.[34,96] Unfortunately, the incidence of renal lesions in cats in the same colony, but without a history of urethral obstruction, was not determined.[34]

A potential consequence of urethral obstruction is damage to the bladder detrusor muscle by prolonged overdistention. Loss of the tight junctions between muscle fibers prevents spread of motor nerve impulses that permit bladder contraction. Thus, even after relief of obstruction, the cat cannot voluntarily empty its bladder, but the bladder can be expressed manually with a good urine stream, indicating that no outflow obstruction exists.[97] Treatment is directed toward keeping the bladder empty, so that the tight junctions can reform, either by frequent manual expression or with an indwelling urinary catheter. Bethanechol, a parasympathomimetic drug, (1.25 to 2.5 mg by mouth every 8 hours) can be tried after a few days of keeping the bladder empty.[98] If the bladder is going to respond to the bethanechol, the response should occur within a few hours of administration. Because bethanechol can increase urethral resistance, it is administered with a urethral relaxant such as phenoxybenzamine (1.25 to 2.5 mg by mouth every 24 hours). If there is no response, either a higher dose of bethanechol is tried with observation for possible side effects (such as abdominal cramps, vomiting, diarrhea, bradycardia), or the drug should be discontinued. The urethra must be patent during administration of parasympathomimetic drugs, or rupture of the bladder could theoretically occur. Time required for return of bladder function varies with degree of injury.

Another reason for inability to urinate after relief of obstruction is outflow resistance. Physical examination shows that even with adequate manual compression, the urine stream is weak. Causes of such outflow resistance include recurrence of intraluminal obstruction, extraluminal obstruction, or urethral spasm.[98] Physical obstructions are ruled out by passage of a catheter or by contrast-enhanced radiography. If urethral spasm is present, drug therapy may be of benefit but has not been evaluated in cats. Extrapolating from other species, drugs to consider include phenoxybenzamine to block urethral alpha adrenergic receptors or diazepam (2.5 mg by mouth every 8 hours) to relieve skeletal muscle spasm. Side effects of phenoxybenzamine such as hypotension are related to alpha adrenergic blockade. The drug should not be used in cats with cardiovascular disease. Side effects of diazepam include sedation or unusual behavior. It must be emphasized that any of these drugs should be used only if indicated and cautiously because of the extremely limited knowledge of dosages and side effects in cats.

Consequences of Therapy

Consequences of therapy include complications associated with urinary catheters and with urethral surgery. Use of urinary catheters during reverse flushing of the urethra can cause urethral injury from mucosal erosions to complete tearing. Care must be taken in manipulation to minimize urethral trauma. Inflammation induced by catheterization may itself result in hematuria and dysuria.

Use of indwelling urinary catheters can result in UTI and urethral and bladder inflammation. Urinary tract infection can occur in spite of prophylactic antibiotics, and infection in cats receiving antibiotics is with more highly antibiotic-resistant organisms.[72] An opportunistic fungal infection of the urine and bladder has also been reported in association with frequent urethral obstruction and antibiotic administration.[99] Indwelling urinary catheters in an open system left in place for 5 days led to a high rate of later urethral obstruction (2 of 10 cats) and inflammatory urethral lesions that persisted up to 90 days in some cats.[73] In spite of these problems, indwelling catheters are necessary in uremic cats whose urine output must be monitored, in cats in which obstruction was difficult to remove and whose urine stream after relief of obstruction is weak, and in cats with detrusor muscle dysfunction who cannot be frequently expressed manually. Our recommendations are that closed drainage systems be used and that antibiotics be given only if signs of infection are present. Otherwise, we recommend a urine culture when the catheter is removed and treatment directed specifically to any organism detected.

Surgical complications of perineal urethrostomy are discussed in Chapter 14.

REFERENCES

1. Osborne C.A., Kruger, J.M., Johnston, G.R., et al.: Feline lower urinary tract disorders. *In* Textbook of Veterinary Internal Medicine. 3rd Ed. Edited by S.J. Ettinger. Philadelphia, W.B. Saunders, 1989, pp. 2057–2082.
2. Osborne, C.A., Caywood, D.D., Johnston, G.R., et al.: Feline perineal urethrostomy. *In* Current Veterinary Therapy X. Edited by R.W. Kirk. Philadelphia, W.B. Saunders, 1989, pp. 1209–1213.
3. Osborne, C.A., Johnston, G.R., Polzin, D.J., et al.: Redefinition of the feline urologic syndrome: Feline lower urinary tract disease with heterogeneous causes. Vet. Clin. North Am. [Sm. Anim. Pract.], 14:409, 1984.
4. Jackson, O.F., and Colles, C.M.: Experimental matrix plug production in male cat urine following a natural case of urolithiasis due to matrix plug. J. Sm. Anim. Pract., 15:701, 1974.

5. Jackson, O.F.: The treatment and subsequent prevention of struvite urolithiasis in cats. J. Sm. Anim. Pract., 12:555, 1971.
6. Sutor, D.J., Wooley, S.E., and Jackson, O.F.: Crystalline material from the feline bladder. Res. Vet. Sci., 11:298, 1970.
7. Carbone, G.: Phosphocrystalluria and urethral obstruction in the cat. J. Am. Vet. Med. Assoc., 147:1195, 1965.
8. Osborne, C.A., Clinton, C.W., Brunkow, H.C., et al.: Epidmiology of naturally occurring feline uroliths and urethral plugs. Vet. Clin. North Am. [Sm. Anim. Pract.], 14:481, 1984.
9. Schwarz, P.D., Greene, R.W., and Patnaik, A.K.: Urinary bladder tumors in the cat: A review of 27 cases. J. Am. Anim. Hosp. Assoc., 21:237, 1985.
10. Filippich, L.J., Read, R.A., and Riesz, G.: Functional urethral obstruction in a cat. Aust. Vet. Practit., 19:202, 1989.
11. Barsanti, J.A., Finco, D.R., Shotts, E.B., et al.: Feline urologic syndrome: Further investigation into etiology. J. Am. Anim. Hosp. Assoc., 18:391, 1982.
12. Martens, J.G., McConnell, S., and Swanson, C.L.: The role of infectious agents in naturally occurring feline urologic syndrome. Vet. Clin. North Am. [Sm. Anim. Pract.], 14:503, 1984.
13. Fabricant, C.G., and Rich, L.J.: Microbial studies of feline urolithiasis. J. Am. Vet. Med. Assoc., 158:976, 1971.
14. Rich, L.J., and Fabricant, C.G.: Experimental production of urolithiasis in male cats. J. Am. Vet. Med. Assoc., 158:974, 1971.
15. Gaskell, R.M., Gaskell, C.J., Page, W., et al.: Studies on a possible viral aetiology for the feline urological syndrome. Vet. Rec., 105:243, 1979.
16. Jackson, O.F.: Feline urolithiasis report. Vet. Rec., 96:390, 1975.
17. Fabricant, C.G.: The feline urologic syndrome induced by infection with a cell-associated herpesvirus. Vet. Clin. North Am. [Sm. Anim. Pract.], 14:493, 1984.
18. Fabricant, C.G., and Gillespie, J.H.: Identification and characterization of a second feline herpesvirus. Infect. Immun., 9:460, 1974.
19. Fabricant, C.G.: Herpesvirus induced feline urolithiasis—a review. Comp. Immunol. Microbiol. Infect. Dis., 1:121, 1979.
20. Fabricant, C.G., and Lein, D.H.: Feline urolithiasis neither induced nor exacerbated by feeding a dry diet. J. Am. Anim. Hosp. Assoc., 20:213, 1984.
21. Fabricant, C.G.: Herpesvirus-induced urolithiasis in specific-pathogen-free male cats. Am. J. Vet. Res., 38:1837, 1977.
22. Reif, J.S., Bovee, K., Gaskell, C.J., et al.: Feline urethral obstruction: A case control study. J. Am. Vet. Med. Assoc., 170:1320, 1977.
23. Barker, J., and Povey, R.C.: The feline urolithiasis syndrome: A review and inquiry into the alleged role of dry cat foods in its etiology. J. Sm. Anim. Pract., 14:445, 1973.
24. Duch, D.S., Hamar, D.W., Chow, F.C., et al.: Study on urine polyelectrolytes of cats with natural and experimental urolithiasis. Biochem. Med., 19:236, 1978.
25. Lewis, L.D., Chow, F.H.C., Taton, G.F., et al.: Effect of various dietary mineral concentration on the occurrence of feline urolithiasis. J. Am. Vet. Med. Assoc., 172:559, 1978.
26. Rich, L.J., Dysart, I., Chow, F.C., et al.: Urethral obstruction in male cats: Experimental production by addition of magnesium and phosphate to diet. Feline Pract., 4:44, 1974.
27. Finco, D.R., Barsanti, J.A., and Crowell, W.A.: Characterization of magnesium-induced disease in the cat and comparison with feline urologic syndrome. Am. J. Vet. Res., 46:391, 1985.
28. Feldman, B.M., Kennedy, R.B., and Schelstraete, M.: Dietary minerals and the feline urologic syndrome. Feline Pract., 7:39, 1977.
29. Chow, F.C., Hamar, D.W., Dysart, I., et al.: Feline urolithiasis/cat foods: Concentration of calcium, magnesium, phosphate and chloride in various cat foods and their relationship to feline urolithiasis. Feline Pract., 5:15, 1975.
30. Graser, D.H., Hamar, D.W., and Lewis, L.D.: The consistency of dietary minerals in commercial cat foods and their relationship to feline urolithiasis. Feline Pract., 11:41, 1981.
31. Dickinson, C.D., and Scott, P.P.: Failure to produce urinary calculi in kittens by the addition of mineral salts, derived from bonemeal, to the diet. Vet. Rec., 68:858, 1956.
32. Sauer, L.S., Hamar, D., and Lewis, L.D.: Effect of dietary mineral composition on urinary mineral concentration and excretion by the cat. Feline Pract., 15:10, 1985.
33. Sauer, L.S., Hamar, D., and Lewis, L.D.: Effect of diet composition on water intake and excretion by the cat. Feline Pract., 15:16, 1985.
34. Lawler, D.F., and Evans, R.H.: Urinary tract disease in cats: Water balance studies, urolith and crystal analyses, and necropsy findings. Vet. Clin. North Am. [Sm. Anim. Pract.], 14:537, 1984.
35. Rich, L.J., and Kirk, R.W.: Feline urethral obstruction: Mineral aspects. Am. J. Vet. Res., 29:2149, 1968.
36. Rich, L.J., and Kirk, R.W.: The relationship of struvite crystals to urethral obstruction in cats. J. Am. Vet. Med. Assoc., 154:153, 1969.
37. Lewis, L.D., and Morris, M.L.: Diet as a causative factor of feline urolithiasis. Vet. Clin. North Am. [Sm. Anim. Pract.], 14:513, 1984.
38. Taton, G.F., Hamar, D.W., and Lewis, L.D.: Evaluation of ammonium chloride as a urinary acidifier in the cat. J. Am. Vet. Med. Assoc., 184:433, 1984.
39. Fennell, C.: Some demographic characteristics of the domestic cat population in Great Britain with particular reference to feeding habits and the incidence of the feline urologic syndrome. J. Sm. Anim. Pract., 16:775, 1975.
40. Walker, A.D., Weaver, A.D., and Anderson, R.S.: An epidemiological survey of the feline urological syndrome. J. Sm. Anim. Pract., 18:283, 1977.
41. Willeberg, P.: Epidemiology of the feline urological syndrome. Adv. Vet. Sci. Comp. Med., 25:311, 1981.
42. Osbaldiston, G.W., and Taussig, R.A.: Clinical report on 46 cases of feline urological syndrome. VM/SAC, 65:461, 1970.
43. Schechter, R.D.: The significance of bacteria in feline cystitis and urolithiasis. J. Am. Vet. Med. Assoc., 156:1567, 1970.
44. Lawler, D.F., Sjolin, D.W., and Collins, J.E.: Incidence rates of feline lower urinary tract disease in the United States. Feline Pract., 15:13, 1985.
45. Tomey, S.L., and Follis, T.B.: Incidence rates of feline urological syndrome (FUS) in the United States. Feline Pract., 8:39, 1978.
46. Willeberg, P.: A case-control study of some fundamental derminants in the epidemiology of the feline urological syndrome. Nord. Vet. Med., 27:1, 1975.
47. Willeberg, P., and Priester, W.A.: Feline urological syndrome: Associations with some time, space, and individual patient factors. Am. J. Vet. Res., 37:975, 1976.
48. Willeberg, P.: Interaction effects of epidemiologic factors in the feline urological syndrome. Nord. Med., 28:193, 1976.
49. Willeberg, P.: Epidemiology of naturally occurring feline urologic syndrome. Vet. Clin. North Am. [Sm. Anim. Pract.], 14:455, 1984.
50. Heron, M.A.: The effect of prepubertal castration of the penile urethra of the cat. J. Am. Vet. Med. Assoc., 160:208, 1972.
51. Meier, F.W.: Urethral obstruction and stenosis in the male cat. J. Am. Vet. Med. Assoc., 137:67, 1960.
52. Foster, S.J.: The "urolithiasis" syndrome in male cats; a statistical analysis of the problems, with clinical observation. J. Sm. Anim. Pract., 8:207, 1967.
53. Dorn, D.R., Saueressig, S., and Schmidt, D.A.: Factors affecting urolithiasis-cystitis-urethritis in cats. Am. J. Vet. Res., 34:433, 1973.
54. Hansen, J.S.: Urachal remnant in the cat: Occurrence and relationship to the feline urological syndrome. VM/SAC, 728:1735, 1977.
55. Johnston, G.R., Feeney, D.A., and Osborne, C.A.: Urethrogra-

phy and cystography in cats. Part II. Abnormal radiographic anatomy and complications. Compend. Contin. Educ. Pract. Vet., 4:931, 1982.

56. Klausner, J.S., Johnston, G.R., and Osborne, C.A.: Diverticula of the urinary bladder. *In* Current Veterinary Therapy VIII. Edited by R.W. Kirk. Philadelphia, W.B. Saunders, 1983, pp. 1093–1095.

57. Osborne, C.A., Kruger, J.M., and Johnston, G.R.: Feline vesicourachal diverticula. *In* Current Veterinary Therapy X. Edited by R.W. Kirk. Philadelphia, W.B. Saunders, 1989, pp. 1153–1157.

58. Johnston, G.R., and Feeney, D.A.: Localization of feline urethral obstruction. Vet. Clin. North Am. [Sm. Anim. Pract.], 14:555, 1984.

59. Cullen, W.C., Fletcher, T.F., and Bradley, W.F.: Morphometry of the male feline urethra. J. Urol., 129:186, 1983.

60. McCully, R.M., and Lieberman, L.L.: Histopathology in a case of feline urolithiasis. Can. Vet. J., 2:52, 1961.

61. Barsanti, J.A., Crowell, W., Losonsky, J., et al.: Complications of bladder distention during retrograde urethrography. Am. J. Vet. Res., 42:819, 1981.

62. Finco, D.R., and Cornelius, L.M.: Characterization and treatment of water, electrolyte, and acid-base imbalances of induced urethral obstruction in the cat. Am. J. Vet. Res., 38:823, 1977.

63. Mehrotra, R.M.L.: An experimental study of the vesical circulation during distention and in cystitis. J. Pathol. Bacteriol., 66:79, 1953.

64. Klahr, S.: Pathophysiology of obstructive uropathy. Kidney Int., 23:414, 1983.

65. Parks, J.: Electrocardiographic abnormalities from serum electrolyte imbalance due to feline urethral obstruction. J. Am. Anim. Hosp. Assoc., 11:102, 1975.

66. Loeb, W.F., and Knipling, G.D.: Glucosuria and pseudoglucosuria in cats with urethral obstruction. Mod. Vet. Pract., 52:40, 1971.

67. Lees, G.E., Simpson, R.B., and Green, R.S.: Results of analyses and bacterial cultures of urine specimens obtained from clinically normal cats by three methods. J. Am. Vet. Med. Assoc., 184:449, 1984.

68. Osborne, C.A., Polzin, D.J., and Johnston, G.R.: Diagnosis of the feline urologic syndrome. Vet. Clin. North Am. [Sm. Anim. Pract.], 14:575, 1984.

69. Raffe, M.R., and Caywood, D.D.: Use of anesthetic agents in cats with obstructive uropathy. Vet. Clin. North Am. [Sm. Anim. Pract.], 14:691, 1984.

70. Riviere, J.E.: Adverse drug reactions in cats with feline urethral obstruction. Vet. Clin. North Am. [Sm. Anim. Pract.], 14:703, 1984.

71. Lees, G.E., Osborne, C.A., Stevens, J.B., et al.: Adverse effects caused by polypropylene and polyvinyl feline urinary catheters. Am. J. Vet. Res., 41:1836, 1980.

72. Lees, G.E., Osborne, C.A., Stevens, J.B., et al.: Adverse effects of open indwelling urethral catheterization in clinically normal male cats. Am. J. Vet. Res., 42:825, 1981.

73. Smith, C.W., Schiller, A.G., Smith, A.R., et al.: Effects of indwelling urinary catheters in male cats. J. Am. Anim. Hosp. Assoc., 17:427, 1981.

74. Lees, G.E., Osborne, C.A.: Use and misuse of indwelling urinary catheters in cats. Vet. Clin. North Am. [Sm. Anim. Pract.], 14:599, 1984.

75. Burrows, C.F., and Bovee, K.C.: Characterization and treatment of acid-base and renal defects due to urethral obstruction in cats. J. Am. Vet. Med. Assoc., 172:801, 1978.

76. Finco, D.R.: Induced feline urethral obstruction: Response of hyperkalemia to relief of obstruction and administration of parenteral electrolyte solution. J. Am. Anim. Hosp. Assoc., 12:198, 1976.

77. Schaer, M.: The use of regular insulin in the treatment of hyperkalemia in cats with urethral obstruction. J. Am. Anim. Hosp. Assoc., 11:106, 1975.

78. Bernard, M.A.: Feline urologic syndrome: A study of seasonal incidence, frequency of repeat visits and comparison of treatments. Can. Vet. J., 19:284, 1978.

79. Barsanti, J.A., Shotts, E.B., Crowell, W.A., et al.: Effect of therapy on susceptibility to urinary tract infection on male cats with indwelling urethral catheters. J. Vet. Int. Med., In press, 1992.

80. Koller, L.C.: Clinical application of DMSO by veterinarians in Oregon and Washington, VM/SAC, 71:591, 1976.

81. Barsanti, J.A., Finco, D.R., Shotts, E.B., et al.: Feline urologic syndrome: Further investigation into therapy. J. Am. Anim. Hosp. Assoc., 18:387, 1982.

82. Dingel, R.M.: Diuretics in FUS treatment. Feline Pract., 5:4, 1975.

83. Harvey, J.W., and Kornick, H.P.: Phenazopyridine toxicosis in the cat. J. Am. Vet. Med. Assoc., 169:327, 1976.

84. Schechter, R.D., Schalm, O.W., and Kaneko, J.J.: Heinz body hemolytic anemia associated with use of urinary antiseptics containing methylene blue in the cat. J. Am. Vet. Med. Assoc., 162:37, 1973.

85. Bovee, K.C., Reif, J.S., Maguire, T.G., et al.: Recurrence of feline urethral obstruction. J. Am. Vet. Med. Assoc., 174:93, 1979.

86. Ching, S.V., Fettman, M.J., Hamar, D.W., et al.: The effect of chronic dietary acidification using ammonium chloride on acid-base and mineral metabolism in the adult cat. J. Nutr., 119:902, 1989.

87. Lewis, L.D., Morris, M.L., and Hand, M.S.: Small Animal Clinical Nutrition III. Topeka, KS, Mark Morris Associates, 1987, pp. 9–30.

88. Finco, D.R.: Efficacy of ethylenediamine dihydrochloride in dogs and cats. Am. J. Vet. Res., 42:670, 1981.

89. Chow, F.H.C., Taton, G.F., Lewis, L.D., et al.: Effect of dietary ammonium chloride, DL-methionine, sodium phosphate and ascorbic acid on urinary pH and electrolyte concentrations of male cats. Feline Pract., 8:29, 1978.

90. Polzin, D.J., and Osborne, C.A.: Medical prophylaxis of feline lower urinary tract disorders. Vet. Clin. North Am. [Sm. Anim. Pract.], 14:661, 1984.

91. Senior, D.F., Sundstrom, B.B., and Wolfson, B.B.: Testing the effects of ammonium chloride and dl-methionine on the urinary pH of cats. Vet. Med., 81:88, 1986.

92. Finco, D.R. Barsanti, J.A., and Brown, S.A.: Ammonium chloride as a urinary acidifier in cats: Efficacy, safety, and rationale for its use. Mod. Vet. Pract., 67:537, 1986.

93. Brown, J.R., and Fox, L.M.: Ammonium chloride/methionine toxicity in kittens. Feline Pract., 14:16, 1984.

94. Dow, S.W., Fettman, M.J., Curtis, C.R., et al.: Hypokalemia in cats: 186 cases. J. Am. Vet. Med. Assoc., 194:1604, 1989.

95. Engle, G.C.: A clinical report on 250 cases of feline urological syndrome. Feline Pract., 7:24, 1977.

96. Hamilton, J.M.: Nephritis in the cat. J. Sm. Anim. Pract., 7:445, 1966.

97. Lees, G.E., and Moreau, P.M.: Management of hypotonic and atonic urinary bladders in cats. Vet. Clin. North Am. [Sm. Anim. Pract.], 14:641, 1984.

98. Moreau, P.M.: Neurogenic disorders of micturition in the dog and cat. Compend. Contin. Educ. Pract. Vet., 4:12, 1982.

99. Doster, A.R., Erickson, E.D., and Chandler, F.W.: Trichosporosis in two cats. J. Am. Vet. Med. Assoc., 190:1184, 1987.

13

Surgical Therapy for Urethral Obstruction in Cats

RELIEF OF URETHRAL OBSTRUCTION

If urethral obstruction in cats cannot be relieved by non-surgical methods (see Chapter 12), surgical techniques for removing or bypassing the obstruction are used. A *perineal urethrostomy* (PU) creates a larger urethral opening just cranial to the caudal edge of the bulbourethral glands. The routine PU procedure does not remove or prevent obstruction of the preprostatic urethra or the bladder trigone. It requires general anesthesia, surgical expertise, delicate instruments, and fine suture material. An intact cat must be castrated during the procedure. If the cat is uremic and a poor candidate for general anesthesia, if equipment and personnel are unavailable, or if the site of the obstruction is more proximal or has not been determined, a temporary *cystostomy catheter* is placed (see Chapter 16), using local and, if necessary, short-acting anesthesia (e.g., intravenous ketamine). The cat is then rehydrated and a diuresis established. After the cat's condition has stabilized, diagnostic testing is performed to localize and identify the cause of such a severe obstruction (see Chapter 12).

PREVENTION OF RECURRENT DISTAL URETHRAL OBSTRUCTION

Perineal Urethrostomy

Indications

A PU is performed to remove a persistent distal urethral obstruction, as just described, and is also recommended if distal urethral obstruction recurs within 6 to 12 months while the cat is on medical management. (See Chapter 12 for discussion of medical and dietary management.) A retrograde cystourethrogram is done before surgery to ensure that there are no abnormalities in the proximal urethra and bladder (e.g., stricture, uroliths, tumor).

The owners are warned that PU will not prevent dysuria or hematuria, but it should avert life-threatening episodes of distal urethral obstruction. The owners are informed that urinary tract infection is a potential complication of PU.

Technique

The cat is positioned in ventral recumbency with its tail over its back (Fig. 13-1A). A pursestring suture is placed in the skin around the anus, and a surgical preparation is done. The Wilson PU technique,[1] with some modifications,[2] is performed. Implantation of a prosthetic shunt into the urethra is not recommended because the implant hinders would healing and induces chronic infection.

An elliptical incision is made around the scrotum and penis (Fig. 13-1B). In an intact male, the scrotum is retracted medially to ensure that the incision is made around the base of the scrotum (Fig. 13-1C). An intact cat is castrated by ligation and severance of the spermatic cords (Fig. 13-1D).

Dissection is continued cranially to the ischiocavernosus muscles, which extend from the medial angle of the ischial tuberosity to the penis (Fig. 13-1E). A hemostat is placed on the middle of each ischiocavernosus muscle and the associated crus of the penis. The hemostat is removed from one of the ischiocavernosus muscles, and a ligature (3–0 gut) is placed in the groove left by the hemostat. The muscle is severed at its insertion on the ischium (Fig. 13-1F). The procedure is repeated on the opposite side.

The penis is retracted dorsally, and the ventral ligament of the penis is palpated between the penis and the dorsal surface of the ischium. The ligament is severed with scissors, which are kept in contact with the ischium to prevent injury to the pelvic urethra (Fig. 13-1G). The loose tissue on the dorsal aspect of the penis is cut. Finger dissection is used ventrally and laterally to free the penis. The dissection is adequate when the bulbourethral glands lie even with the skin with minimal retraction on the penis.

A transverse cut is made through the retractor penis muscle and urethra 2 cm caudal to the bulbourethral glands (Fig. 13-1H). A 20-gauge intravenous catheter or a 3.5 F gauge urethral catheter is inserted through the opening to demarcate the urethra. The retractor penis muscle is dissected from the dorsal aspect of the penis and severed at its origin near the bulbourethral glands.

The catheter is removed, and the urethra is incised along the dorsal midline, using fine tenotomy or iris scissors (Fig. 13-1I). The incision extends to the cranial edge of the bulbourethral glands (Fig. 13-1J). The catheter is replaced in the urethra, and the bladder is flushed with warm saline to remove residual sand and proteinaceous material.

Control of bleeding with a tourniquet makes the urethra more distinct and prevents accumulation of blood clots around the urethra. To make a tourniquet, a 0–gut suture material or umbilical tape is passed through a piece of rubber tubing and then around the penis 1 to 2 cm cranial to the bulbourethral glands (Fig. 13-1K).

A mattress suture, using 3–0 absorbable suture material, is placed through the periurethral tissue and the subcutaneous fascia to help relieve tension on the urethra to skin closure (Fig. 13-1L). Proper orientation of the bulbourethral glands and the ischiocavernosus muscles is maintained to prevent inadvertent 360° rotation of the urethra. The urethra mucosa is apposed to the skin with 4–0 monofilament nonabsorbable suture material (e.g., nylon or polypropylene) on a swedged-taper needle. Synthetic absorbable sutures are not used because absorption of these sutures at an air-tissue interface causes an inflammatory reaction with induration

and, in some instances, granuloma formation.[3] Four sutures are preplaced through the urethra and skin at 11:00, 1:00, 10:00, and 2:00 positions (Fig. 13-1M). The 11:00 suture is tied first, using a surgeon's knot to appose the skin and urethral mucosa. The 1:00 suture is tied followed by the other two sutures in a similar fashion. Care is taken to appose the urethral mucosa directly to the skin. The catheter is removed.

Simple interrupted sutures are continued on both sides of the urethra 3 mm apart for approximately 3 cm. The needle passes through the urethral mucosa and a portion of corpus spongiosum and emerges through the skin. Including the corpus spongiosum within the suture bite reduces postoperative hemorrhage from this vascular structure. The tourniquet is removed. A 3–0 gut ligature is placed around the penis just distal to the last suture. The penis is severed distal to the ligature (Fig. 13-1N).

If there is seeping hemorrhage from the proximal surgical area, a drain can be placed between the urethra and ischium and exited through a stab incision lateral to the skin incision. The drain is anchored to the skin. The drain prevents accumulation of blood clots around the urethra.

A final urethra to skin suture is placed at each corner of the severed urethra. The remaining skin incision is closed (Fig. 13-1O).

SALVAGE OF A RUPTURED OR STRICTURED URETHRA

Fortunately, urethral rupture or stricture in association with urethral obstruction is uncommon. It can be caused by devascularization and necrosis, traumatic catheter-

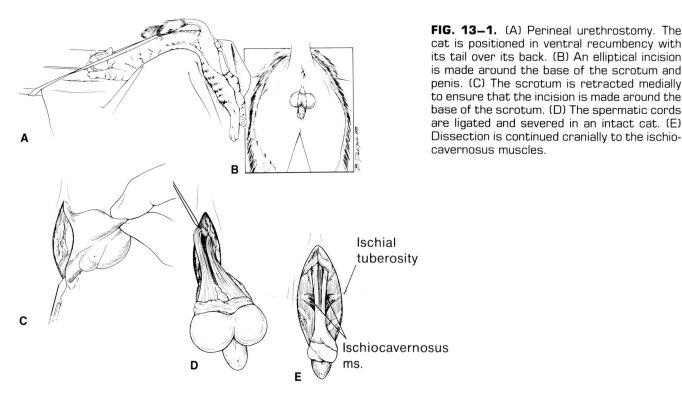

FIG. 13–1. (A) Perineal urethrostomy. The cat is positioned in ventral recumbency with its tail over its back. (B) An elliptical incision is made around the base of the scrotum and penis. (C) The scrotum is retracted medially to ensure that the incision is made around the base of the scrotum. (D) The spermatic cords are ligated and severed in an intact cat. (E) Dissection is continued cranially to the ischiocavernosus muscles.

Ischial tuberosity

Ischiocavernosus ms.

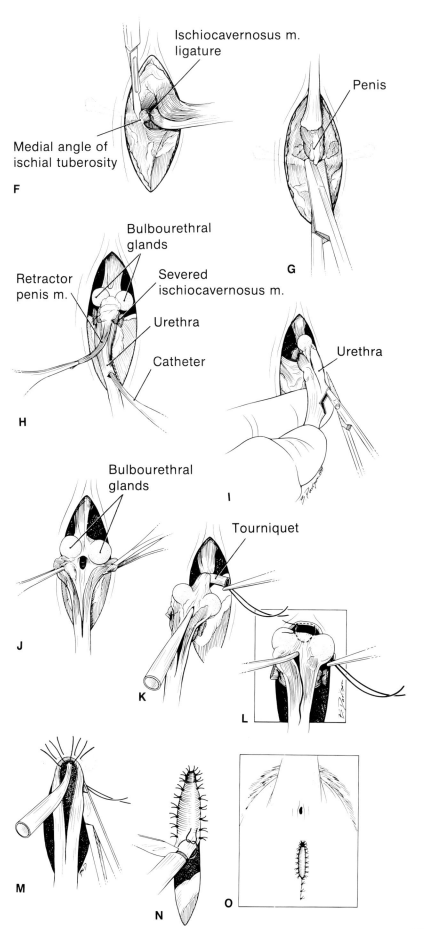

Ischiocavernosus m.
ligature

Medial angle of
ischial tuberosity

F

Penis

G

Retractor
penis m.

Bulbourethral
glands

Severed
ischiocavernosus m.

Urethra

Catheter

H

Urethra

I

Bulbourethral
glands

J

Tourniquet

K

L

M

N

O

FIG. 13—1. (*Cont.*) (F) After the ischiocavernosus muscle is ligated, the muscle is severed at its junction with the medial angle of the ischial tuberosity. (G) The penis is retracted dorsally. The ventral ligament of the penis is severed between the penis and dorsal surface of the ischium. (H) A transverse cut is made through the urethra 2 cm from the caudal edge of the bulbourethral glands. A catheter is inserted through the opening to help demarcate the urethra. The retractor penis muscle is dissected from the urethra. (I) The catheter is removed. The urethra is incised along the dorsal midline, using fine tenotomy or iris scissors.

FIG. 13—1. (*Cont.*) (J) The incision extends to the caudal edge of the bulbourethral glands. (K) The catheter is replaced in the urethra, and a tourniquet is passed around the penis 1 to 2 cm cranial to the bulbourethral glands. (L) A mattress suture is placed between the periurethral tissue, at the caudal edge of bulbourethral glands, and the subcutaneous fascia to help relieve tension. (M) The bulbourethral glands are positioned beneath the skin. Four sutures are preplaced through the cut edge of the urethra and the skin. (N) The preplaced sutures are tied, and the catheter is removed. Urethra to skin sutures are continued for 3 cm. The tourniquet is removed. A ligature is placed around the penis, and the penis is severed distal to the ligature. (O) Urethra to skin sutures are placed at each corner of the severed urethra. The skin to skin sutures are completed.

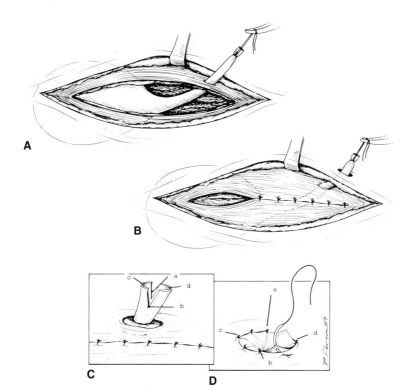

A

B

C

D

FIG. 13–2. (A) Prepubic urethrostomy. After a paramedian caudal abdominal incision and isolation of the preprostatic urethra, the urethra is doubly ligated and severed, just cranial to the prostate. A stab incision is made through the linea alba in a caudoventral direction from the bladder. The ends of the suture and the severed end of the proximal urethra are passed through the incision. (B) A circular piece of skin (0.5 cm diameter) is excised on the midline in a site that will continue the caudoventral course of the urethra. The urethra is passed through the stoma. The subcutaneous fascia and skin of the paramedian incision are closed. (C and D) The damaged end of the urethra is severed, and the healthy urethra is incised to make equal cranial and caudal flaps. The first two sutures are placed through the junction of the urethral flaps (a and b) and through the skin with 5–0 monofilament nonabsorbable suture material in a simple interrupted pattern. The cranial and caudal sutures are placed (c and d). Four more sutures are placed alternating with the first four.

ization, or excessive traction on the penis during a perineal urethrostomy. The urethra may also be damaged by external trauma (e.g., automobile accident). If the rupture or stricture occurs caudal to the prostate, a PU may be possible. Insufficient urethral length for a PU necessitates a urethrostomy cranial or ventral to the pubis, i.e., a *prepubic urethrostomy.* Urinary continence can be maintained after a prepubic urethrostomy if 3 to 4 cm of urethra remain.

Lacerations and incomplete ruptures of the urethra could be sutured if the surrounding urethral tissue is healthy. Urine should be temporarily diverted by a cystostomy catheter (see Chapter 16). If the proximal urethra is destroyed, a *permanent cystostomy* or *trigone-colonic anastomosis* is considered (see Chapter 31). A cystostomy causes incontinence. Trigone-colonic anastomosis preserves continence but induces electrolyte and acid-base abnormalities, necessitating continual monitoring.

Prepubic Urethrostomy

A paramedian abdominal incision (1 cm from midline) is started at the pubis and extended cranially for 6 cm.[4] The bladder is emptied by cystocentesis and elevated from the incision with the ventral ligament intact. The attachment of the ventral ligament to the urethra is severed. The fat around the urethra is divided on the midline. The urethra is isolated, starting 1.5 cm from the bladder neck and continuing caudally to the cranial prostate (approximately 3.5 cm), taking care to preserve the blood supply. The prostate may not be apparent in a castrated male.

The vasa deferentia are ligated and severed near the prostate. The urethra is double ligated and severed just cranial to the prostate. The suture ends on the proximal urethra are left long, so they can be passed through the abdominal stab incision. The bladder is replaced into the abdomen.

In a cat with large inguinal fat pads, it may be preferable to preserve more urethral length by severing the urethra caudal to the prostate. This would make it possible to position the urethrostomy caudal to the inguinal fat pads and ventral to the pubis. To access the postprostatic urethra, a pubic osteostomy (see Fig. 10-4) is necessary.[5]

The location of the stab incision through the linea alba is determined by the urethral length. It is placed as far caudally as possible without creating tension on the urethra-skin anastomosis. The suture ends and the proximal urethra are passed through the incision (Fig. 13-2A). The paramedian incision through the rectus muscle is closed. A circular piece of skin (0.5 cm diameter) is excised on the midline in a site that will continue the caudoventral course of the urethra (Fig. 13-2B). Allowance is made for cranial movement of the skin, when the cat assumes a normal walking position instead of the splayed-out position on the operating table. The urethra is passed through the midline stoma. To prevent unnecessary tension on the urethra to skin closure, the subcutaneous fascia and skin of the paramedian skin incision are closed before suturing the urethra to the skin.

The damaged end of the urethra is severed, and the healthy urethra is incised into equal cranial and caudal flaps (i.e., "fish-mouth," Fig. 13-2C). The flaps are sutured to the skin with 5–0 monofilament synthetic nonabsorbable suture material in a simple interrupted pattern. The first two sutures are placed at the junction of the flaps, and then the cranial and caudal sutures are placed. Four more sutures are placed alternating with the first four (Fig. 13-2D).

REFERENCES

1. Wilson, G.P., and Harrison, J.W.: Perineal urethrostomy in cats. J. Am. Vet. Med. Assoc., *159*:1769, 1971.
2. Johnston, D.E.: Feline urethrostomy—a critique and new method. J. Sm. Anim. Pract., *15*:1, 1974.
3. Bartone, F., Shore, N., Newland, J., et al.: The best suture for hypospadias? Urology, *29*:517, 1987.
4. Mendham, J.H.: A description and evaluation of antepubic urethrostomy in the male cat. J. Sm. Anim. Pract., *11*:709, 1970.
5. Ellison, G.W., Lewis, D.D., Boren, F.C.: Subpubic urethrostomy to salvage a failed perineal urethrostomy in a cat. Compend. Contin. Educ. Pract. Vet., *8*:946, 1989.

14

Postoperative Management and Surgical Complications of Feline Urethral Obstruction

POSTOPERATIVE MANAGEMENT

An Elizabethan collar is placed on the cat to prevent self-mutilation of the incision site (see Fig. 11-1). Litter is removed from the litterbox and replaced with shredded newspaper. An indwelling urethral catheter is not used because it may injure the urethra and induce stricture.[1] The incision is not cleansed unless blood clots obstruct urine flow.

Postobstructive diuresis is managed as described in Chapter 12. Sutures are removed atraumatically in 7 to 10 days using tranquilization, if necessary. Owners may need to keep the coat of long-haired cats clipped near the urethrostomy to prevent urine soilage.

The owner is instructed to return the cat every 6 months for urinalysis and urine bacteriologic culture because cats with perineal urethrostomy or prepubic urethrostomy are predisposed to bacterial cystitis.[1-4]

EARLY POSTOPERATIVE COMPLICATIONS OF PERINEAL URETHROSTOMY

Hemorrhage

Postoperative hemorrhage is minimized by including corpus spongiosum within the urethral sutures. If hemorrhage occurs after surgery, pressure on the incision site may control it. Usually, hemorrhage is not life-threatening and stops without reoperation. The cat's mucous membrane color and hematocrit should be monitored. If the hemorrhage is serious and persists, the cat is anesthetized, and the source of hemorrhage is identified and ligated.

Anuria

A cat may be anuric after perineal urethrostomy for several reasons. If the bladder was distended before surgery for a prolonged period, the detrusor muscle may have been damaged. For treatment of a hypotonic bladder, see Chapter 12.

Urethral Obstruction

A cat with primary urethral obstruction should have a palpably full bladder. The urethral opening is inspected. If the urethra is obstructed with blood clots, the urethral opening is gently cleansed and a urethral catheter passed. If the penis is inadvertently twisted 360° during surgery and sutured into a rotated position, the urethra will be occluded. Catheterization is impossible, and reoperation is necessary. Obstruction can be prevented by maintaining proper orientation of the bulbourethral glands and ischiocavernosus muscles during surgery.

Renal Failure

If the cat had renal disease before surgery or if the cat was dehydrated and hypotensive during surgery, acute renal failure may develop. A urethral catheter should be passed to rule out urethral obstruction and any residual urine collected for urinalysis. A urine specific gravity greater than 1.030 suggests prerenal causes of renal failure. Appropriate measures to correct dehydration, hypotension, and hypovolemia should be taken. For further differentiation and treatment of acute and chronic renal failure, see Chapter 1.

LATE POSTOPERATIVE COMPLICATIONS OF PERINEAL URETHROSTOMY

Cystitis

The incidence of bacterial cystitis after Wilson perineal urethrostomy (PU) in cats is 19 to 30%[1,2,4] compared with a 2% incidence in feline urologic syndrome cats without PU.[5] The cystitis is often asymptomatic; thus, urine bacteriologic cultures are recommended every 6 months.

Dysuria

To determine the cause of dysuria, the perineal region should be examined carefully for overlooked sutures. A urethral catheter is passed to assess urethral patency. Obstructing sand can be removed after application of topical anesthetic and massage of the urethrostomy. Urine is obtained by cystocentesis and submitted for bacteriologic culture. If urine bacteriologic cultures are positive, appropriate antibiotic therapy is started. If the urine culture is negative, the cat may be having a recurrence of feline urologic syndrome. Although the PU prevents urethral obstruction, it does not preclude recurrence of feline urologic syndrome. Management of this syndrome is discussed in Chapter 12. Persistent dysuria necessitates a contrast-enhanced cystogram and urethrogram to look for other causes of lower urinary tract disease (e.g., uroliths, neoplasia).

Stricture

Strictures occur most frequently at the junction of the urethra and the skin.[6] Strictures occurred in 12% (6 of 52) of cats after perineal urethrostomy using the Wilson technique. Five of these cats had indwelling catheters after surgery.[1] In a later review of 35 cats, there were no strictures 2 years after Wilson PU.[2] Stricture formation can best be prevented by careful attention to surgical technique and gentle tissue handling.

Operative Errors

The most common errors made during surgery are as follows:

1. *Failure to dissect far enough cranially so that the bulbourethral glands are flush with the skin.* When this is not done, tension can cause retraction of the stoma and subsequent stricture formation. The ischiocavernosus muscles and pubic ligaments must be severed to free the penis sufficiently.
2. *Failure to extend the urethral incision to the cranial edge of the bulbourethral glands.* The urethra widens at the bulbourethral glands, which makes the new stoma larger.
3. *Improper placement of urethra to skin sutures.* If the urethral mucosa is not directly apposed to the skin, primary wound healing does not occur. Granulation tissue produced during second intention healing can occlude the urethral opening.
4. *Traumatic placement of the sutures.* Tearing of the urethra by indelicate technique or by a cutting needle induces granulation, which may proliferate over the urethral opening.

Nonoperative Causes of Strictures

Nonoperative causes include the following:

1. *Lacerations of the urethra.* The urethra can be torn during attempts to unblock the urethra. If the urethra

remains obstructed after a few attempts to relieve the obstruction, a PU or cystostomy should be done, rather than cause further trauma to the urethra.
2. *Self-mutilation.* If the cat removes the Elizabethan collar, it may damage the surgical incision by licking it with its rough tongue. If the cat refuses to eat with the collar in place, it can be removed while the cat eats and then replaced.
3. *Retained suture.* The ends of the sutures around the urethral stoma should be cut long enough to make them easy to identify at the time of suture removal. A suture granuloma can form around a retained suture.

Correction of Stricture

Occasionally, a minor stricture involving the most distal part of the urethra can be corrected by gently dilating the urethra with small forceps.

Usually, however, additional surgery is necessary. The urethral lumen is identified by a catheter, if possible. A circular skin incision is made around the urethrostomy site. The penis is dissected from any attachments within the pelvis (e.g., fibrous tissue, ischiocavernosus muscles, pubic ligaments). The dorsal urethra is incised further cranially, so that healthy urethra can be sutured to the skin. The corpus cavernosum is ligated and the penis and urethra severed just cranial to the stricture. The urethral mucosa to skin apposition is the same as described for PU.

In the rare instance in which the majority of the postprostatic urethra is strictured or damaged, a prepubic urethrostomy can be performed (see Fig. 13-2).

Urinary Incontinence

Urinary incontinence is an unusual complication following PU. The specific cause has not been identified. Sharp dissection and identification and protection of the urethral branches of the pudendal nerve during surgery have been advocated to preserve urethral function.[7] The results of one study, however, indicated that extensive blunt dissection of the urethra, except for the dorsal 5% of the urethral circumference, did not alter neuromuscular function of the lower urinary tract.[8]

Wound Dehiscence

Minor wound dehiscence occurs when the sutures are pulled too tightly and lacerate the urethral mucosa. The dehiscence is not treated, and the sutures are removed routinely. Stricture may be more likely at the site of dehiscence.

Major wound dehiscence may result from urine leakage into the subcutaneous space. This can be caused by urethral lacerations or improper apposition of urethral mucosa to skin. Initially, the perineal region around the incision may be swollen, discolored, and warm. Urine may seep from the wound. If urine leakage is severe, the cat can develop postrenal uremia. The wound is managed as an open wound. It is debrided, lavaged, and allowed to heal by granulation. A cystostomy catheter is placed (see Chapter 16) to prevent further urine contamination of the wound. Urethral stricture may develop and is managed as described previously.

Pararectal Abscess

If dissection extends too far dorsally, the rectum can be injured. Leakage of feces contaminates the wound and causes an abscess. Treatment requires dissection and identification of the rectal damage, debridement, and closure with simple interrupted absorbable sutures. The area is lavaged and drains are placed.

COMPLICATIONS OF PREPUBIC URETHROSTOMY

Experience with complications specific for prepubic urethrostomy is limited because the procedure is done infrequently. Similar complications can occur following prepubic urethrostomy as with PU, including urethral obstruction, subcutaneous urine leakage, and bacterial cystitis.[3]

Anuria after prepubic urethrostomy can result from a kinked urethra, in addition to the causes discussed with perineal urethrostomy. If the tunnel through the abdominal wall and skin is not oriented in a smooth, caudoventral line, the urethra may become occluded. The cat has difficulty urinating, even though a flexible catheter may pass easily. A contrast urethrogram and cystogram delineate the kinked area. Surgical creation of a new stoma is necessary to realign the urethra.

Dribbling often occurs for a few days after prepubic urethrostomy. The resultant urine dermatitis resolves once the dribbling stops. Incontinence persisted in 9% (3 of 32) of cats in a retrospective study.[3] Potential reasons for incontinence include inadequate residual urethral length and damage to nerves supplying the urethra.

REFERENCES

1. Smith, C.W., and Schiller, A.G.: Perineal urethrostomy in a cat: A retrospective study of complications. J. Am. Anim. Hosp. Assoc., 14:225, 1978.
2. Gregory, C.R., and Vasseur, P.B.: Long-term examination of cats with perineal urethrostomy. Vet. Surg., 12:210, 1983.
3. Mendham, J.H.: A description and evaluation of antepubic urethrostomy in the male cat. J. Sm. Anim. Pract., 11:709, 1970.
4. Osborne, C.A., Caywood, D.D., Johnston, G.R., et al.: Feline perineal urethrostomy. A potential cause of hematuria, dysuria, and urethral obstruction. In Current Veterinary Therapy X. Edited by R.W. Kirk. Philadelphia, W.B. Saunders, 1989, p. 1209.
5. Barsanti, J.A., Finco, D.R., Shotts, E.B., et al.: Feline urologic syndrome: Further investigation into etiology. J. Am. Anim. Hosp. Assoc., 18:391, 1982.
6. Kusba, J.K., and Lipowitz, A.J.: Repair of strictures following perineal urethrostomy in the cat. J. Am. Anim. Hosp. Assoc., 18:308, 1982.
7. Griffin, D.W., Gregory, C.R., and Kitchell, R.L.: Preservation of striated urethral sphincter function with use of a surgical technique for perineal urethrostomy in cats. J. Am. Vet. Med. Assoc., 194:1057, 1989.
8. Sackman, J.E., Sims, M.H., and Krahwinkel, D.J.: Urodynamic evaluation of lower urinary tract function in cats after perineal urethrostomy with minimal and extensive dissection. Vet. Surg., 20:55, 1991.

Section Five

Canine Urethral Obstruction

15

Diagnosis and Medical Management of Canine Urethral Obstruction

The pathophysiology, diagnosis, and therapy of urethral obstruction is quite similar in dogs and cats (see Chapter 12). This chapter focuses on aspects of urethral obstruction that are different in dogs.

CAUSES

The general categories of causes of obstruction of the canine urethra are the same as those in cats (see Table 12-1). How common each cause is, however, differs in the two species. For example, urethral plugs are uncommon in dogs (Table 15–1). As in cats, urethral obstruction is more common in males. In male dogs, however, the most common cause of obstruction is urolithiasis. As in cats uroliths are more likely to cause urethral obstruction in males than females because of the longer, less distensible male urethra. In female dogs, the most common cause of urethral obstruction is urethral neoplasia. Neoplasia of the bladder neck may also obstruct urine outflow into the urethra.

PATHOPHYSIOLOGY

The usual site of obstruction by uroliths in male dogs is at the os penis (Fig. 15–1). The urethra passes through the ventral groove of the os penis, which restricts the ability of the urethra to dilate. Otherwise, the site of obstruction varies with the cause.

The clinical and biochemical changes that occur subsequent to urethral obstruction are similar in dogs and cats (see Chapter 12). Urinary tract infection, however, is much more common in dogs with urolithiasis than in cats. Such infection may be the cause or effect of urolithiasis (see Chapter 18).

DIAGNOSIS

As with cats, affected dogs try to urinate frequently. They often strain during urination but produce little urine. In male dogs, a few drops of urine may be noted at the preputial orifice. If the obstruction is not detected and relieved promptly, signs of uremia develop.

The first diagnostic step for a dysuric dog is to determine whether the bladder is distended. This can usually be done by physical examination. As in cats, finding a distended, tense bladder, which may be painful, is indicative of urethral obstruction. In male dogs, the urethra is palpated from the os penis to the scrotum and in the perineal area. Calculi often feel like small, firm, round pebbles. Rectal palpation is performed in male and female dogs, to check the size and location of the prostate gland in males and to palpate the pelvic urethra in males and females. A vaginal examination should be performed in female dogs to evaluate the urethral orifice. The rest of the physical examination helps to determine the duration and severity of the obstruction (see Chapter 12).

Blood is obtained for a complete blood count and serum biochemical analysis, including blood urea nitrogen, creatinine, and electrolytes. In dogs with urolithiasis, serum calcium and phosphorus concentrations should also be measured. Urine is obtained either by cystocentesis or by passing a catheter by the obstruc-

---

TABLE 15–1. POTENTIAL CAUSES OF URETHRAL OBSTRUCTION IN DOGS

Intraluminal	Extraluminal	Functional
Uroliths	Neoplasia	Reflex
Neoplasia	Strictures	dyssynergia
Urethral	Prostatomegaly	Muscle
plugs	Inflammatory swelling	spasm

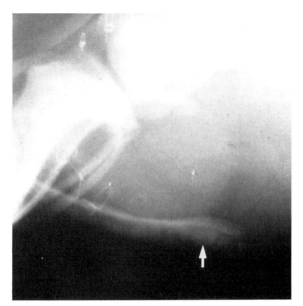

FIG. 15–1. Survey lateral radiograph of the distal urethra of a dog showing multiple calculi lodged in the urethra as it courses through the os penis. The arrow points to the largest of the calculi. (The rear legs are pulled cranially.)

tion. If cystocentesis is performed, as much urine as possible is removed to decompress the bladder (see Chapter 12). A complete urinalysis and both qualitative and quantitative urine cultures are indicated in all dogs with urethral obstruction.

Radiography is often performed in dogs with urethral obstruction before removing or bypassing the obstruction, unless the dog's condition is medically unstable as a result of uremia and hyperkalemia. Survey radiographs of the abdomen and perineal area are made so that the kidneys, bladder, and entire urethral length can be examined for the presence of radiopaque calculi. If no cause of obstruction is visualized, a retrograde cystourethrogram is indicated (see Figs. 6-41 to 6-46). Ultrasonography is often useful in determining the cause of prostatomegaly (see Chapters 4 and 27) and in identifying bladder masses (see Figs. 6-37, 6-52, 6-54). Ultrasonography is less useful for visualizing the urethra.

If the dog's condition is unstable, the location and nature of the obstruction is noted during attempted passage of a urinary catheter. A small-gauge catheter, relative to the dog's size, is used initially to determine if the catheter can bypass the obstruction and relieve bladder distention. If a small-gauge catheter passes easily, a larger-gauge catheter, more appropriate to the size of the dog, may be passed to determine the approximate site and character of the obstruction.

TREATMENT

As in cats, symptomatic therapy is directed toward relieving the obstruction and institution of fluid therapy to reverse uremia and electrolyte and acid-base disorders. Specific therapy is directed to the cause of ob-

struction and is covered in appropriate chapters (see Chapters 18, 27, and 30).

Relief of Obstruction

As already noted, passage of a small-gauge catheter past the obstruction may be used to relieve the obstruction temporarily, as fluid therapy is begun to stabilize the dog's condition and as diagnostic efforts are begun to determine the cause of the obstruction. Urinary catheters can abrade, lacerate, and even puncture the urethral wall if not used gently. One should never attempt to force a catheter past an obstruction. If a small-gauge catheter cannot be passed easily, cystocentesis may be used to decompress the bladder to allow time for initial fluid therapy and diagnostic tests to be accomplished.

Hydropropulsion

If the cause of the obstruction is found to be a urolith, an attempt may be made to push the urolith back into the bladder, using a stream of sterile fluid after dilating the urethra (hydropropulsion, Fig. 15-2).[1,2] The purpose is to relieve the obstruction, allowing time for fluid therapy to resolve fluid and electrolyte disorders, and to permit later removal of the urolith by cystotomy, rather than urethral surgery. Hydropropulsion should not be used if one suspects a tear in the wall of the urethra or urinary bladder.

Hydropropulsion usually requires sedation or general anesthesia, unless the dog is severely depressed from uremia. Sedation relieves urethral spasm and pain. Remember to administer all sedatives and anesthetics cautiously, considering uremia and hyperkalemia (see Chapter 8).

At least two people are needed to perform hydropropulsion. Equipment required includes a sterile urethral catheter, sterile teat cannula, sterile fluid (such as saline) and sterile aqueous lubricant. It may be necessary to relieve bladder distention by cystocentesis before hydropropulsion, since hydropropulsion involves injection of more fluid into the bladder. During hydropropulsion, one person performs a rectal palpation and occludes the pelvic urethra by applying digital pressure across the urethra against the pelvic symphysis. This person, or an assistant, holds the penis out of the sheath. The other person cleans the penis at the urethral orifice. A 60-ml syringe is half filled with sterile saline into which an equal amount of sterile aqueous lubricant (Surgilube, E. Fougera and Co, Melville, NY 11747) is drawn and mixed. A lubricated, sterile, bovine teat cannula, or similar instrument, is inserted into the distal urethra. The urethral orifice is manually occluded around the cannula. The saline is injected into the urethra so that the urethra is distended. Once the urethra is fully distended, as detected by rectal palpation and by back pressure on the syringe plunger, the person performing rectal occlusion of the urethra releases the occlusion as the person with the syringe continues to inject fluid. The goal is for the fluid to push the urolith through the distended urethra into the bladder. Alternatively, pressure may be

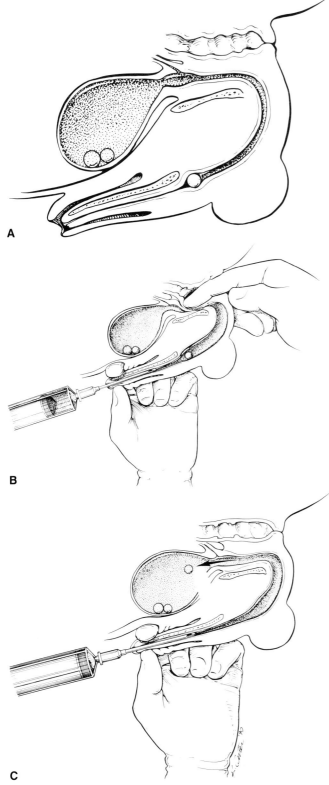

A

B

C

FIG. 15–2. The technique of hydropropulsion. (A) A urethral calculus has lodged behind the os penis producing urethral obstruction. (B) The urethra has been manually occluded at the urethral orifice around a teat cannula and in the pelvic canal via rectal palpation. The urethra has been distended with sterile saline injection. (C) Pressure on the pelvic urethra is removed while injection is continued, pushing the urethral calculus back into the bladder.

released at the urethral orifice by removing the teat cannula in an attempt to flush small calculi out the urethral orifice. Which procedure to attempt should be based on the size of the urolith(s). If hydropropulsion successfully moves the urolith(s) into the bladder, the catheter should be advanced to the bladder and the bladder emptied. Whether the catheter is left in place depends on the severity of uremia, as in cats (see Chapter 12).

If hydropropulsion is unsuccessful in moving the obstructing urolith, one must consider whether further attempts will result in iatrogenic urethral trauma. It may be preferable to perform a urethrotomy or tube cystostomy (see Chapter 16), rather than persist in attempts to move the calculus by hydropropulsion or catheter pressure.

Hydropropulsion can also be performed in female dogs, by occluding the distal urethral orifice around the catheter per vagina.[1] Concomitant rectal occlusion of the urethra is usually not performed because of the short length of the female urethra. A balloon-tipped cardiovascular catheter is very useful in female dogs, if available. Inflation of the balloon, after insertion of the catheter into the distal urethra, prevents reflux of fluid out of the urethral orifice and allows increased intraurethral pressure to push the urolith into the bladder.

Fluid Therapy

For dogs that are uremic, intravenous fluid therapy as well as relief of obstruction is important for survival. A balanced, alkalinizing electrolyte solution such as lactated Ringer's is usually used. The amount of fluid to administer is based on the severity of dehydration, uremia, and hyperkalemia. Approximately 5% body weight is given if the signs are mild, 8% if moderate, and 12% if severe. This amount is administered over 2 to 4 hours with a maximum rate of 88 ml/kg/hr. These are general guidelines. Actual amounts and rates must be individualized for each dog, based on vital signs, concomitant disease processes (such as cardiac disease), mental status, urine output, and blood chemistry changes.

After the initial fluid amount is administered, the dog's condition usually improves if urine output has been established. At this point, the rate and amount of fluid administration can be reduced. Sufficient fluids are given to meet maintenance needs (estimated at 66 ml/kg/day) plus correct any detected dehydration. Food and water should be offered once vomiting from uremia stops. Fluid therapy is generally continued until azotemia is resolved or minimal, and serum electrolytes are normal. As in cats, a postobstructive diuresis may occur (see Chapter 12).

Antibiotic therapy for urinary tract infection should be based on results of urine culture. Therapy can usually be delayed until culture results are returned, unless signs of systemic infection such as fever and leukocytosis are present. Choice of antibiotic is usually based on the organism isolated (Table 15-2).[3,4] If surgery is required, and the urine is known to be infected, intravenous antibiotics during surgery may be beneficial to prevent bacteremia. Nephrotoxic antibiotics such as

TABLE 15–2. COMMONLY USED ANTIBIOTICS IN URINARY TRACT INFECTIONS*

Bacteria Isolated or Suspected	Antibiotic of Choice
Staphylococcus spp	Penicillin, ampicillin, amoxicillin
Streptococcus spp	Penicillin, ampicillin, amoxicillin
Eschericia coli	Trimethoprim/sulfa, enrofloxacin
Proteus mirabilis	Penicillin, ampicillin, amoxicillin, enrofloxacin
Pseudomonas aeruginosa	Tetracycline
Klebsiella pneumoniae	Cephalosporin, enrofloxacin
Enterobacter spp	Trimethoprim/sulfa, enrofloxacin

* The choice of antibiotic should be based on the organism isolated from urine culture.[3,4]

aminoglycosides should be avoided unless the organism isolated is resistant to less toxic drugs. As in cats, indwelling urethral catheters lead to infection.[5,6] Use of antibiotics does not prevent such infections and may lead to infection with resistant organisms. If the dog's condition permits, antibiotic therapy is avoided until the indwelling catheter is removed.

CONSEQUENCES

The consequences of urethral obstruction in dogs are similar to those in cats (see Chapter 12). Drug dosages for treatment, however, are different.

If bladder function has been impaired by overdistention, optimal therapy is to keep the bladder empty, by frequent manual expression, intermittent urethral catheterization, or indwelling urethral catheterization, depending on the dog's size, sex, and nature. As in cats, bethanechol can be tried as adjunctive therapy, as long as the obstruction has been removed. Bethanechol is contraindicated in the presence of continuing complete or partial obstruction. The dosage of bethanechol in dogs is 5 to 15 mg by mouth every 8 hours.[7] As in cats,

bethanechol is usually administered with an alpha adrenergic antagonist such as phenoxybenzamine (0.25 mg/kg by mouth every 12 hours or 0.5 mg/kg by mouth every 24 hours).[7] As in cats, time required for return of bladder function varies with degree of injury.

In dogs with urethral spasm, diazepam may be used in conjunction with phenoxybenzamine to relax the urethra. The recommended dosage in dogs for this purpose is 0.2 mg/kg by mouth every 8 hours. Efficacy is unproved.[7]

PREVENTION OF RECURRENCE

Prevention of recurrence depends on the cause of urethral obstruction. With uroliths, prevention of recurrence depends on identification of urolith type to alter predisposing factors (see Chapter 18). With prostatomegaly, both treatment and prevention depend on identification of the underlying prostatic disease (see Chapters 2 and 27). For neoplasia, treatment and prevention depend on identification of the type of neoplasia (see Chapter 30).

REFERENCES

1. Osborne, C.A., and Polzin, D.J.: Nonsurgical management of canine obstructive urolithopathy. Vet. Clin. North Am. [Sm. Anim. Pract.], *16*:333, 1986.
2. Piermattei, D.L., and Osborne, C.A.: Nonsurgical removal of calculi from the urethra of male dogs. J. Am. Vet. Med. Assoc., *159*:1755, 1971.
3. Ling, G.V.: Management of urinary tract infections. *In* Current Veterinary Therapy IX. Edited by R.W. Kirk. Philadelphia, W.B. Saunders, 1986, pp. 1174–1177.
4. Rey, A.M., Gums, J.G., and Grauer, K.: The new antimicrobial agents. Postgrad. Med., *88*:64, 1990.
5. Barsanti, J.A., Blue, J., and Edmunds, J.: Urinary tract infection due to indwelling bladder catheters in dogs and cats. J. Am. Vet. Med. Assoc., *187*:384, 1985.
6. Lippert, A.C., Fulton, R.B., and Parr, A.M.: Nosocomial infection surveillance in a small animal intensive care unit. J. Am. Anim. Hosp. Assoc., *24*:627, 1988.
7. Moreau, P.M., and Lappin, M.R.: Pharmacologic maintenance of urinary incontinence. *In* Current Veterinary Therapy X. Edited by R.W. Kirk. Philadelphia, W.B. Saunders, 1989, pp. 1214–1222.

16

Surgical Therapy for Urethral Obstruction in Dogs

Surgical procedures for correction of urethral obstruction can be temporary or permanent. A *urethrotomy*, i.e., a temporary opening into the urethra, is used to remove calculi or bypass temporarily a more distal obstruction, e.g., stricture, fractured os penis, or neoplasia (Fig. 16–1). A *urethrostomy* is a permanent opening into the urethra. Nonsurgical techniques for relieving urethral obstruction are discussed in Chapter 15.

A *prescrotal urethrotomy* is used to bypass or remove an obstruction distal to the scrotum. Calculi most frequently lodge in the urethra just caudal to the os penis and can be retrieved through a prescrotal urethrotomy with alternate flushing between the end of the urethra and the urethrotomy site. More proximal calculi often can be flushed into the urinary bladder and later removed by cystotomy. Prescrotal urethrotomy is preferable to perineal urethrotomy because the prescrotal urethra is more superficial and less vascular than the perineal urethra.

If a urethral obstruction cannot be easily bypassed or removed by prescrotal urethrotomy and the dog is a poor anesthetic and surgical risk, a *cystostomy catheter* can be placed to bypass the obstruction temporarily until corrective surgery can be performed.

When a dog with urethral obstruction is azotemic and hyperkalemic, the minimal anesthesia necessary for restraint is given before performing a urethrotomy or placing a cystostomy catheter. A local anesthetic is used in a calm or depressed dog. In the more excitable dog, oxymorphone (0.1 to 0.2 mg/kg IV) can be used. The narcotic effect is then reversed with naloxone (0.02 mg/kg IV) after the procedure. Management of postrenal azotemia is discussed in Chapter 15.

When a dog with urethral calculi is a good anesthetic risk, *prescrotal urethrotomy can be combined with cystotomy* to enable removal of calculi lodged in the perineal or pelvic urethra (Fig. 16–2).[1] A catheter is placed through the prescrotal urethrotomy, and calculi are flushed into the bladder and recovered through the cystotomy incision. Alternatively, the calculi can be flushed distally using a catheter placed into the proximal urethra via the cystotomy incision.

A *scrotal urethrostomy* is performed when there is irreparable injury, stricture, or neoplasia to the more distal urethra. It is selected instead of a prescrotal urethrostomy because the scrotal urethra is wider than the prescrotal urethra. Scrotal urethrostomy necessitates castration, but urethrostomy at any site makes a dog infertile. Scrotal urethrostomy is also indicated for dogs that are recurrent stone-formers because of persistent urinary tract infection, metabolic abnormalities, inability of owner to follow prevention recommendations, or unknown factors. It allows the passage of a 0.5-cm calculus in a medium-sized dog. Scrotal urethrostomy can be combined with cystotomy as already described for removal of perineal and pelvic urethral calculi. The risk of urinary tract infection may be increased after scrotal urethrostomy because of changes in urethral anatomy.[2]

Perineal urethrostomy is rarely done and is reserved for dogs with neoplasia or irreparable damage to the scrotal and distal perineal urethra (see Chapter 31). Perineal urethrostomy is not indicated for recurrent stone-formers because it is less cosmetic and causes more bleeding and urine scalding than a scrotal urethrostomy. Perineal urethrostomy was shown to predispose dogs to urinary tract infections.[3]

Obstruction of the membranous or prostatic urethra by stricture or neoplasia is difficult to manage. Prostatectomy is used to excise strictures of the prostatic urethra, but there is a risk of urinary incontinence (see Chapter 28). Balloon dilation of the prostatic urethra is used in humans but has not been described in dogs. A short stricture of the membranous urethra (less than 1 cm) can be excised followed by primary anastomosis of the urethra. Urinary diversion and management of urethral tumors is discussed in Section 7.

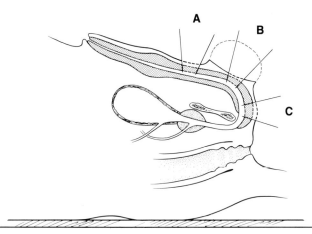

FIG. 16–1. Urethrotomy and urethrostomy sites in the male dog. (A) Prescrotal urethrotomy; (B) scrotal urethrostomy; (C) perineal urethrotomy or urethrostomy (rarely done). Dog is in dorsal recumbency.

TEMPORARY BYPASS OF URETHRAL OBSTRUCTION

Prescrotal Urethrotomy[4]

The area between the scrotum and the middle of the prepuce is prepared and draped for surgery. The skin incision extends from just caudal to the prepuce to just cranial to the scrotum (Fig. 16–3A, insert). Extension of the incision onto the scrotum increases the likelihood of excoriation of the site, prolapse of the testes through the incision, or both.

Subcutaneous tissue is dissected to the level of the retractor penile muscle (Fig. 16–3A). The grayish corpus spongiosum and the white, fibrous-covered corpora cavernosa should be identified. If the corpora cavernosa is the most visible midline structure, the penis is rotated between thumb and forefinger to bring the retractor penile muscle and corpus spongiosum to midline. The retractor penile muscle is retracted laterally (Fig. 16–3B).

Hemorrhage is minimized by careful attention to the anatomy of the urethra and penis. A cross section of the penis and urethra at the level of the prescrotal urethra shows the urethra surrounded by the corpus spongiosum. The paired bodies of the corpora cavernosa lie lateral to the urethra (Fig. 16–4). An exact midline incision avoids damage to the very vascular corpora cavernosa, which would cause considerable hemorrhage. A longitudinal incision is made into the corpus spongiosum and urethra (Fig. 16–3C). The urethral mucosa lining is shiny and pinkish white and contrasts with the surrounding corpus spongiosum. If urethral calculi are present, they are removed and saved for mineral analysis. A catheter is passed into the proximal urethra to identify additional uroliths or obstruction. The catheter is also passed distally to assess patency and to dislodge calculi within the penile urethra, if present. After the catheter is removed, the urethrotomy is left open. The dog will urinate from both the urethrotomy and the terminal urethra for up to 2 weeks. The wounds heal com-

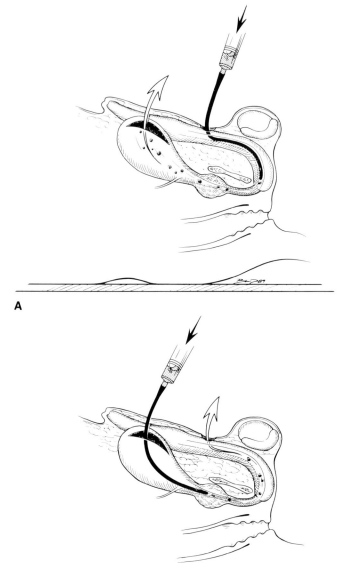

FIG. 16–2. Removal of calculi from perineal urethra. (A) Calculi are flushed from the prescrotal urethrotomy site into the bladder. (B) Calculi are flushed from the urethra out through the prescrotal urethrotomy.

pletely by second intention and epithelialization in 2 to 4 weeks.[4]

Although primary closure of the urethra reduces postoperative hemorrhage,[5,6] it requires more operative time, gentle tissue handling, and delicate instruments to prevent postoperative stricture formation. Thus, a prescrotal urethrotomy is not routinely sutured. Closure is indicated in an anemic dog or in a dog with coagulopathy (e.g., a Doberman pinscher with von Willebrand's disease), unless the urethra was traumatized during surgery or by uroliths. The urethrotomy is sutured with 4–0 or 5–0 surgical gut in a simple interrupted pattern (Fig. 16–3C, insert). The suture material penetrates the mucosa

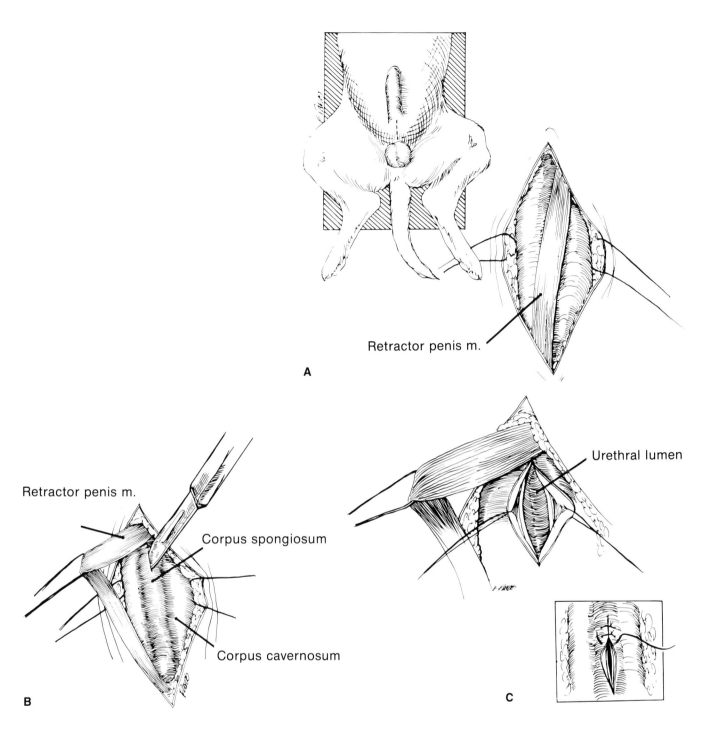

Retractor penis m.

A

Retractor penis m.

Corpus spongiosum

Corpus cavernosum

B

Urethral lumen

C

FIG. 16–3. Prescrotal urethrotomy. (A) Skin incision extends from just caudal to prepuce to just cranial to scrotum (insert). Subcutaneous tissue is dissected to level of retractor penile muscle. (B) Retractor penile muscle is retracted laterally. Longitudinal incision is made into corpus spongiosum and urethra. Retention sutures can be placed in corpus spongiosum to aid in identification of urethra. (C) The urethrotomy can be closed with 4–0 or 5–0 synthetic absorbable suture material in simple interrupted pattern (insert). Usually, however, the urethrotomy is left open to heal by second intention (see text). (From Stone, E.A.: Urologic surgery—an update. *In* Nephrology and Urology. Edited by E.B. Breitschwerdt. New York, Churchill Livingstone, 1986, pp. 75–88; with permission.)

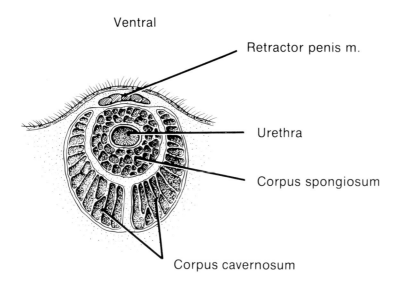

Ventral

Retractor penis m.

Urethra

Corpus spongiosum

Corpus cavernosum

Dorsal

FIG. 16—4. Cross-section of penis and urethra at level of prescrotal urethra (dog in dorsal recumbency). Urethra is surrounded by corpus spongiosum. Paired corpora cavernosa lie lateral and dorsal to urethra.

to approximate the urethral edges accurately. The subcutaneous and skin closure is routine.

If the catheter remains within the urethra for monitoring urine output, it is secured to the skin (Fig. 16–5) and connected to a closed urinary collection system. After catheter removal, the urethrotomy is not sutured.

Catheter Cystostomy[4]

A size 8 gauge Foley catheter, with an inflatable bulb, works well as a cystostomy catheter to bypass a urethral obstruction temporarily. It is also used to divert urine from a healing urethral anastomosis and to keep the bladder decompressed. The catheter must be placed through a surgical incision in the body wall, rather than percutaneously with a stylet because a dog's bladder is too mobile for accurate placement and retention of a percutaneously placed cystostomy catheter.[7]

After aseptic preparation and draping, a 1- to 2-cm skin and abdominal wall incision is made between the pubis and the umbilicus, on the midline in female dogs and lateral to the prepuce in male dogs (Fig. 16–6A). To place a cystostomy catheter during a laparotomy, a stab incision is made through the skin and abdominal wall lateral to the laparotomy incision. After either approach, the bladder is located. Two retention sutures and a pursestring suture of synthetic absorbable suture material are placed through the serosal and muscular layers of the cranial ventral bladder wall. A stab incision is made through the bladder wall within the pursestring suture (Fig. 16–6B).

A Foley catheter is inserted into the bladder and the bulb inflated with sterile saline (Fig. 16–6C). Omentum

is incorporated into the pursestring as it is gently tightened and tied (Fig. 16–6D). The retention sutures are passed through the linea alba or ventral fascia and tied. The abdominal wall and skin incisions are closed. The catheter is secured to the skin. The catheter is connected to a closed drainage system. The bulb on the Foley catheter can be deflated and removed percutaneously after 5 to 7 days. Within 24 hours after removal, the stoma should seal, and any urine leakage from the stoma site should cease.[6]

Rarely, a permanent cystostomy catheter is placed to drain urine in an animal with inoperable stricture or

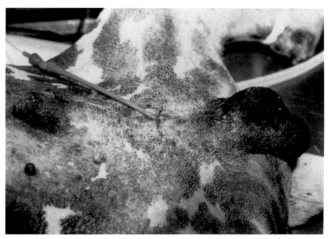

FIG. 16—5. If catheter is to remain within urethra for monitoring urine output, it is secured to the skin and connected to a closed urinary collection system.

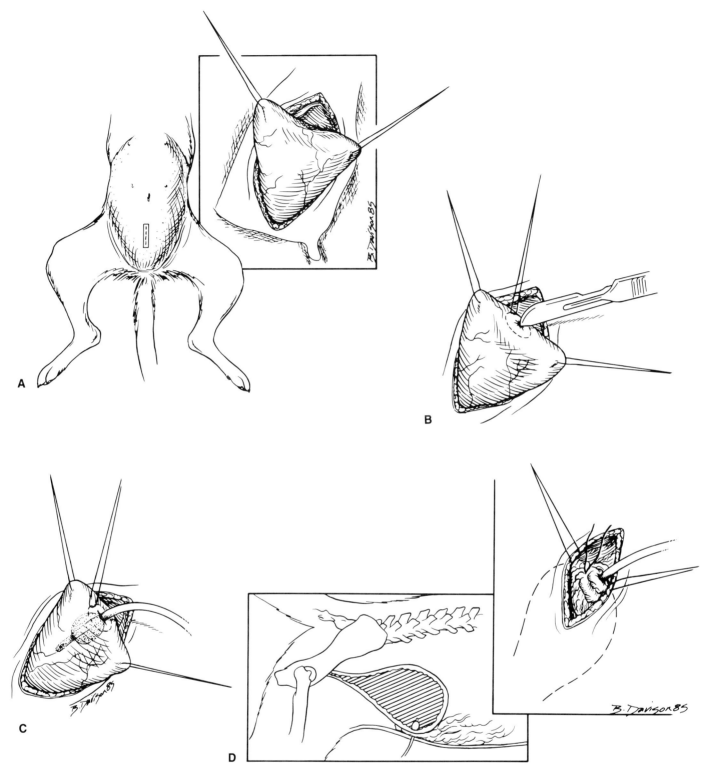

FIG. 16—6. Cystostomy catheter. (A) A 1- to 2-cm skin incision is made between pubis and umbilicus, on the midline in female dogs. The incision is continued through body wall. Bladder is exteriorized, and two retention sutures are placed. (B) Purse-string suture is placed through serosa and muscular layers of cranial ventral bladder wall. Stab incision is made through bladder wall within the pursestring suture. (C) A size 8 gauge catheter is inserted into bladder and inflated with sterile saline. (D) Omentum is incorporated into the pursestring as it is tightened gently and tied. The retention sutures are passed through linea alba or ventral fascia and tied. (From Stone, E.A., Urologic surgery—an update. *In* Nephrology and Urology. Edited by E.B. Breitschwerdt. New York, Churchill Livingstone, 1986, pp. 75–88; with permission.)

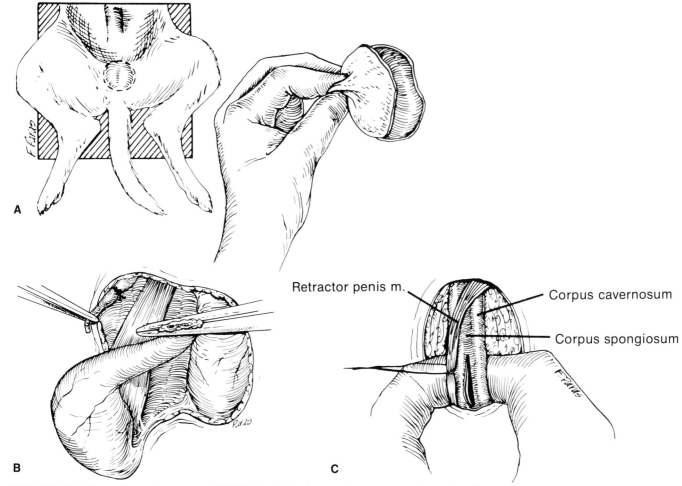

FIG. 16–7. Scrotal urethrostomy. (A) Skin is incised around scrotum at junction of scrotal and inguinal skin. (B) If dog is intact, a routine castration is done. (C) Subcutaneous tissue is dissected from retractor penile muscle, which is retracted laterally. A midline incision is made in the corpus spongiosum. (D) Urethral incision is extended caudally to point where the urethra courses in a dorsal-ventral (or vertical) plane. A catheter can be passed to identify this area. (E) The tunica albuginea, which covers each corpus cavernosum, is sutured to the subcutaneous fascia with absorbable suture material (a). Urethral mucosa is sutured to skin with 4–0 nonabsorbable monofilament suture material (b). (F) Urethra to skin sutures are continued cranially for about 2 cm. Remaining skin incision is apposed. (From Stone, E.A., Urologic surgery—an update. *In* Nephrology and Urology. Edited by E.B. Breitschwerdt. New York, Churchill Livingstone, 1986, pp. 75–88; with permission.)

tumor of the prostatic or membranous urethra. For this palliative procedure, a de Pezzer (mushroom) catheter (see Fig. 7–4) is inserted surgically, as already described, and not removed.

PERMANENT BYPASS OF URETHRAL OBSTRUCTION

Scrotal Urethrostomy[4]

To begin the scrotal urethrostomy, a skin incision is made around the scrotum at the junction of the scrotal and inguinal skin (Fig. 16–7A). If the incision extends too far laterally, there will be excessive tension on the urethra to skin closure. The scrotal skin is retracted to one side. In an intact dog, the subcutaneous tissue is dissected to the spermatic cord, and the dog is castrated routinely (Fig. 16–7B). The dissection is continued dorsally to the penis. The thumb and forefinger are used to stabilize the penis and hold the retractor penile muscle and the grayish corpus spongiosum on the midline (Fig. 16–7C). The retractor penile muscle is retracted laterally.

A longitudinal incision is made into the corpus spongiosum and urethra. As with the prescrotal urethrotomy procedure (Fig. 16–3), an exact ventral midline incision avoids damage to the very vascular corpora cavernosa. The urethral incision is extended caudally to the point where the urethra courses in a dorsal-ventral (or vertical) plane. A catheter can be passed to identify this area (Fig. 16–7D). Calculi can then exit without having

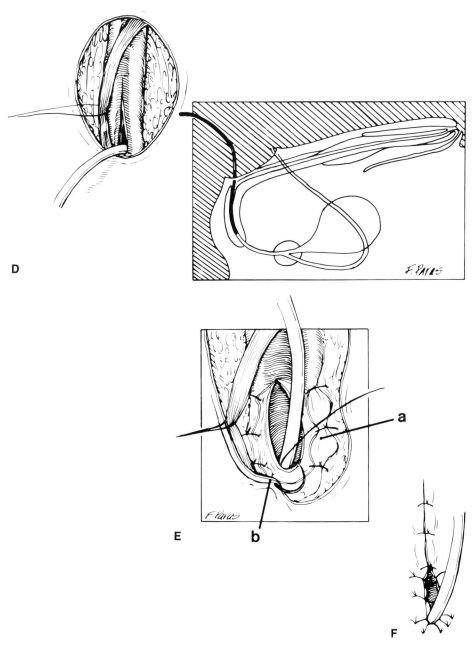

D

E   b

a

F

(*Legend appears on facing page.*)

to pass through the urethra as it curves into a cranial-caudal (or horizontal) plane.

The tunica albuginea, which surrounds each corpus cavernosum, is sutured to the subcutaneous fascia beneath the skin edges with absorbable suture material (Fig. 16–7E). This step helps prevent tension on the urethra to skin suture line. The urethral mucosa is sutured to the skin with 4–0 nonabsorbable monofilament suture material, including some of the corpus spongiosum in each suture bite (Fig. 16–7F). The four most caudal sutures are placed first to align the urethral opening with the skin. The urethra to skin sutures are continued cranially for about 2 cm. The remaining skin incision is apposed. Sutures are removed in 7 to 10 days.

REPAIR OF URETHRAL STRICTURES

Excision of Penile Urethral Strictures

A method for repairing short penile urethral strictures (less than 5 cm in length) has been described,[1] but clinical results have not been reported. A skin incision is made over the strictured area. The retractor penile muscle, if still present, is retracted laterally. The corpus spongiosum is incised over the stricture. One half the circumference of the strictured area of the urethra is excised. The incision is not closed. A cystostomy catheter is placed to divert urine until the urethra heals by second intention (2 to 4 weeks depending on the length of the excision).[1]

Excision and Anastomosis of Strictured Membranous Urethra

The membranous urethra, located between the prostate and the proximal penile urethra, is approached through a pubic and ischiatic osteotomy (see Fig. 10–4). A urethral catheter is placed to help locate the stricture. The length of the stricture is measured to ascertain that it can be excised and the urethra anastomosed without tension (approximately 1 cm length in a 10-kg dog). The urethra is sharply excised on each side of the stricture. The edges of the urethra are joined with simple interrupted absorbable sutures, which penetrate the mucosa to ensure accurate apposition. A cystostomy catheter is placed to divert urine. The urethral catheter is left in place for 2 days to allow the urethral mucosa to seal. The cystostomy catheter is removed in 5 to 7 days.

REFERENCES

1. Stone, E.A.: Surgical management of urolithiasis. Compend. Contin. Educ. Pract. Vet., 3:627, 1981.
2. Bilbrey, S.A., Birchard, S.J., Smeak, D.J.: Scrotal urethrostomy: A retrospective review of 38 dogs (1973 through 1988). J. Am. Anim. Hosp. Assoc., 27:560, 1991.
3. Bergmeister, M.: Perineal urethrostomy in canine urolithiasis. A review of 38 cases in the years from 1979–84. Munchen, Ludwig-Maximilians-Universitat. Dissertation, 1986.
4. Stone, E.A.: Urologic surgery—an update. In Nephrology and Urology. Edited by E.B. Breitschwerdt. New York, Churchill Livingstone, 1986, pp. 75–88.
5. Waldron, D.R., Hedlund, C.S., Tangner, C.H., et al.: The canine urethra. A comparison of first and second intention healing. Vet. Surg., 14:213, 1985.
6. Weber, W.J., Boothe, H.W., Brassard, J.A., et al.: Comparison of the healing of prescrotal urethrotomy incisions in the dog: Sutured versus nonsutured. Am. J. Vet. Res., 46:1309, 1985.
7. Dhein, C.R., Person, M.W., Leathers, C.W., et al.: Prepubic (suprapubic) catheterization of the dog. J. Am. Anim. Hosp. Assoc., 25:261, 1989.

17

Postoperative Management and Surgical Complications of Canine Urethral Obstruction

POSTOPERATIVE MANAGEMENT

Urinary catheters are not routinely maintained after a urethrotomy or urethrostomy. If a catheter has been placed for monitoring urine output, it is connected to a closed collection system.

An Elizabethan collar or side brace is used if necessary to curb licking of the incision. To prevent urine scalding, petroleum jelly can be applied to the skin around the urethrotomy or urethrostomy.

If calculi have been retrieved, they are submitted for quantitative mineral analysis and appropriate measures taken to prevent recurrence (see Chapter 18). Plans are made to diagnose and remove any additional calculi.

A cystostomy catheter is connected to a closed collection system, and the collection bag is emptied as needed to prevent overflow or reflux into the collection line. The cystostomy catheter should remain in place for at least 5 to 7 days to prevent urine leakage following removal. The catheter can be temporarily occluded to assess urine outflow through the urethra before it is removed.

Dogs are not routinely started on antibiotic therapy while there is an indwelling urinary catheter. The urine is cultured and appropriate therapy started after the catheter is removed. Scrotal urethrostomy and perineal urethrostomy may predispose dogs to urinary tract infection.[1,2] Urine should be cultured every six months or if the dog has hematuria or dysuria.

COMPLICATIONS OF URETHROTOMY AND URETHROSTOMY

Hemorrhage

Blood may drip from a urethrotomy or urethrostomy incision for 7 to 10 days after surgery. The dog should be kept away from female dogs in estrus. It may be necessary to tranquilize an excitable dog. The bleeding can be a nuisance to the owner, but it is rarely critical. The hematocrit is monitored if there is any concern about the severity of blood loss.

Hematoma can form in the preputial area after scrotal urethrostomy,[1] particularly in combination with cystotomy (Fig. 17–1). This complication is avoided by including corpus spongiosum in the urethra to skin sutures. Usually, the swelling subsides with warm compresses, but, occasionally, surgical drainage is required.

Urethral Stricture

Stricture After Prescrotal Urethrotomy

Urethral stricture is more common after improper closure of a urethrotomy than after a urethrotomy that has healed by second intention. The stricture is identified by urethral catheterization and retrograde urethrography. A stricture after a prescrotal urethrotomy is best treated with a scrotal urethrostomy. If the dog is a breeding animal, an attempt can be made to excise the stricture as described in Chapter 16.

Stricture After Scrotal Urethrostomy

Stricture following scrotal urethrostomy is uncommon.[1] An attempt is made to dilate the stoma with hemostats. If this is unsuccessful, a new urethrostomy is made more proximally, using a similar technique as for a scrotal urethrostomy.

Urethral Fistula

Urethral fistula is a rare complication of urethrotomy (Fig. 17–2), which may be caused by the skin incision healing faster than the urethra. For repair, the skin over the fistula is excised, including some normal skin. The fibrous tissue tract to the urethra is excised, and the

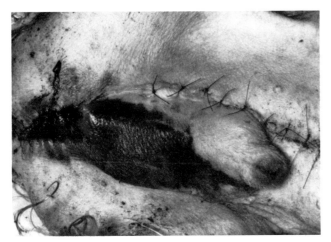

FIG. 17-1. Dog with parapreputial hematoma after a scrotal urethrostomy and cystotomy.

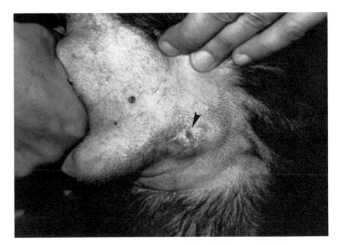

FIG. 17-2. Dog with urethral fistula (arrow) after a prescrotal urethrotomy.

urethra is left open to heal. Urine is diverted from the urethra by a cystostomy catheter until the urethra heals (2 to 4 weeks).

COMPLICATIONS OF CATHETER CYSTOSTOMY

Catheter Dislodgment

Catheter dislodgment can best be prevented by securely anchoring the catheter in position and placing a self-restraint device on the dog (see Chapter 12). When the catheter becomes dislodged within the first four days, urine may leak into the abdomen. The animal should be monitored closely for signs of urine accumulation in the abdomen (e.g., abdominal distention, pain). An abdominocentesis is performed if there is any evidence of fluid accumulation. The blood urea nitrogen or serum creatinine concentration is measured. A cystogram is not routinely performed because the increased bladder pressure during injection of contrast material may force open a sealed cystostomy site.

If the bladder is not leaking and urine diversion is still needed, minimal anesthesia necessary for analgesia is administered. After a surgical preparation, the skin and body wall sutures are removed, and ventral wall of the bladder is exteriorized, and a new catheter placed as previously described (see Fig. 16–6).

If the cystostomy site is leaking, surgical repair is needed. In a uremic animal that is a poor anesthetic risk, a peritoneal catheter is placed to drain the urine from the abdomen while the animal is diuresed (see Chapter 21 and Fig. 21–1). After the animal is stabilized, the abdomen is explored, lavaged with warm saline, and the cystostomy is closed or a new cystostomy catheter placed.

Urine Extravasation

Subcutaneous urine leakage causes severe cellulitis. If a cystostomy catheter partially pulls out, one of the holes of the catheter can become lodged between the body wall and the skin, allowing urine to leak from the bladder into the subcutaneous space.

For treatment, the area is thoroughly debrided. If there is sufficient skin, the wound can be closed over drains. Otherwise, the wound is bandaged and left open to granulate.

REFERENCES

1. Bilbrey, S.A., Birchard, S.J., Smeak, D.J.: Scrotal urethrostomy: A retrospective review of 38 dogs (1973 through 1988). J. Am. Anim. Hosp. Assoc., 27:560, 1991.
2. Bergmeister, M.: Perineal urethrostomy in canine urolithiasis. A review of 38 cases in the years from 1979–84. Munchen, Ludwig-Maximilians-Universitat, Dissertation, 1986.

Section Six

Urolithiasis

18

Diagnosis and Medical Therapy of Urolithiasis

Urolithiasis refers to the occurrence of "stones" within the urine collecting system (Fig. 18–1). Such stones cause uroepithelial inflammation and renal pelvic, ureteral, and urethral obstruction (Fig. 12–6) and predispose to urinary tract infection (UTI). Urinary stones are organized aggregations of crystals embedded in a small amount of organic matrix. Usually one type of crystal is dominant, although other crystals found in urine may become trapped within the urolith as it forms. It is extremely important diagnostically to determine the dominant mineral in the uroliths removed from a dog or cat to prevent recurrence of uroliths in that animal effectively.

Uroliths form because the amount of the major crystal involved exceeds its solubility in urine. Thus, the urine is supersaturated with this type of crystal and it precipitates. Various characteristics of urine affect the solubility of the crystalloid material, including concentration of the crystalloid, urine pH, presence of crystallization inhibitors, and the proteinaceous matrix. The characteristics of urine that affect the crystalloid vary with the type of crystal.

There are two major clinical questions related to uroliths. One is what type of urolith is present. Many different minerals, which can form crystals, are present in urine. Most animals, however, form uroliths of one type and are prone to recurrence of this same type. The most common types of uroliths in dogs and cats are listed in Tables 18–1 and 18–2. The predisposing factors to occurrence of each type of urolith are different. These factors are important, both in medical therapy and in prevention of recurrence. The pathophysiology of formation of each type of urolith is discussed for these reasons.

Another important question is where the uroliths are located. Uroliths can form in both the renal pelvis and the urinary bladder. Uroliths are transported through the ureters and urethra. Uroliths may obstruct urine flow in the renal pelvis, ureters, and urethra, depending on their size. Clinical signs vary with urolith location. Animals may have uroliths at more than one site. This chapter reviews the clinical signs related to urolith location.

Diagnosis of urolithiasis is based on clinical signs, radiography, blood chemistry, and, most importantly, quantitative analysis of the urolith. Some types of uroliths may be dissolved with medical therapy if the uroliths are in the bladder. Nephroliths are more difficult to treat effectively medically, and uroliths in the ureter or urethra cannot be dissolved unless they move or are moved into the bladder. This chapter discusses diagnosis, medical therapy, and consequences of urolithiasis. Surgical therapy is discussed in Chapter 19.

PATHOPHYSIOLOGY

As already noted, certain components of normal urine may precipitate in urine as crystals if the urine becomes supersaturated with them. If these crystal complexes grow and remain within the urinary tract, they form uroliths. Urolithiasis should not be considered as a single "disease" because the causes of formation, treatment, and prevention of recurrence of different types of uroliths are quite different. In discussing urolithiasis in a clinical case, it is always best to state the type of urolith such as "struvite urolithiasis." This section describes the causes for formation for the most common types of uroliths. Some uroliths, referred to as *mixed*, contain more than one type of mineral.

Most types of uroliths in dogs have been noted to have a breed predisposition. In urate and cystine calculi, the underlying genetic defect predisposing to calculi formation is at least partially understood. For other calculi, a breed predilection and even familial incidence are recorded, but the underlying defect or defects remain unknown.[1]

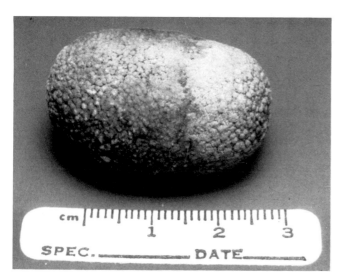

FIG. 18–1. Urolith removed from a dog's bladder. The outer core was composed of 100% struvite, while the inner core was composed of 100% urate. The dog also had hepatic atrophy secondary to a congenital portovascular shunt.

Struvite

The most common type of urolith in dogs and cats is magnesium ammonium phosphate hexahydrate, commonly referred to as struvite after the man who performed the first analysis (Fig. 18–1). Struvite uroliths may form secondary to UTI or may develop in sterile urine. Struvite uroliths can affect an animal at any age.

Infection-Induced Struvite Uroliths

Urinary tract infection with bacteria that produce urease (staphylococci, *Proteus* spp) leads to urine alkalinization as well as increased concentrations of ammonium and phosphate.[2] Struvite becomes progressively less soluble as urine pH increases above 6.5. This combi-

nation of factors leads to formation of struvite uroliths. Infection-induced struvite uroliths are the most common form of struvite uroliths in dogs. Although any breed can be affected, a higher incidence has been noted in miniature schnauzers, dachshunds, poodles, Scottish terriers, beagles, Pekingese, and Welsh corgis.[3] Females have a higher incidence than males.[3]

Struvite uroliths can form within 2 to 8 weeks following onset of infection with urease-producing organisms.[4] Infection-associated struvite uroliths have produced urethral obstruction in young puppies.[5,6]

Sterile Struvite Uroliths

Sterile struvite uroliths are the most common form of struvite uroliths in cats. The etiology of sterile struvite uroliths is poorly understood. Both dietary and metabolic factors that could increase urine pH or increase concentrations of magnesium, ammonium, or phosphate have been theorized. In the absence of urease, however, an increase in urine pH is generally associated with a decrease in ammonium. In fact, many cats and dogs with sterile struvite uroliths have acidic urine. This illustrates the complexity of multiple ion interactions in urolith formation.

Sterile struvite uroliths in cats are often quite small and shaped like wafers or disks (Fig. 18–2). Because of their small size, they are often difficult to detect with survey radiographs, requiring contrast cystography or ultrasonography for visualization (Fig. 18–3).

Calcium Oxalate Uroliths

Calcium oxalate uroliths are more common in male dogs than female dogs, at a mean age of 8 to 9 years.[7,8] Any breed may be affected, but a higher incidence has been reported in Dalmatians, Lhasa apsos, miniature schnauzers, miniature poodles, Shih tzus, and Yorkshire terriers.[7–9] Calcium oxalate uroliths are relatively uncommon in cats, but there is a trend to an increasing inci-

TABLE 18–1. MOST COMMON TYPES OF UROLITHS IN DOGS

Type	Approximate Percentage
Struvite (magnesium ammonium phosphate hexahydrate)	60
Calcium oxalate (monohydrate or dihydrate)	15
Calcium phosphate	2
Urate	5
Cystine	2
Silica	2
Other (mixed)	14

Data from Osborne, C. A., Polzin, D. J., Johnston, G. R., et al.: Canine urolithiasis. *In* Textbook of Veterinary Internal Medicine. Edited by S. J. Ettinger. Philadelphia, W. B. Saunders, 1989, pp. 2083–2107.

TABLE 18–2. MOST COMMON TYPES OF UROLITHS IN CATS

Type	Approximate Percentage
Struvite (magnesium ammonium phosphate hexahydrate)	80–90
Calcium oxalate (monohydrate or dihydrate)	2–7
Calcium phosphate	2
Urate	1–3
Matrix	5

Data from Osborne, C. A., Kruger, J. M., Johnston, G. R., et al.: Feline lower urinary tract disorders. *In* Textbook of Veterinary Internal Medicine. Edited by S. J. Ettinger. Philadelphia, W. B. Saunders, 1989, pp. 2057–2082; and Ling, G. V., Franti, C. E., Ruby, A. L., et al.: Epizootiologic evaluation and quantitative analysis of urinary calculi from 150 cats. J. Am. Vet. Med. Assoc., *196:* 1459, 1990.

FIG. 18–2. Small struvite urolith removed surgically from a cat's bladder. The urine was sterile.

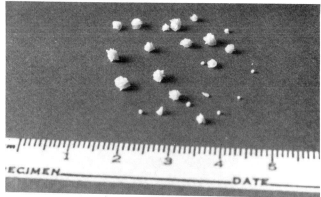

FIG. 18–4. Multiple calcium oxalate uroliths removed from the bladder and urethra of a female cat.

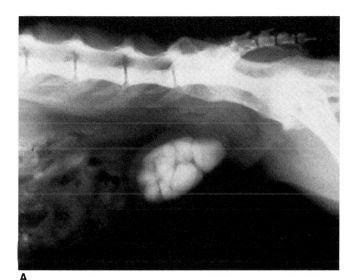

A

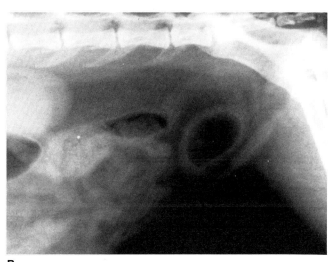

B

FIG. 18–3. Lateral radiographs from two cats. (A) Numerous large radiopaque uroliths in a cat with staphylococcal urinary tract infection. (B) Single small urolith on a pneumocystogram in a cat with sterile urine. Both cats have thickened bladder walls.

dence as dietary changes are made to control struvite crystalluria (Fig. 18–4). The solubility of calcium oxalate is not markedly affected by pH.

The pathogenesis of calcium oxalate urolithiasis is poorly understood in companion animals. Only more recently with the advent of quantitative urolith analysis has the frequency of calcium stones been recognized in dogs and cats. To date, hypercalciuria is thought to be an important factor in formation. Hypercalciuria may occur in the presence or absence of hypercalcemia.

Calcium Oxalate Uroliths Associated with Hypercalcemia

Hypercalcemia results in hypercalciuria, which can lead to formation of calcium uroliths. Major causes of significant hypercalcemia include primary hyperparathyroidism, pseudohyperparathyroidism, and vitamin D intoxication.

Calcium oxalate uroliths associated with hypercalcemia are uncommon in comparison with calcium oxalate uroliths associated with normocalcemia. Nevertheless, measurement of serum calcium in all animals with calcium-containing uroliths is important in determining the underlying cause and in preventing recurrence.

Calcium Oxalate Uroliths Associated with Normocalcemia

Most dogs and cats with calcium oxalate uroliths are normocalcemic. Two major causes have been theorized for hypercalciuria with normocalcemia: increased intestinal absorption of calcium (absorptive hypercalciuria) and decreased renal reabsorption of calcium (renal-leak hypercalciuria). With absorptive hypercalciuria, there is a tendency to increased serum calcium, which suppresses parathyroid hormone (PTH) production. Urine calcium concentrations become normal with fasting. With renal-leak hypercalciuria, there is a tendency to decreased serum calcium, which stimulates PTH production. Urine calcium concentrations do not change with fasting. Preliminary studies in dogs indicate that either absorptive hypercalciuria or renal-leak hypercalciuria can occur in dogs with normocalcemic calcium oxalate uroliths.[2]

Urate Uroliths

Urate uroliths include those composed of uric acid, ammonium urate (also known as ammonium biurate and ammonium acid urate), and sodium urate (sodium acid urate). In dogs, 90% of urate calculi are ammonium urate in type (Fig. 18–5).[2] Dalmatian dogs are genetically predisposed to urate uroliths; however, 40% of urate uroliths occur in other breeds.[10] Also, although urates are the most common urolith in Dalmatians, approximately 25% of Dalmatians with uroliths have uroliths of another type.[10] Urate uroliths are more common in males than females. Urate uroliths can occur at any age, but are most frequent between the ages of 3 to 6 years.

Urate Uroliths in Dalmatians

The ability of the liver of Dalmations to oxidize uric acid to allantoin is intermediate between other dogs and humans as a result of a homozygous recessive gene in Dalmations.[2,11] This leads to a urine uric acid concentration in Dalmatians that is approximately 10 times the concentration in other dogs.[12] Although all Dalmatians excrete high concentrations of urate in urine, only a small percentage develop calculi, indicating that unknown factors are also important. Whether stone-forming Dalmatians excrete more urate than nonstone-formers is controversial,[2] owing to variability in measurement of urine urate in dogs.[11]

Urate Uroliths in Non-Dalmatians

The major defined cause of urate uroliths in non-Dalmatians is a portosystemic shunt. Calculi secondary to shunts occur in both males and females and are usually detected at a young age (< 3 years). Shunts, in which blood bypasses the liver, are associated with hepatic atrophy and dysfunction. This leads to hyperammonemia and hyperuricemia, which in turn leads to increased urine concentrations of ammonia and uric acid. Ammonium biurate crystals are common in dogs with portovascular shunts; however, calculi are not common. Similar to Dalmatians, other factors besides ammonium urate urine concentrations are probably involved in calculi formation.

Occasionally, urate calculi occur in non-Dalmatian dogs that do not have portosystemic shunts. The mechanism for formation of urate uroliths in these dogs has not been well defined, but a few of those studied have had hyperuricemia. Prolonged consumption of severely protein restricted diets and other causes of hepatic dysfunction such as cirrhosis have been associated, although rarely, with urate uroliths in dogs.[2]

Calcium Phosphate Uroliths

The most common forms of calcium phosphate uroliths are hydroxyapatite and carbonate-apatite. Because this type of urolith is uncommon, less is known about its pathogenesis. Hypercalciuria, as in calcium oxalate uroliths, is thought to be an important factor. Calcium phosphates are less soluble in alkaline urine.

Cystine Uroliths

Cystine uroliths are associated with cystinuria (Fig. 18–6). Cystine is a nonessential amino acid, which is normally reabsorbed in the renal proximal tubule. It is the least soluble of the naturally occurring amino acids.[2] Its solubility decreases markedly at pH less than 7.5. Cystinuria is caused by a genetic inability to reabsorb cystine and other amino aids from the proximal tubule. Other than the predisposition to formation of calculi, cystinuria is medically innocuous. Many breeds of dogs have been reported with cystine uroliths, but dachshunds and English bulldogs have been especially prev-

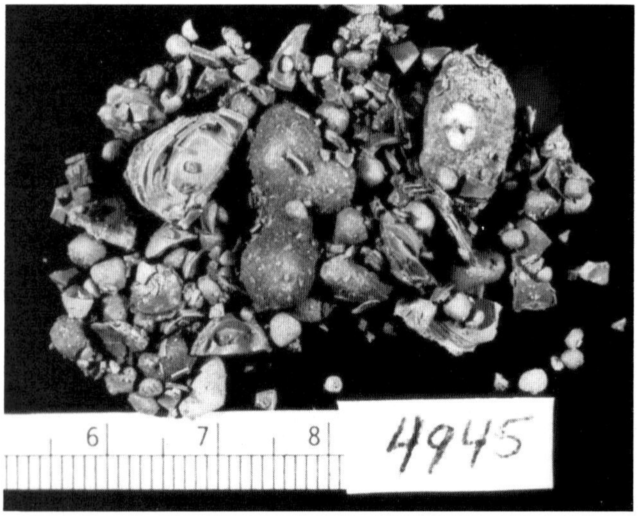

FIG. 18–5. Numerous urate uroliths.

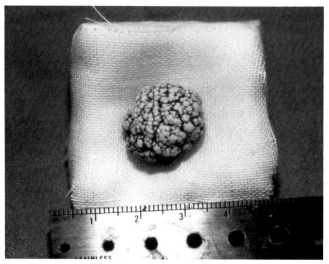

FIG. 18–6. Cystine urolith from the bladder of a dachshund.

alent. The average age of detection of cystine uroliths is 3 to 5 years.[13]

Not all cystinuric dogs form calculi, so other factors are probably important. It is known that cystine is less soluble in acid urine. Cystine uroliths are much more common in males than females,[9,14,15] even though cystinuria is occasionally found in females. The genetic mode of inheritance of cystinuria is unknown; both sex-linked and autosomal recessive patterns have been suggested.[13,16]

Silica Uroliths

Most silica uroliths are shaped like a child's jacks (jackstones). Calcium oxalate uroliths, however, also occasionally have the configuration of jacks. Silica uroliths have not been found in the kidney to date.[2]

The etiology of silica uroliths is unknown, but diets containing large amounts of corn gluten or soybean hulls are strongly suspected. Male dogs are most commonly affected.[9] The most frequent breed has been the German shepherd dog.[2]

CLINICAL SIGNS

The clinical signs associated with uroliths vary more with the location of the urolith than with the type of urolith. Uroliths can occur in animals of any age, although the majority occur in middle-aged adults.[14] In puppies, the most common presentation has been urethral obstruction in males.[5,14] Considering all age groups, the most frequent site of uroliths is the bladder.[15] No association has been noted between type of urolith and location in dogs.[15] Nephroliths in cats, however, tend to be predominantly calcium oxalate, whereas cystoliths in cats are predominantly struvite.[2]

Nephroliths

Occasionally, nephroliths cause hematuria, either gross or microscopic, or vague malaise. If the stone becomes quite large or produces hydronephrosis through pelvic or ureteral obstruction, an enlarged kidney may be palpable. Most nephroliths produce no clinical signs directly, however. Their silent presence damages normal tissue, predisposing to chronic inflammation and bacterial infection. If renal infection is severe, signs of systemic illness, such as anorexia, depression, and fever, may develop. As the urolith grows, it also displaces normal tissue (Fig. 18–7) and, if bilateral, can result in chronic renal failure. Polyuria and polydipsia may be noted with either pyelonephritis or renal failure.

Most nephroliths are identified on abdominal radiographs, which have been made in animals with uroliths in the bladder, urethra, or both; in animals with chronic or relapsing urinary tract infection; or in animals with chronic renal failure of unknown etiology (see Fig. 6–12). They may be identified incidentally on abdominal radiographs taken for an unrelated purpose.

Calcium uroliths in the kidneys of cats are often clin-

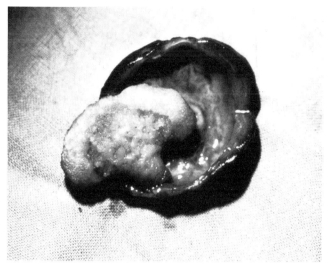

FIG. 18–7. Nephrolith that through its growth destroyed most of the renal tissue.

ically silent for years. Surgery should be performed in cats with nephroliths only if hematuria, UTI, declining renal function, changes in renal size and shape, or increasing nephrolith size are found on repeat examinations.[2]

Ureteroliths

Ureteroliths are uncommonly described in dogs and cats. In the few cases seen by the authors, either the animal was asymptomatic, or the predominant sign was abdominal pain. Others have described hematuria.[17] Prolonged partial obstruction can cause hydroureter and hydronephrosis (see Fig. 6–20).

Cystoliths

Some cystoliths are asymptomatic, being detected by abdominal palpation or abdominal radiography (see Fig. 6–35). Other cystoliths produce signs related to lower urinary tract inflammation, e.g., dysuria and hematuria. Struvite cystoliths can result from bacterial cystitis. Any type of cystolith can predispose UTI, which produces similar clinical signs.

Urethroliths

Urethral calculi are one of the predominant causes of urethral obstruction (see Chapters 12 and 15). The obstruction may be complete or partial, depending on the size and number of uroliths present. The most prominent initial clinical sign is dysuria. Hematuria may also be noted. If the obstruction is complete and not relieved promptly, postrenal uremia develops. A paradoxical type of incontinence occurs as increased pressure cranial to the obstruction forces drops of urine past the obstruction and out the urethral orifice.

DIAGNOSIS

Uroliths are determined to be present by palpation or by radiography. The mineral composition of the urolith can be definitively determined only by quantitative stone analysis. An educated guess as to the composition of the urolith can be made by considering signalment, history of previous stone formation, urinalysis, urine culture, serum calcium concentration, and radiodensity of the urolith.

Palpation

Cystoliths are often palpable, especially if the bladder is only mildly distended or empty. The bladder should be thoroughly palpated in all dogs and cats presented for dysuria or hematuria. If the bladder is full, voluntary urination should be observed. After the animal finishes voiding, the bladder should be repalpated. If it is still full, urethral obstruction may be present. If it is empty, it may be palpated for calculi as well as other abnormal masses. Cystoliths are more easily palpated in dogs than cats because the most common type of urolith in cats, sterile struvite, is often of small size.

Urethroliths are often palpable in dogs but not in cats. In male dogs, urethroliths are commonly felt in the urethra just caudal to the os penis. Calculi may also be felt in the perineal and pelvic urethra. In female dogs, urethral calculi may be felt by palpation of the urethra per rectum. Nephroliths and ureteroliths are not palpable.

Radiography

Whenever a urolith is detected by palpation in the lower urinary tract, abdominal radiographs should be taken to check the rest of the urinary tract for calculi. Abdominal radiographs are also indicated in animals that have chronic or rapidly relapsing urinary tract infections or hematuria or pyuria of unknown etiology, any of which may be secondary to urolithiasis.

The radiodensity of a urolith varies somewhat with its mineral composition (Table 18–3). Radiodensity is relative, however. Most uroliths in dogs and cats have some degree of radiodensity, although it may be minimal. Within one mineral type, radiodensity is suffi-

ciently variable that it alone cannot be used to predict the type of urolith. Radiodense uroliths can be seen with survey radiographs (see Figs. 6–12, 6–35). To visualize radiolucent uroliths, contrast-enhanced radiography (retrograde urethrography, cystography, excretory urography) or ultrasonography is required (see Figs. 6–17, 6–28, 6–36, 6–43).

Uroliths always have the potential of moving within the urinary tract. If several days have elapsed between radiography and surgery to remove uroliths, it is always a good idea to repeat the radiographs to recheck urolith location. One may find that some of the calculi that were in the bladder 1 week ago have moved into the urethra. If a cystotomy only is performed, calculi will be missed.

Urinalysis/Urine Culture

Many parts of the urinalysis are important. The urine specific gravity should be evaluated for evidence of concentrating ability as a preliminary index of renal function (see Chapter 1). A urine specific gravity between 1.008 and 1.030 in the face of dehydration or azotemia would be suggestive of renal dysfunction. A careful radiographic search for nephroliths would be indicated.

An alkaline urine pH would be one factor that suggests that calculi are struvite, although calcium phosphate uroliths also form in alkaline urine. Urate and cystine calculi are associated with acidic urine. The urine pH with calcium oxalate uroliths is variable.

If crystalluria is noted, the type of crystal is an important clue in determining the type of urolith (see Figs. 5–3, 12–4; Figs. 18–8, 18–9). The presence of one type of crystal in urine, however, does not guarantee that the urolith is composed of the same type of mineral. All the facts about the case must be considered in forming an educated guess as to the type of urolith.

Urinary tract inflammation or hemorrhage can occur with any type of urolith. With struvite uroliths, UTI predisposes to urolith development. Damage to the mucosa of the urinary tract by other types of uroliths results in inflammation and hemorrhage as well as bacterial infection.

A culture of urine should always be performed on dogs with urolithiasis and in cats with evidence of pyuria or bacteriuria on urinalysis. Finding staphylococci or *Proteus* on urine culture in association with alkaline urine would strongly suggest that calculi present were struvite. Other calculi are not associated with infection with specific organisms. Many infections with other calculi are caused by *Escherichia coli*, the most common urinary pathogen.

Hematology

A complete blood count is performed to detect evidence of a systemic inflammatory response. An inflammatory leukogram in an animal with calculi would suggest bacterial pyelonephritis or bacterial prostatitis. Cystic calculi and bacterial cystitis are usually not associated with a systemic inflammatory response. Urethral calculi may

---

TABLE 18–3. RADIODENSITY OF COMMON URINARY CALCULI

Type of Calculus	Radiodensity
Struvite	
Infection type	Radiodense
Sterile	Variable
Calcium oxalate	Radiodense
Urate	Relatively radiolucent
Calcium phosphate	Radiodense
Cystine	Relatively radiolucent
Silica	Variable, usually radiodense

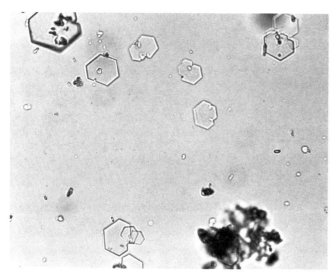

FIG. 18—8. Cystine crystals in urine (Courtesy of Dr. Robert Duncan, Department of Pathology, College of Veterinary Medicine, University of Georgia, Athens, GA.)

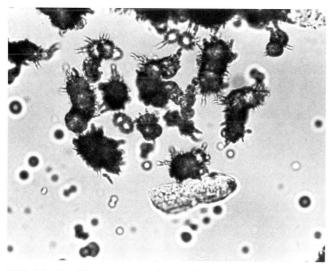

FIG. 18—9. Biurate crystals in urine.

be associated with a stress leukogram if urethral obstruction and postrenal uremia are present. Urethral calculi producing partial or complete obstruction and in conjunction with UTI can result in bacteremia and leukocytosis. This may be caused by bacteria crossing through damaged and ischemic lower urinary tract tissue into the blood stream.

Blood Chemistry

Measurement of blood urea nitrogen (BUN), serum creatinine, serum electrolytes, serum calcium and phosphorus, and liver enzymes and measures of liver function (BUN, glucose, albumin) are indicated in all animals with uroliths.

Serum creatinine and BUN concentrations, in con-

junction with urine specific gravity, help estimate renal function in animals without urethral obstruction (see Chapter 3) and help estimate severity and duration of obstruction in animals with urethral obstruction. Serum electrolytes (sodium, potassium, chloride, total CO_2) are indicated in animals with urethral obstruction. Acid-base status can also be useful in animals with persistently alkaline urine that is not associated with urease-producing bacteria.

Serum calcium is measured to detect hypercalcemia, which would be suggestive of calcium-containing calculi. Serum phosphorus is evaluated in conjunction with calcium to help determine potential causes of hypercalcemia.

Increased hepatic enzymes or a low BUN, glucose, or albumin concentration is suggestive of hepatic disease or hepatic dysfunction. In an animal with uroliths and these blood chemistry abnormalities, especially if the uroliths are fairly radiolucent, urate calculi would be most likely. Further liver function tests and portography to identify shunts would be indicated. The history of the animal's illness should also be reviewed to determine whether behavioral abnormalities consistent with hepatic encephalopathy had been noted.

Urolith Analysis

To perform analysis of a urolith, one must have a urolith to submit for analysis. Uroliths are usually recovered from the urinary tract at surgery (see Chapter 19). With increasing emphasis on medical dissolution of uroliths, however, nonsurgical retrieval of uroliths should be attempted. Occasionally, small uroliths are passed in the urine. In female dogs and cats, these may become trapped in the vagina or in the coat around the vulva, from which they can be retrieved and submitted for analysis. Any calculi removed by urethral flushing in males should also be submitted for analysis. In dogs and cats of either sex, straining of voided urine may detect small uroliths trapped in the sieve.

There are two types of stone analysis available to clinicians: qualitative and quantitative. Qualitative analysis, such as with the Oxford Stone Analysis Kit, is too inaccurate to be of clinical use.[18-20] All uroliths should be analyzed quantitatively by one of several methods, the most frequently used being optical crystallography and x-ray diffraction. A few laboratories providing quantitative analysis to veterinarians are listed in Table 18–4. A proper quantitative analysis should give all the mineral components of the urolith by percentage and by location (center, middle, outer portion of the urolith).

Uroliths may also trap bacteria as they form, and these bacteria often remain viable. Laboratories that analyze uroliths can also culture them at an additional cost.[21] The center of the urolith is used for culture. The urolith must be at least 5 mm in size to enable culturing the center without surface contamination.[21] We usually reserve urolith culture for struvite calculi in dogs without urinary infection with staphylococci or *Proteus*. In these animals, we are trying to ensure that the calculi are sterile and not induced by infection.

TABLE 18–4. LABORATORIES THAT PROVIDE
QUANTITATIVE ANALYSIS OF
UROLITHS FOR VETERINARIANS

Urinary Stone Analysis Laboratory
Room 3106 Medical Sciences Building
Department of Medicine
School of Veterinary Medicine
Davis, CA 95616

Minnesota Urolith Center
College of Veterinary Medicine
University of Minnesota
St. Paul, Minnesota 55108

Urolithiasis Laboratory
Baylor College of Medicine
Division of Urology
PO Box 25375
Houston, TX 77005

LC Herring and Co
PO Box 2191
Orlando, FL 32707

MEDICAL THERAPY

One aspect of medical therapy of uroliths is directed toward eliminating the uroliths by prompting their dissolution, rather than by surgical removal. Medical therapy is always indicated in preventing recurrence of uroliths after either surgical removal or medical dissolution. Medical therapy is also indicated to control associated UTI.

Medical Dissolution of Uroliths

Medical dissolution is based on the principle that undersaturation of fluid with the mineral components of a crystal will prompt dissolution of the crystal in that fluid. In relationship to uroliths, if the characteristics of urine can be changed appropriately, the urine can be made undersaturated with the mineral components in the urolith, and the urolith will begin to undergo dissolution. Because uroliths must be bathed in urine for dissolution to be possible, dissolution is most successful for uroliths in the bladder. Nephroliths may also be dissolved if renal function is adequate in the affected kidney. A longer time is required to dissolve nephroliths. Ureteroliths and urethroliths cannot be dissolved medically unless they move or are moved into the bladder. Dissolution of cystoliths requires 2 to 4 months. If urethroliths in male dogs are retropulsed into the bladder and the dog placed on dissolution therapy, the risk of recurrent obstruction from calculi moving back into the urethra exists during the weeks of medical dissolution.

Methods for dissolving calculi have been established for struvite calculi in dogs and cats and urate and cystine calculi in dogs but not for calcium or silica-containing uroliths. Therapy for dissolution differs with each type of urolith. Thus, the type of urolith must be known on the basis of quantitative analysis, or a highly educated guess must be made based on clinical findings. If the treatment decision is based on an educated guess and the urolith does not dissolve as expected, the guess may be wrong, or the urolith may contain more than one type of mineral. Surgical removal and quantitative analysis is indicated if there is minimal decrease in urolith size after 2 months of medical therapy.

Animals that are being treated medically to dissolve calculi must be evaluated frequently. These evaluations should include complete blood count, biochemical profiles, urinalysis, urine culture, and radiography. The evaluations are performed at 4-week intervals, unless the animal's condition warrants more frequent evaluations.

The decision as to whether to use medical or surgical therapy for urolithiasis should be individualized to each animal. The decision must consider the location and type of urolith, the age and sex of the animal and the severity of its clinical signs, the presence of other diseases, the anesthetic risk, and the owner's desires and willingness to comply with the stringent requirements of medical dissolution. Size and number of uroliths do not seem to affect the efficacy of medical therapy.[22] Cost is often not significantly different. The expense of surgical therapy is anesthesia and surgery, whereas the expense of medical therapy is special diets, medication, and medical re-evaluations that must include radiography to monitor urolith size. In certain situations, surgery is the preferred method of therapy. These are listed in Chapter 19.

Infection-Induced Struvite Uroliths

Dissolution of struvite uroliths, which have formed secondary to infection with urea-splitting organisms, requires control of the infection and reduction of urine concentrations of ammonium, magnesium, and phosphate.

By eliminating infection, urine pH shifts from alkaline to acid, thus increasing struvite solubility. Infection is eliminated by administration of an appropriate antimicrobial agent. The antibiotic is chosen by knowledge of the causative organism by urine culture and by antibiotic sensitivity testing. Most staphylococci and *Proteus* spp are sensitive to ampicillin, amoxicillin, and penicillin (see Table 15–2), unless they have become resistant through prior exposure. Antibiotics should be administered at full dosage for 2 weeks beyond the time that the uroliths are no longer radiographically visible. As already noted, urinalysis and urine culture should be performed on each recheck evaluation during medical dissolution to ensure that the infection is being controlled.

Prescription diets are usually used to reduce the concentration of mineral constituents of struvite. Prescription diet canine s/d (Prescription Diets, Hill's Pet Products, Inc., Topeka, KS 66601) is formulated to be restricted in protein (to reduce urine urea concentration), magnesium, phosphorus, and calcium (to reduce urine mineral concentration and maintain calcium/phosphorus balance). The diet contains supplemental salt to stimulate polydipsia and polyuria. The diet is also formulated to result in acid urine. Contraindications to the use of this diet include any conditions in which salt should not be supplemented including edema, ascites, hypertension, heart failure, and liver failure, and in animals with hypoalbuminemia (Table 18–5).[2,12] The diet should be instituted slowly over weeks in animals in renal failure to be sure hypertension does not develop. The diet is not recommended in growing dogs, in reproducing dogs, in dogs treated surgically, or for prevention of recurrence (long-term use).[23]

If the owner is appropriately feeding only canine s/d, there should be a reduction in BUN concentration, a urine specific gravity of less than 1.016, and a urine pH of less than 6.6. If such changes are not evident, the owner may not be complying with the dietary recommendations. Serum albumin concentrations also often fall. Concentrations of serum alkaline phosphatase often increase. These changes have been associated primarily with the reduced protein concentration in the diet. The animal's body weight, serum albumin, and serum alkaline phosphatase should be monitored during therapy. BUN should also be monitored to determine owner compliance with the diet. Clinicopathologic changes have reversed when the diet was discontinued.[24]

In cats, the corresponding diet is feline s/d (Prescription Diets, Hill's Pet Products). Feline s/d is restricted in magnesium, phosphorus, and calcium (but not protein) and supplemented with salt. It is also designed to result in a urine pH of about 6.0. It has similar contraindications as listed for canine s/d. It should also not be fed if metabolic acidosis is present.[23]

To dissolve calculi, only the prescription diet can be fed with no supplements. The diet must be fed for 2 to 4 weeks after calculi are no longer visible radiographically. Urinary acidifiers are contraindicated when using these already acidifying diets. Because of the different nutritional requirements of cats and dogs, the species-appropriate food must be fed. Note again that these diets should not be fed to growing dogs or cats. Surgery is the appropriate therapy for immature animals with struvite calculi.

In dogs, infection-induced struvite uroliths have re-

quired a mean of 3 months of medical therapy to dissolve, with a range of 2 weeks to 7 months.[2] In cats, infection-induced struvite uroliths are relatively uncommon, but the time required for dissolution in three cats ranged from 9 to 13 weeks.[25]

Sterile Struvite Uroliths

Prescription diets are the primary mode of therapy for sterile struvite uroliths. Canine s/d is used in dogs and feline s/d in cats. The same precautions and contraindications exist as already noted. Sterile struvite uroliths generally dissolve faster than those associated with infection. In dogs, the mean time of dissolution was 6 weeks, with a range of 1 to 3 months.[2] In cats, sterile struvite uroliths dissolved in a mean of 5 weeks, with a range of 2 to 20 weeks.[25,26]

Urate Uroliths Unassociated with Portovascular Shunts

Medical dissolution of urate calculi involves using drugs, which decrease formation of uric acid; alkalinizing the urine; and modifying the diet. Because urate uroliths are difficult to visualize radiographically, therapy should be continued for 1 month beyond the time the uroliths can no longer be visualized by radiography.[2,27] The time required for dissolution has ranged from 8 to 11 weeks.

These recommendations are for dogs only. They have not been evaluated for safety or efficacy in cats. Surgery remains the recommended therapy for urate uroliths in cats.

Allopurinol decreases the formation of urate by inhibiting the enzyme xanthine oxidase, which normally converts xanthine to uric acid. The dosage is 30 mg/kg/day divided into two or three doses.[2] Although no adverse effects have been described in dogs, many adverse effects occur in humans, including further decline in renal function in individuals with underlying renal insufficiency.

Urine alkalinization is usually achieved with sodium bicarbonate. The dosage given should maintain a urine pH of approximately 7.0. The initial dosage is 2 grains/kg/day (approximately 125 mg/kg/day) in two to three doses. The owner can then monitor urine pH with pH paper so that appropriate dosage adjustments can be made. Dosages as high as 600 mg/kg/day may be needed.[12] One quarter of a teaspoon of sodium bicarbonate powder contains approximately 1 g.

The goal of dietary modification is to reduce uric acid intake, which is primarily contained in purine-containing glandular organs (e.g., kidney, liver). Prescription diet u/d (Prescription Diets, Hill's Pet Products) has been recommended by some,[2] whereas others have recommended prescription diet s/d.[10,27] Both diets are similarly protein restricted. The advantage of u/d is that it tends to produce more alkaline urine, whereas s/d acidifies the urine. The advantage of s/d is that it is high in sodium to induce diuresis. A perfect prescription diet that would combine these advantages is not available.

TABLE 18–5. CONTRAINDICATIONS TO USE OF SUPPLEMENTAL SALT EITHER IN THE DIET OR ADDED TO THE DIET

Hepatic failure
Cardiac failure
Edema/ascites
Hypertension
Renal failure*

* Renal failure is a relative contraindication because animals with renal failure may be hypertensive and those with glomerular disease are prone to edema. Institute salt supplementation gradually over weeks in animals with renal failure after measuring blood pressure. Also, discontinue salt supplementation gradually in animals with renal failure, as their ability to adapt to sudden changes is limited.

Sodium bicarbonate could be added to s/d. Salt (⅓ teaspoon/10 kg/day; 200 mg/kg/day) or water could be added to u/d. Remember the contraindications to the use of salt (see Table 18–5).

Urate Uroliths Associated with Portovascular Shunts

Surgical correction of the shunt should be performed. It is still unknown whether such therapy alone results in dissolution of urate uroliths. The safety and efficacy of allopurinol in dogs with hepatic dysfunction are unknown. Most dogs to date have been treated surgically.

Cystine Uroliths

Medical dissolution of cystine uroliths involves drugs to decrease formation of cystine, urine alkalinization, and dietary modification. Dissolution requires 2 to 4 months.[28] Drug therapy is thought to be more important than diet or alkalinization.[13]

N-(2-mercaptopropionyl)-glycine (Thiola, Mission Pharmacal Co, San Antonio, TX 78296) (2-MPG) decreases the concentration of cystine in urine by combining with cystine to form a disulfide of cysteine, which is much more soluble than cystine. This drug is less toxic than D-penicillamine, which acts similarly. The dosage of both drugs is 30 mg/kg/day given once a day or divided into 2 equal doses.[29] The optimal dosage of 2-MPG for dogs is still unknown and may vary with individuals.[28] These drugs can cause nonpruritic vesicular skin lesions, vomiting, fever, Coombs' positive hemolytic anemia, and lymphadenopathy (Fig. 18–10).[29]

Sodium bicarbonate or potassium citrate (Urocit-K, Mission Pharmacal Co) is given orally to alkalinize the urine to a pH of approximately 7.0.

Reducing dietary protein has been recommended via feeding prescription diet u/d.[29] Others have noted that low protein intake has little effect on urine cystine, at least in humans.[12,13] At present, the effect of low protein diets on cystine excretion in dogs remains unknown.

Urine volume can be increased by adding water to whatever diet is fed or by salting the food (⅓ tsp/10 kg/day) to increase water intake. The goal is to maintain urine specific gravity at less than 1.025. The client's ability to manage a dog with polyuria and polydipsia should be considered before instituting this therapy. Remember that salt should not be supplemented in animals with heart disease, liver disease, edema or ascites of any cause, and hypertension. Salt supplementation should be instituted gradually in dogs with renal failure (see Table 18–5).

Prevention of Recurrence of Uroliths

Uroliths always tend to recur if preventive measures are not instituted. The factors that predisposed the animal to calculi formation are not addressed by surgical therapy. Although the principles of prevention are the same as those for medical dissolution, preventive measures must be safe for lifelong use (Table 18–6). Because preventive measures are not always easy or inexpensive for the client to maintain, it should always be the client's

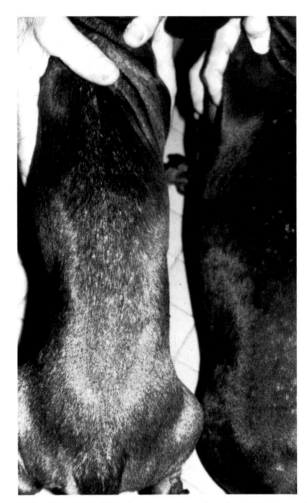

FIG. 18–10. Skin lesions that developed in two dachshunds being treated with D-penicillamine. The dogs' coats returned to normal when the drug was discontinued.

choice whether to comply or not. It is unfair to the client and the animal not to discuss the importance of preventive measures in all animals with uroliths. Multiple recurrences of uroliths often can and should be avoided with appropriate care based on the type of calculus identified.

Infection-Induced Struvite Uroliths

The most important factor in preventing recurrence is to eliminate infection first and then monitor for recurrence of infection. To be sure infection has been eliminated and not just suppressed, urine cultures should be performed at each re-evaluation during calculi dissolution. Antibiotic therapy should be continuous throughout dissolution and for 2 weeks beyond the last radiographic evidence of uroliths. If uroliths have been treated surgically, antibiotics should be continued for 4 weeks postoperatively. Approximately 1 week after discontinuing antibiotics and every month thereafter for 2 months, a urinalysis and urine culture should be performed to detect any recurrence of infection. In addition, the owner should monitor urine pH several times a week on urine collected in the morning prior to feeding

TABLE 18–6. COMMON DOSAGES OF
MEDICATIONS USED IN
DISSOLUTION AND PREVENTION
OF RECURRENCE OF UROLITHS*

Medication	Dosage
Sodium bicarbonate†	120–200 mg/kg/day (1 g = ¼ tsp)
Salt	200 mg/kg/day (2 g = ⅓ tsp)*
Allopurinol	30 mg/kg/day divided tid for dissolution 10 mg/kg/day for prevention
Penicillamine	30 mg/kg/day divided bid
2-Methylproprionyl-glycine	30 mg/kg/day once or divided bid
Hydrochlorothiazide	4–8 mg/kg/day divided bid
Potassium citrate†	15–60 mEq/day divided bid or 100–150 mg/kg/day divided bid
Ammonium chloride‡	200 mg/kg/day divided with meals
DL-methionine‡	600 mg/day divided with meals

* See text for specific indications and contraindications.
† These are used to alkalinize the urine. The doses given are approximate. These should be used to effect: to produce a urine pH of >7.0.
‡ These are used to acidify urine. The doses given are approximate. These should be used to effect: to produce a urine pH of 6–6.5.

(to avoid the postprandial alkaline tide). If the owner notes a urine pH greater than 7.5, the owner should return the dog as soon as possible for urinalysis and urine culture because infection with urea-splitting organisms may have begun.

Sterile Struvite Uroliths

Prevention of recurrence of sterile struvite uroliths is more difficult than infection-induced struvite uroliths because the cause is less well understood. To date, most emphasis has been placed on diet or use of urinary acidifiers. Less proof is available to date that such therapy is beneficial.

In cats, feline c/d (Prescription Diets, Hill's Pet Products, Inc) is generally used to try to prevent recurrence of sterile struvite uroliths. Feline c/d is restricted in magnesium, phosphorus, and calcium and tends to promote acid urine. It is not restricted in protein and sodium content and is similar to regular cat foods. Alternatively, urinary acidifiers can be used in conjunction with regular cat foods. Dosages are 600 mg/cat/day for d,l-methionine or ammonium chloride.[25] These are relatively high dosages. As noted in Chapter 12, there is concern for long-term use of acidifying diets as well as acidifiers.[30] Feline c/d was also associated with hypokalemia in cats, especially if renal dysfunction was present.[31] The amount of potassium in cat foods has been increased to avoid this problem.

In dogs, canine c/d (Prescription Diets, Hill's Pet Products, Inc) has been recommended to prevent recurrence of sterile struvite uroliths.[23] Canine c/d is mildly restricted in protein as well as being restricted in magnesium, phosphorus, and calcium. It promotes acidic urine. It is also restricted in sodium, which diminishes its efficacy in promoting diuresis. The efficacy of this type of diet is unknown.[2] Another option is to increase urine volume by salting the animal's regular food (about ⅓ tsp/10 kg/day) or by mixing water with the food to achieve a urine specific gravity of less than 1.025. Additional water may be eliminated in the feces so it is important to measure urine specific gravity to ascertain that increased water intake is increasing urine output. In addition, urinary acidifiers can be given to maintain a urine pH of less than 6.5.

Calcium Oxalate Uroliths

Because the importance and frequency of calcium-containing uroliths has only relatively recently been recognized, less is known about their prevention. Because this is a common type of urolith in humans, many recommendations have been extrapolated from human medicine. Methods of prevention currently focus on diet, use of diuretics, and use of citrate. If these uroliths are associated with hypercalcemia, however, the most important part of prevention is identification and successful therapy of the cause of the hypercalcemia. The most common cause of hypercalcemia associated with calcium oxalate uroliths is hyperparathyroidism.[2]

General dietary recommendations are to avoid excessive sodium or protein intake and not to restrict intake of phosphorus or magnesium. Diets designed for struvite uroliths (s/d, c/d) should *not* be used. Prescription diets k/d or u/d could be fed because they are restricted in sodium and protein and do not promote aciduria. These diets are not ideal, however, since they are phosphorus-restricted. Another option is to feed regular foods (not high protein). Supplemental salt should not be used to induce diuresis.

Thiazide diuretics have been used in humans to prevent calcium oxalate uroliths because they increase renal calcium absorption. For this reason, they should never be used in animals that are hypercalcemic. Animals whose hypercalciuria is caused by intestinal hyperabsorption of calcium may be predisposed to hypercalcemia with this therapy. Serum calcium must be monitored when thiazide diuretics are used for prevention. One reported dosage of chlorothiazide was 35 mg/kg/day divided into 2 doses.[2] Efficacy of thiazide diuretics to prevent calcium oxalate uroliths in dogs is unknown.[2]

Citrates prevent the formation of calcium oxalate crystals by chelating with calcium to form soluble salts. Citrates also alkalinize urine. Potassium citrate (Urocit-K, Mission Pharmacal Co) is usually used in humans. Efficacy in dogs is unknown, but a suggested dosage is 100 to 150 mg/kg/day divided into two doses.[8] A urine pH of at least 7.0 suggests that adequate urine citrate concentrations have been achieved. Side effects of potassium citrate have not been noted in dogs to date.

Urate Uroliths

Prevention is similar to medical dissolution. Dietary modifications and urine alkalinization should be continued. Urine should be examined for urate crystals. If hyperuricuria persists despite dietary therapy, allopurinol at a dosage of 10 to 20 mg/kg/day divided into two doses can be administered.[2] Note that this dose is less than the dose used for medical dissolution.

Cystine Uroliths

Prevention of recurrence of cystine uroliths is identical to therapy given for medical dissolution. Side effects reported with long-term use of 2-MPG (over 1 year) include skin lesions, which may resolve with dosage reduction, and abnormal urine odor.[28]

Calcium Phosphate Uroliths

There are currently no established methods for prevention of calcium phosphate uroliths. The guidelines for prevention of calcium oxalate uroliths should be followed. If these uroliths are associated with hypercalcemia, the cause of the hypercalcemia should be identified and treated.

Silica Uroliths

Since the cause of formation of silica uroliths is unknown, no specific guidelines are available for preventing recurrence. Some general guidelines are to change diets to one based on meat rather than plant proteins. In particular, diets with soybean hulls or corn gluten should be avoided.[2] As long as there are no diseases associated with salt retention, the diet can be salted to induce diuresis. The goal is a urine specific gravity of less than 1.030. The amount of salt to achieve this goal is variable from 500 mg to 10 g.[2] Urinary acidifiers and acidifying prescription diets should be avoided.

Treatment of Associated Urinary Tract Infection

The treatment of UTI required with infection-induced struvite uroliths has already been covered under "Medical Therapy" and "Prevention of Recurrence of Uroliths." Urinary tract infection may also occur with all other types of urinary calculi as a result of the tissue injury to the urinary tract that they induce. In all dogs with uroliths and in cats with suggestive urinalysis findings, urine obtained preferably by cystocentesis should be cultured. If an associated urinary tract infection is present, the causative organism should be identified. An appropriate antimicrobial agent is chosen, based on the identity of the organism (see Table 15–2), in association with antimicrobial sensitivity testing.

If the animal's urinalysis indicates infection and it is systemically ill or requires emergency surgery, antibiotic therapy should be begun before return of the results of urine culture. If the calculi are thought to be struvite, and the animal has not been on antimicrobial therapy recently, ampicillin or amoxicillin are drugs of choice. If the calculi are other than struvite, *Escherichia coli* is the most common organism. Trimethoprim/sulfa or enrofloxacin would be reasonable choices for oral therapy, pending culture results. Chloramphenicol or a first-generation cephalosporin would be reasonable for intravenous use during surgery or in animals appearing septic. Aminoglycosides could also be considered for parenteral use (subcutaneous or intramuscular administration) as long as renal function was not impaired and treated animals were monitored for nephrotoxicity.

If an animal has been placed on antibiotic therapy and a sensitivity test result indicates that the organism is not sensitive to the antimicrobial being given, a repeat urinalysis is indicated to check for efficacy in vivo before changing drugs, if the animal seems to be improving. Because of high urinary concentrations of most antimicrobials, sensitivity tests based on serum concentrations of drugs are often inaccurate in predicting in vivo response. Whenever a drug is instituted, a urinalysis and urine culture is indicated in 3 to 7 days to be sure the drug is efficacious.

Once an efficacious antibiotic is known, that drug should be continued for at least 4 weeks postoperatively or, with medical dissolution, for at least 2 weeks beyond the date that uroliths are last visualized radiographically. A drug that can be safely used for this period of time is essential. Aminoglycosides should be avoided.

To be sure the infection was eliminated and not merely suppressed, a urinalysis and urine culture should be performed approximately 1 week after therapy is stopped and monthly for 1 or 2 months.

REFERENCES

1. Osborne, C.A., Clinton, C.W., Bamman, L.K., et al.: Prevalence of canine uroliths. Vet. Clin. North Am. [Sm. Anim. Pract.], *16*:27, 1986.
2. Osborne, C.A., Polzin, D.J., Johnston, G.R., et al.: Canine urolithiasis. *In* Textbook of Veterinary Internal Medicine. Edited by S.J. Ettinger. Philadelphia, W.B. Saunders, 1989, pp. 2083–2107.
3. Osborne, C.A., Klausner, J.S., Polzin, D.J., et al.: Etiopathogenesis of canine struvite urolithiasis. Vet. Clin. North Am. [Sm. Anim. Pract.], *16*:67, 1986.
4. Klausner, J.S., Osborne, C.A., O'Leary, T.P., et al.: Experimental induction of struvite uroliths in miniature schnauzer and beagle dogs. Invest. Urol., *18*:127, 1980.
5. Hardy, R.M., Osborne, C.A., Cassidy, F.C., et al.: Urolithiasis in immature dogs. Vet. Med. Sm. Anim. Clin., *67*:1025, 1972.
6. Brown, C.C., Gibson, K.L., and Kreeger, J.M.: Obstructive urolithiasis in a 6-week-old puppy. J. Am. Anim. Hosp. Assoc., *24*:466, 1988.
7. Osborne, C.A., Poffenbarger, E.M., and Klausner, J.S.: Etiopathogenesis, clinical manifestations, and management of canine calcium oxalate urolithiasis. Vet. Clin. North Am. [Sm. Anim. Pract.], *16*:133, 1986.
8. Lulich, J.P., Osborne, C.A., Parker, M.L., et al.: Canine calcium oxalate urolithiasis. *In* Current Veterinary Therapy X. Edited by R.W. Kirk. Philadelphia, W.B. Saunders, 1989, pp. 1182–1188.
9. Ling, G.V., and Ruby, A.L.: Canine uroliths: Analysis of data derived from 813 specimens. Vet. Clin. North Am. [Sm. Anim. Pract.], *16*:303, 1986.

10. Senior, D.F.: Medical management of urate uroliths. *In* Current Veterinary Therapy X. Edited by R.W. Kirk. Philadelphia, W.B. Saunders, 1989, pp. 1178–1181.
11. Schaible, R.H.: Genetic predisposition to purine uroliths in Dalmatian dogs. Vet. Clin. North Am. [Sm. Anim. Pract.], *16:*127, 1986.
12. Senior, D.F.: Canine urolithiasis. *In* Nephrology and Urology. Edited by E.B. Breitschwerdt. New York, Churchill Livingstone, 1986, pp. 1–24.
13. Bovee, K.C.: Canine cystine urolithiasis. Vet. Clin. North Am. [Sm. Anim. Pract.], *16:*211, 1986.
14. Brown, N.O., Parks, J.L., and Greene, R.W.: Canine urolithiasis: Retrospective analysis of 438 cases. J. Am. Vet. Med. Assoc., *170:*415, 1977.
15. Bovee, K.C.: Genetic and metabolic diseases of the kidney. *In* Canine Nephrology. Edited by K.C. Bovee. Media, PA, Harwal Pub., 1984, pp. 339–354.
16. Brand, E., Cahill, G.F., and Kassell, B.: Canine cystinuria. J. Biol. Chem., *133:*431, 1940.
17. Kruger, J.M., and Osborne, C.A.: Etiopathogenesis of uric acid and ammonium urate uroliths in non-Dalmatian dogs. Vet. Clin. North Am. [Sm. Anim. Pract.], *16:*87, 1986.
18. Osborne, C.A., Clinton, C.W., Moran, H.C., et al.: Comparison of qualitative and quantitative analyses of canine uroliths. Vet. Clin. North Am. [Sm. Anim. Pract.], *16:*317, 1986.
19. Ruby, A.L., and Ling, G.F.: Methods of analysis of canine uroliths. Vet. Clin. North Am. [Sm. Anim. Pract.], *16:*293, 1986.
20. Bovee, K.C., and McGuire, T.: Qualitative and quantitative analysis of uroliths in dogs: Definitive determination of chemical type. J. Am. Vet. Med. Assoc., *185:*983, 1984.
21. Ruby, A.L., and Ling, G.V.: Bacterial culture of uroliths. Vet. Clin. North Am. [Sm. Anim. Pract.], *16:*325, 1986.
22. Osborne, C.A., Polzin, D.J., Kruger, J.M., et al.: Medical dissolution of canine struvite uroliths. Vet. Clin. North Am. [Sm. Anim. Pract.], *16:*349, 1986.
23. Lewis, L.D., Morris, M.L., and Hand, M.S.: Small Animal Clinical Nutrition. Topeka, KS, Morris Animal Associates, 1987, pp. A2-1–A2-8.
24. Osborne, C.A., Polzin, D.J., Kruger, J.M., et al.: Medical dissolution and prevention of canine struvite uroliths. *In* Current Veterinary Therapy IX. Edited by R.W. Kirk. Philadelphia, W.B. Saunders, 1986, pp. 1177–1187.
25. Osborne, C.A., Kruger, J.M., Johnston, G.R., et al.: Feline lower urinary tract disorders. *In* Textbook of Veterinary Internal Medicine. Edited by S.J. Ettinger. Philadelphia, W.B. Saunders, 1989, pp. 2057–2082.
26. Osborne, C.A., Kruger, J.M., Polzin, D.J., et al.: Medical dissolution and prevention of feline struvite uroliths. *In* Current Veterinary Therapy IX. Edited by R.W. Kirk. Philadelphia, W.B. Saunders, 1986, pp. 1188–1195.
27. Osborne, C.A., Kruger, J.M., Johnston, G.R., et al.: Dissolution of canine ammonium urate uroliths. Vet. Clin. North Am. [Sm. Anim. Pract.], *16:*375, 1986.
28. Hoppe, A., Denneberg, T., and Kagedal, B.: Treatment of normal and cystinuric dogs with 2-mercaptoproprionylglycine. Am. J. Vet. Res., *49:*923, 1988.
29. Osborne, C.A., Hoppe, A., and O'Brien, T.D.: Medical dissolution and prevention of cystine urolithiasis. *In* Current Veterinary Therapy X. Edited by R.W. Kirk. Philadelphia, W.B. Saunders, 1989, pp. 1189–1193.
30. Ching, S.V., Fettman, M.J., Hamar, D.W., et al.: The effect of chronic dietary acidification using ammonium chloride on acid-base and mineral metabolism in the adult cat. J. Nutr., *119:*902, 1989.
31. Dow, S.W., Fettman, M.J., Curtis, C.R., et al.: Hypokalemia in cats: 186 cases. J. Am. Vet. Med. Assoc., *194:*1604, 1989.
32. Ling, G.V., Franti, C.E., Ruby, A.L., et al.: Epizootiologic evaluation and quantitative analysis of urinary calculi from 150 cats. J. Am. Vet. Med. Assoc., *196:*1459, 1990.

19

Surgical Therapy for Urolithiasis

Surgical removal of uroliths is indicated in many instances,[1,2] including the following:

1. *Uroliths in immature dogs.* Prolonged low protein diets may retard growth, and the effects of low magnesium intake in a growing animal are unknown.
2. *Urinary tract obstruction.* Uroliths causing obstruction of the renal pelvis, ureter, or urethra are removed to treat and prevent postrenal uremia and to prevent further compromise of renal function. Removal of calculi from the urethra by catheterization and hydropropulsion should be attempted before resorting to urethral surgery (see Chapter 15). After retropulsion of calculi into the bladder of male dogs, cystotomy is indicated to prevent rapid reobstruction of the urethra.
3. *Concomitant presence of urinary tract anomalies.* Diverticulum of the urinary bladder, patent urachus, and urethral stricture may increase the susceptibility of the urinary tract to infections. Surgical correction may reduce incidence of urinary tract infection (UTI) and calculi formation.
4. *Unknown or unpredictable urolith composition.* The most accurate method for determining urolith composition is by quantitative analysis.
5. *Failure of medical therapy.* Medical therapy is most efficacious for certain types of bladder uroliths. Failure may be caused by inaccurate assumption of urolith composition, lack of owner compliance, inability to control UTI, or poor renal function (in the instance of nephroliths).
6. *Owner preference.* Some owners will not feed their dogs calculolytic diets, and some dogs will not eat the diet. The costs of surgical removal and medical dissolution are often comparable.

NEPHROTOMY

Surgical removal of nephroliths is indicated when there is uncontrollable infection, obstruction of the renal pelvis, progressive enlargement of nephroliths, or deterioration of renal function. The presence of nephroliths may cause persistent infection and destruction of renal parenchyma. Once the nephroliths are removed, there is potential for compensatory hypertrophy and improved renal function even in a diseased kidney.

Preoperative Evaluation

The diagnosis and medical therapy of nephroliths are discussed in Chapter 18. A thorough evaluation of renal function is done before surgical removal. In a nonazotemic dog, 24-hour endogenous creatinine clearance or subcutaneous exogenous creatinine clearance (see Chapter 5) can be used to measure glomerular filtration rate (GFR) of the entire renal mass and determine subclinical renal dysfunction. At referral centers, renal scintigraphy using technetium 99m dimercaptosuccinic acid (Tc99mDPTA), which is totally filtered by the renal glomeruli, can be used to determine single-kidney GFR and the relative contribution of each kidney.

Osmotic diuresis with mannitol is initiated before surgery to increase GFR, renal blood flow, and urine output and to help protect renal function during surgery.[3,4] An infusion of mannitol (0.25 to 0.5 g/kg of body weight) is given as a 20% solution during a 3- to 5-minute period. Urine output is monitored to evaluate the diuretic effect. After diuresis starts, a maintenance infusion of 5 to 10% mannitol in a balanced electrolyte solution can be continued to promote diuresis for 12 to 24 hours.[5]

Nephrotomy Versus Nephrectomy

A nephrectomy (removal of kidney) is performed when there is a nonfunctional, infected kidney on one side and a contralateral functional kidney. A nephrotomy (incision into kidney to remove nephroliths) is indicated for a noninfected kidney with marginal or better renal function.

Bilateral Nephroliths

Bilateral nephroliths are removed in one or two operations. The safest approach is to operate on one kidney, allow the animal and kidney to recover for 4 to 6 weeks, and then operate on the second kidney. In an azotemic animal, this management plan is always used. In a non-azotemic animal, if the expense of two operations discourages an owner from pursuing any treatment, we assume there is sufficient reserve renal function to allow removal of nephroliths from both kidneys during one operation. When there is concern regarding unilateral versus bilateral nephrotomy and nephrotomy versus nephrectomy, it may be necessary to refer the animal for determination of single-kidney GFR by radionuclide scans.

Bisection Nephrotomy Versus Pyelolithotomy

Surgical removal of nephroliths is done through a *bisection nephrotomy* or a *pyelolithotomy*. For a bisection nephrotomy, a longitudinal midline sagittal incision is made through the convex lateral surface of the kidney. A bisection nephrotomy is used to remove large nephroliths within a normal-sized renal pelvis or to remove multiple calculi within the diverticula. The procedure decreases function, at least temporarily, in the operated kidney. The amount of functional loss is probably determined by the surgical technique and suture materials used for the bisection nephrotomy, in addition to the preoperative status of the kidney.[6-8] A pyelolithotomy incision is made through the relatively avascular dorsolateral renal pelvis. It spares more renal parenchyma than bisection nephrotomy, but the technique can be used only to remove large calculi from a kidney with a greatly dilated renal pelvis.[9]

Bisection Nephrotomy[10]

A midline abdominal incision enables the surgeon to examine both kidneys and to explore the abdomen, if necessary. The incision extends caudally from the xiphoid process to at least the umbilicus. For examination of the urinary bladder, the abdominal incision is extended to the pubis. The approach to the kidneys from a midline incision is described in Figs. 10–1 and 10–2. After the kidney is located, a small hole is cut in the cranial part of the peritoneum covering the ventral surface of the kidney. The index finger is inserted into this hole, and the cranial pole of the kidney is elevated. Additional peritoneal and sublumbar fascial attachments are incised as needed to gain access to the renal vessels. The caudal pole of the kidney can remain within the peritoneal covering, since complete mobilization is usually not necessary.

A paracostal incision (see Fig. 10–5) is used if only one kidney needs surgery and abdominal exploration is unnecessary. The peritoneum does not need to be incised because the kidney remains in its retroperitoneal position with this approach. The kidney is elevated from the incision with umbilical tapes (Fig. 19–1).

With either approach, the cranial pole of the kidney

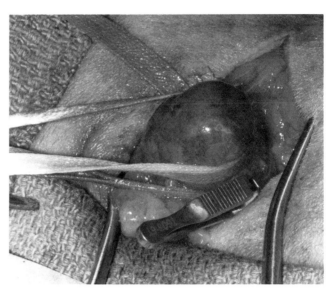

FIG. 19–1. Approach to right kidney through a paracostal incision. Kidney is elevated using umbilical tapes around the cranial and caudal poles. A vascular clamp is positioned on the renal artery.

is grasped and elevated. The renal vessels enter the kidney in the cranioventral region of the renal hilus. A moistened gauze sponge can be used to remove gently some of the fat surrounding the vessels. The renal artery, located on the craniodorsal surface of the renal vein, is identified. The primary renal artery divides into dorsal and ventral branches at varying distances from the aorta. Double or triple renal arteries are found in 12% of left renal arteries and 0.5% of right renal arteries in dogs.[11,12] If a single renal artery divides into dorsal and ventral branches near the aorta, it may appear to be a double artery.

A small mosquito hemostat or right-angle vascular clamp is used to separate the renal artery from the renal vein. A vascular clamp or a tourniquet is placed on the renal artery. Double or triple renal arteries and dorsal and ventral branches of a single renal artery can be clamped separately (Fig. 19–2A). Hemostats should not be used for temporary occlusion because they damage the vessel. The duration of ischemia to the normothermic canine kidney should not exceed 20 minutes.[4]

Occlusion of the renal artery and not the renal vein permits venous drainage of the kidney and increases pliability of the kidney. Occlusion of both the renal artery and the vein is not recommended because the kidney may slowly distend with blood from numerous small collateral arteries. The origins of these arteries include ovarian, uterine, ureteral, diaphragmatic, adrenal, lumbar, spermatic, phrenicoabdominal, and caudal mesenteric suprarenal arteries. In addition, because it is easier to separate the renal artery from the dorsal surface of the renal vein than to dissect completely around the renal vein, damage to the ureter and the renal vessels, nerves, and lymphatics is less likely.

After occlusion of the renal artery, the kidney is immobilized between the surgeon's thumb and forefinger. The renal capsule is incised sharply with a scalpel for

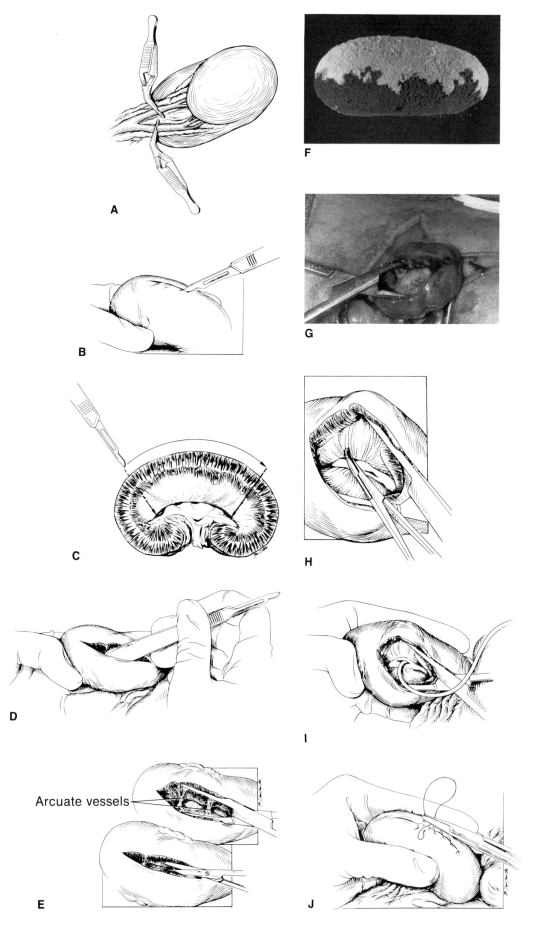

Arcuate vessels

approximately two thirds the length of the kidney (Fig. 19–2B). The incision should not extend over the cortical areas of the cranial and caudal poles of the kidney because this may cause additional parenchymal damage without increasing access to the renal pelvis (Fig. 19–2C).

The renal parenchyma is dissected bluntly with the scalpel handle or a blunt osteotome (Fig. 19–2D). This technique is preferable to sharp incision because it lessens damage to small veins and arteries and the renal hilus.

The cut edges of the kidney are gently separated with hemostats. If arcuate or interlobar vessels are spanning the incision, they are ligated and severed (Fig. 19–2E). These vessels are confronted because of the asymmetry of the blood supply to the canine kidney. The dorsal and ventral renal artery branches divide the kidney roughly into halves, with no arterial anastomoses between the dorsal and ventral segments. The avascular line that divides the dorsal and ventral halves (the intersegmental line), however, is undulating and seldom on the midline (Fig. 19–2F). Thus, a midline incision often traverses arcuate or even interlobar branches of the renal artery. A more complex technique, which involves identifying and incising between the dorsal and ventral segments of the kidney (intersegmental or anatrophic nephrotomy), has been described.[13] A study in normal dogs concluded that the reduction in GFR was similar after bisection and intersegmental nephrotomies[8]; therefore, bisection nephrotomy is recommended.

After the renal pelvis is opened, nephroliths are removed with forceps, taking care not to fragment the calculi (Fig. 19–2G). Urine or tissue can be taken for bacteriologic culture. Each diverticulum is systematically explored with a small mosquito forceps to ensure removal of all nephroliths (Fig. 19–2H). A 3.5 Fr gauge soft catheter and syringe is used to flush the diverticula with warm saline. The catheter is passed down the ureter to check for obstruction (Fig. 19–2I).

The two sides of the incision are apposed with digital pressure, while a simple continuous suture pattern is placed in the renal capsule (Fig. 19–2J). Size 4–0 po-lydioxanone suture material on a taper needle is recommended because it glides easily through the tissue and has minimal inflammatory reaction during absorption.[14] Mattress sutures through the renal parenchyma cause additional destruction of nephrons and are not needed.

The vascular clamp or tourniquet is removed, and the source of any hemorrhage from the kidney is identified. A bleeding collateral or capsular vessel can be controlled with ligation, or additional capsular sutures can be placed. Bleeding from a vessel within the parenchyma can usually be controlled by digital compression of the kidney. If an interlobar artery has been transected, it might be necessary to reclamp the renal artery and apply digital pressure for an additional 5 to 10 minutes.

The kidney is repositioned in its original site. The ureter is identified to ascertain that the kidney is not rotated. If the kidney is mobile, tacking sutures are placed between the renal capsule and the body wall to prevent rotation in the early postoperative period. Abdominal closure is routine.

Pyelolithotomy

For a pyelolithotomy, the kidney can be approached from a paracostal or midline incision. Through a paracostal incision, the kidney is retracted ventrally to expose the dorsal surface of the renal pelvis. From a midline incision, the uppermost (i.e., ventral) surface of the renal pelvis is obscured by the renal vessels (Fig. 19–3A). The peritoneal covering is cut, rather than torn, from the surface of the kidney because tearing the peritoneum causes more hemorrhage. The kidney is rotated over and toward the midline so that the dorsal surface is uppermost (Fig. 19–3B). The dilated renal pelvis and proximal ureter are incised longitudinally. Vascular occlusion is not necessary because the pelvis is relatively avascular. The nephrolith is gently removed from the pelvis and proximal ureter (Fig. 19–3C). A 3.5 Fr gauge soft catheter is passed into the diverticula, and saline is flushed (Fig. 19–3D). The catheter is passed distally into

◄

FIG. 19–2. Bisection nephrotomy. (A) Left kidney has been approached through a midline abdominal incision. Vascular clamps are placed on dorsal and ventral renal artery branches when the renal artery divides near the aorta. (B) Renal capsule is incised sharply with a scalpel blade for approximately two thirds the length of the kidney. (C) Midline sagittal section of canine kidney. The nephrotomy incision is made over the renal pelvis and does not extend over cortical areas of the cranial and caudal poles. (D) Renal parenchyma is dissected bluntly with the scalpel handle or a blunt osteotome. (E) If arcuate or interlobar vessels are spanning the incision, they are ligated and severed. (F) Corrosion cast of renal artery distribution. A light-colored material was injected into the dorsal branch of the renal artery and a dark-colored material into the ventral branch of the renal artery. The intersegmental avascular line is undulating and not on the midline. (G) Following a bisection nephrotomy, the cut edges of the kidney are gently separated, and a nephrolith is grasped with hemostats. (H) Each diverticulum is systematically explored with a small mosquito forceps to ensure removal of all nephroliths. (I) A 3.5 Fr gauge soft catheter is passed down the ureter to check for obstruction. (J) The two sides of the incision are apposed with digital pressure while a simple continuous suture pattern is placed in the renal capsule. (From Stone, E.A.: Canine nephrotomy. Compend. Contin. Educ. Pract. Vet., *9*:883, 1987; with permission.)

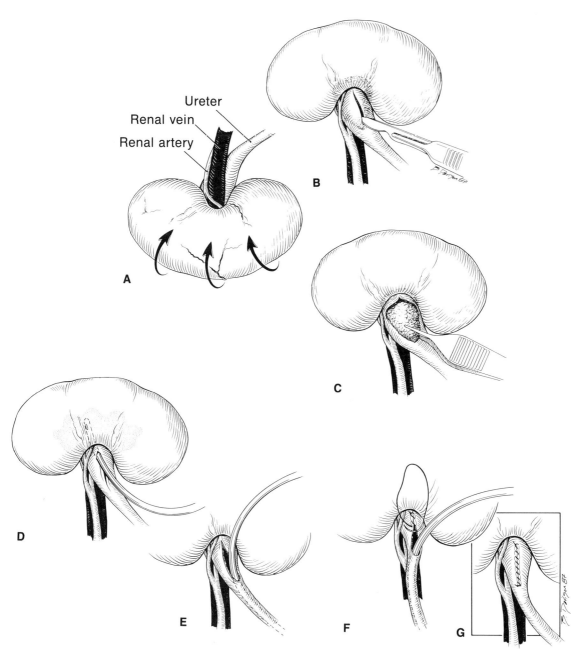

Ureter
Renal vein
Renal artery

A

B

C

D

E

F

G

FIG. 19–3. Pyelolithotomy. (A) Right kidney from a midline incision with surgeon standing on right side of the animal. Renal vessels lie ventral to the renal pelvis and ureter. The kidney must be rotated for access to the renal pelvis. (B) After the dorsal surface of renal pelvis is exposed, a longitudinal incision is made in the dilated renal pelvis and proximal ureter. (C) The calculus is gently lifted from the pelvis. (D) A small catheter is used to flush diverticula. (E) Catheter is passed distally into ureter to check for obstruction. (F) Catheter is left in place as the simple continuous closure is started. (G) Closure is complete.

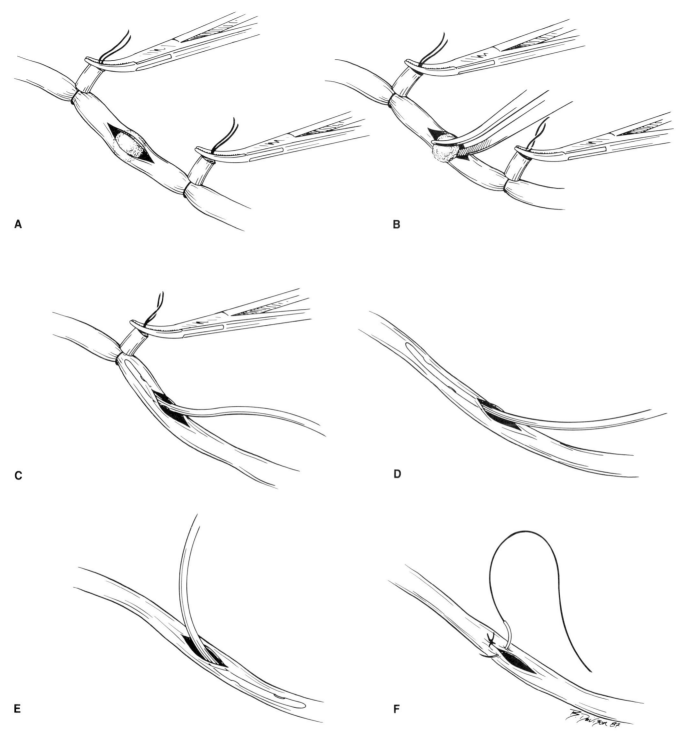

FIG. 19–4. Ureterotomy. (A) Tourniquets made from umbilical tape or silk suture looped through rubber tubing are placed around the ureter above and below the calculus. A longitudinal incision is made directly over the calculus. (B) Calculus is gently lifted from ureter. (C) Catheter is passed proximally with tourniquet in place, and ureter is flushed with saline. (D) Tourniquet is removed, and catheter is passed further proximally. Saline is instilled as catheter is passed. (E) Catheter is inserted distally to check for obstruction. (F) Closure of the ureteral incision is with 5–0 absorbable sutures in a simple interrupted pattern.

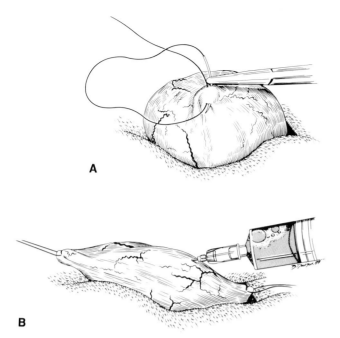

A

B

FIG. 19–5. Cystotomy. (A) A retention suture is placed in the cranial bladder wall. (B) Urine is aspirated from bladder using a 22-gauge needle and syringe.

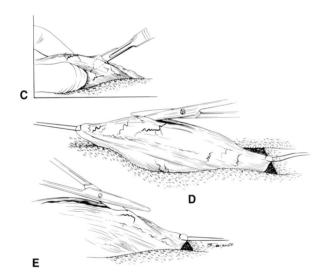

C

D

E

FIG. 19–5. (*Cont.*) (C) A stab incision is made into the bladder with a scalpel blade. (D,E) Incision is extended cranially and caudally with scissors.

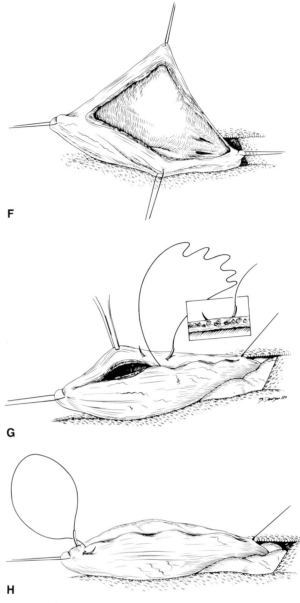

F

G

H

FIG. 19–5. (*Cont.*) (F) Retention sutures are placed lateral to the incised edges to open the bladder. If there are no indications for examining the trigone of the urinary bladder, the incision does not need to extend as far caudally as depicted here. (G) For closure with a Cushing pattern, the knot is made caudal to end of incision. After the knot is tied, one end is left long to be grasped by a hemostat. The needle does not enter the lumen (insert). (H) Final knot is tied cranial to the end of the incision.

the ureter (Fig. 19–3E), and the ureter is flushed. The catheter is retained initially to help the surgeon begin the closure (Fig. 19–3F). The pyelotomy incision is closed with 5–0 synthetic absorbable suture in a simple continuous pattern (Fig. 19–3G). An attempt is made to avoid placing suture material in the lumen of the pelvis and ureter. Unless the wall of the pelvis and ureter is thickened, however, it is usually necessary to penetrate the lumen to obtain a good seal.

URETEROTOMY

Ureteral calculi are rarely diagnosed in dogs and cats. An asymptomatic ureteral calculus is monitored by serial radiographs to see if it will advance into the bladder. A ureterotomy is performed to remove a stationary calculus or if hydroureter and hydronephrosis have developed.

The ureter is gently isolated, taking care to preserve

the vasculature and adventitia surrounding the ureter. Umbilical tape or silk suture is passed in a loop through a short piece of rubber tubing and used as a tourniquet above and below the calculus. The tourniquet stabilizes the ureter and prevents urine leakage into the abdominal cavity (Fig. 19–4A). The tourniquet also prevents calculus fragments from ascending or descending. A longitudinal incision is made directly over the calculus, and the calculus is gently lifted from the ureter (Fig. 19–4B). The catheter is passed proximally with the tourniquet in place, and the ureter is flushed with saline (Fig. 19–4C). The tourniquet is removed, and the catheter is passed further proximally, instilling saline as it is passed (Fig. 19–4D). Suction is used to remove urine and saline and prevent contamination of the abdomen. The catheter is inserted distally to check for obstruction (Fig. 19–4E). The incision is closed with 5–0 absorbable sutures in a simple interrupted pattern (Fig. 19–4F).

CYSTOTOMY

A caudal midline incision is made in cats or female dogs; a parapreputial incision is made in male dogs (see Fig. 10–3). After the bladder is located, a retention suture is placed in the cranial bladder wall (Fig. 19–5A). The bladder is isolated from the abdomen with moistened lap pads or towels. A ventral cystotomy incision is recommended because it provides better access to the trigone and the proximal urethra than a dorsal cystotomy, and the risk of leakage or adhesions is similar.[15] The length of the incision is determined by the size of the cystic calculi and the extent of the planned exploration of the bladder interior. Retention sutures are placed at the caudal end of the proposed incision.

Urine is aspirated from the bladder using a 22-gauge needle and syringe (Fig. 19–5B). The urine is submitted for urinalysis and bacteriologic culture, if these tests have not yet been done or if they need to be repeated. A stab incision is made into the bladder with a scalpel blade (Fig. 19–5C). The incision is extended cranially and caudally with scissors (Fig. 19–5D,E). Retention sutures are placed lateral to the incised edges to open the bladder. Calculi are removed with forceps or a bladder spoon. The bladder mucosa is inspected, and abnormal appearing areas are biopsied. If the incision is extended into the trigone, the ureteral openings will be visible (Fig. 19–5F). The trigone is flushed with saline. A catheter is passed into the urethra to dislodge any urethral calculi. Urethral calculi can often be dislodged by flushing the urethra alternately from the bladder and the urethral opening (see Fig. 16–2).

The incision is closed in one layer, using an inverting pattern in a bladder wall of normal thickness or a simple interrupted pattern in a thickened wall. The suture material does not enter the lumen of the bladder, and braided nonabsorbable suture material should not be used. Selection of suture material is discussed in Chapter 7.

For an inverting Cushing pattern, the closure begins caudal to the end of the incision (Fig. 19–5G). After the knot is tied, one end is left long to be grasped by a hemostat. The caudal retention suture can then be removed. The needle does not enter the lumen, and each bite of the needle overlaps the previous bite on the opposite side by about 50% of its length. An assistant can use a hemostat to invert the incised edges of the bladder gently as the suture is pulled snug. The final knot is placed cranial to the end of the incision (Fig. 19–5H), and the needle is passed perpendicular to the incision. After the closure is completed, only the knots are visible. The purpose of this pattern is to invert the incision and leave little exposed suture to induce adhesion formation. The cranial retention suture is removed. The abdomen is lavaged with warm saline, and the abdominal wall is closed routinely.

REFERENCES

1. Osborne, C.A., Klausner, J.S., Abdullahi, S., et al.: Medical dissolution and prevention of canine struvite uroliths. *In* Current Veterinary Therapy VIII. Edited by R.W. Kirk. Philadelphia, W.B. Saunders, 1983, pp. 1066–1072.
2. Stone, E.A.: Urologic surgery—an update. *In* Nephrology and Urology. Edited by E.B. Breitschwerdt. New York, Churchill Livingstone, 1986, pp. 75–88.
3. Morris, C.R., Alexander, E.A., Burns, F.J., et al.: Restoration and maintenance of glomerular filtration by mannitol during hypoperfusion of the kidney. J. Clin. Invest., *51:*1555, 1972.
4. Selkurt, E.E.: The changes in renal clearance following complete ischemia of the kidney. Am. J. Physiol., *144:*395, 1945.
5. Bovee, K.C., Rosin, A., and Hart, B.L.: Pathophysiology and therapeutics of urinary tract disorders. *In* Textbook of Small Animal Surgery. Edited by D.H. Slatter. Philadelphia, W.B. Saunders, 1985, pp. 1732–1754.
6. Gahring, D.R., Crowe, D.T., Powers, T.E., et al.: Comparative renal function studies of nephrotomy closure with and without sutures in dogs. J. Am. Vet. Med. Assoc., *171:*537, 1977.
7. Fitzpatrick, J.M., Sleight, M.W., Braack, A., et al.: Intrarenal access: Effects on renal function and morphology. Br. J. Urol., *52:*409, 1980.
8. Stone, E.A., Metcalf, M.R., and Robertson, J.L.: Glomerular filtration rate morphology after nephrotomy: A comparison of intersegmental and bisection nephrotomy (abstr). Vet. Surg., *19:*76, 1990.
9. Greenwood, K.M., and Rawlings, C.A.: Removal of canine renal calculi by pyelolithotomy. Vet. Surg., *10:*12, 1981.
10. Stone, E.A.: Canine nephrotomy. Compend. Contin. Educ. Pract. Vet., *9:*883, 1987.
11. Reis, R.H., and Tepe, P.: Variations in the pattern of renal vessels and their relation to the type of posterior vena cava in the dog (Canis familiaris). Am. J. Anat., *99:*1, 1956.
12. Shively, M.J.: Origin and branching of renal arteries in the dog. J. Am. Vet. Med. Assoc., *173:*986, 1978.
13. King, W.W.: Renal wound healing histologic and histochemical sequences in the repair of intersegmental nephrotomies. Invest. Urol., *11:*278, 1974.
14. Ray, J.A., Doggi, N., Regula, D., et al.: Polydioxanone (PDS), a novel monofilament synthetic absorbable suture. Surg. Gynecol. Obstet., *153:*497, 1981.
15. Desch, J.P., and Wagner, S.D.: Urinary bladder incisions in dogs. Comparison of ventral and dorsal. Vet. Surg., *15:*153, 1986.

20

Postoperative Management and Surgical Complications of Urolithiasis

POSTOPERATIVE MANAGEMENT

Retrieved calculi are submitted for quantitative analysis and for bacteriologic culture if the urine is sterile. If the animal had multiple calculi, radiographs are taken after surgery to document complete removal.

Intravenous fluid therapy (e.g., lactated Ringer's solution) is continued at a rate of 3 ml/kg body weight for 12 to 24 hours after surgery. Urination is monitored by observation and palpation. The flow of urine helps wash out blood clots and prevent obstruction. Fluid therapy is continued until the animal can maintain hydration by oral intake. The bladder is kept decompressed by allowing frequent urination, preferably, or by placement of an indwelling catheter.

If urine output decreases below 1.5 ml/kg/hr, the catheter is checked for patency, urine specific gravity is determined, and the animal is examined for signs of hypotension, hypovolemia, and dehydration. If urine output remains low once these abnormalities are corrected, a diuretic can be administered to increase urine output (see Chapter 8).

Treatment of urinary tract infection and prevention of calculi recurrence are discussed in Chapter 18. If a dog continues to have recurrence of calculi and urethral obstruction, a scrotal urethrostomy is performed (see Fig. 16–7) to allow small uroliths (0.2 to 0.5 cm, depending on dog's size) to pass from the urethra.

SURGICAL COMPLICATIONS

Hemorrhage

Minor hematuria is common after nephrotomy or cystotomy. The animal's hematocrit is monitored to assess blood loss. A dog with persistent hematuria should be evaluated for bleeding disorders.

Ureteral Stricture

Unilateral ureteral stricture following a ureterotomy in an animal with a normal opposite kidney could cause hydronephrosis with no clinical signs. If a narrowed ureteral lumen is detected on an excretory urogram, additional excretory urograms to follow changes are recommended. Persistence of a narrowed area suggests a ureteral stricture, which should be explored surgically, with resection of the strictured area and primary ureteral anastomosis or nephroureterectomy.

Urinary Bladder Granuloma

Granuloma formation can be induced by closure of a cystotomy incision with braided nonabsorbable suture material.[1] It has not been observed with other suture materials. The granuloma should be excised and the bladder closed with absorbable suture material. See Chapter 7 for discussion of suture materials.

REFERENCE

1. Pearl, G.S., and Someren, A.: Suture granuloma simulating bladder neoplasm. Urology, *15:*304, 1980.

Section Seven

Urinary Tract Trauma

21

Diagnosis and Medical Therapy of Urinary Tract Trauma

The organs of the urinary tract can be injured by blunt trauma (e.g., from automobiles, kicks, falls) or by penetrating trauma (e.g., from bullets, bites, fractured bone fragments). Damage may not be apparent immediately after trauma, but the owner should be forewarned of the possibility of urinary tract injury that could require further diagnostic workup and treatment. The potential for urinary incontinence secondary to neurologic injury must also be considered.

Urinary bladder rupture following automobile trauma is the most common form of urinary tract trauma. Iatrogenic damage can also occur; e.g., the bladder may be punctured during urinary catheterization, or a needle hole may leak after cystocentesis of devitalized bladder. Severe trauma to the abdominal wall may cause herniation of the bladder ventrally or into the femoral or inguinal canal. Damage to the kidneys and proximal ureters is much less common because these organs are protected by the rib cage and abdominal musculature, but they can be damaged by blunt trauma or penetrating objects such as a broken rib or a bullet. The ureter is occasionally damaged by accidental ligation during ovariohysterectomy. Urethral trauma occurs more frequently in male dogs. The pelvic urethra may be avulsed from the bladder or lacerated by bone fragments. In the perineal region, direct blunt trauma can injure and devascularize the urethra. A fractured os penis may lacerate the penile urethra.

CLINICAL SIGNS

Emergency diagnosis and treatment of life-threatening conditions such as shock and hemorrhage take precedence over evaluation of the urinary tract. Urologic injury should be suspected when there has been trauma to the abdomen, pelvis, or perineum. Signs of forceful injury include femoral or pelvic fracture, crush injury of the chest, or severe bruising of the abdomen. Clinical signs of urinary tract trauma vary with the organ injured and the duration of injury. Hematuria or dysuria are often present, but an animal with urinary tract trauma may void clear urine. Physical examination can be unreliable in diagnosing abdominal trauma and is usually nonspecific for urinary tract trauma.

Ascites

Hemoperitoneum

Because each kidney receives 12% of cardiac output, severe hemoperitoneum and shock quickly develop after avulsion of the renal pedicle, laceration of a major renal vessel, or shattering of the kidney. Exsanguination and death can rapidly ensue. Blood accumulates more slowly with minor or moderate damage to the kidney or bladder.

Uroperitoneum

Injury to the distal ureter, bladder, or proximal urethra can cause leakage of urine into the abdomen. Urine from a damaged renal pelvis or proximal ureter remains in the retroperitoneal space unless the peritoneum is torn. Sterile urine causes minimal irritation to the peritoneum, but infected urine can induce peritonitis. Injury to the bladder can vary from a small tear to a complete rupture. Signs may not be apparent for a few days, depending on the size of the hole. Small bladder tears may seal on their own. If the animal is anuric because of dehydration or hypovolemia, abdominal distention with urine may not develop until the animal is rehydrated and urine production has resumed.

Hematuria

Animals with urologic injury do not always have hematuria, and hematuria is common with any blunt abdominal trauma. Thus, hematuria is an unreliable sign of significant urologic injury. Persistence of hematuria, however, is an indication for radiographic evaluation of the urinary tract. Likewise, the absence of hematuria should not preclude radiographic studies, if other signs or diagnostic tests are suggestive of injury.

Bruising and Swelling

Clipping the hair of the abdomen and perineum allows thorough visual examination of the skin. A painful lumbar mass or bruise suggests possible renal trauma. Urine extravasation from a damaged urethra may cause perineal, scrotal, or preputial discoloration and swelling. If urine extravasation continues, necrosis and sloughing of the skin can occur.

Uremia

Prerenal causes for uremia such as dehydration and primary renal causes such as chronic renal failure must always be considered. See Chapter 3 for differentiating prerenal, renal, and postrenal causes of azotemia. An animal with a bladder rupture may become uremic within 48 hours. Experimentally, death from uremia occurred 2 to 4 days after urinary bladder rupture.[1] If urethral or bladder outlet obstruction occurs secondary to scar formation, uremia may develop weeks to months after trauma.

DIAGNOSTIC TESTS

Laboratory Tests

Increased serum concentrations of urea, creatinine, and potassium in a traumatized animal indicate renal failure, but they are not pathognomonic for urinary tract injury. As mentioned for uremia, prerenal and renal causes must also be considered.

The hematocrit may be increased because of vomiting and insufficient water intake, but extensive blood loss may mask hemoconcentration by decreasing the number of red blood cells.

Urine specific gravity is measured to help determine renal function. Microscopic analysis of urine sediment following trauma frequently reveals red blood cells. If bacteria are present, the risk of peritonitis from abdominal urine is greatly increased.

Cystocentesis is difficult when there is fluid in the abdomen because the bladder can be hard to palpate, and retrieval of yellow fluid does not confirm that the needle is in the bladder. The animal should be allowed to void voluntarily and the urine collected for a urinalysis. If there is any suspicion of urethral injury, the urethra should not be catheterized.

Abdominocentesis

Abdominocentesis is performed to obtain fluid for evaluation. Before abdominocentesis, the animal is allowed to urinate, if possible. After aseptic preparation, a 22-gauge needle attached to a 10-ml syringe is inserted into the abdomen through the umbilicus in a caudal direction. Alternatively, a butterfly catheter and syringe can be used. Fluid creatinine, urea nitrogen, and protein concentrations are determined, and a cell count and differential are performed. Diagnostic peritoneal lavage[2,3] is not done for evaluation of suspected uroperitoneum because it dilutes the creatinine and urea in the retrieved fluid. It is used to detect peritonitis or leakage from abdominal viscera in animals that do not have ascites.

To determine if the fluid retrieved is urine, the fluid urea or creatinine concentrations are compared with peripheral blood concentrations. With uroperitoneum, urea and creatinine concentrations are higher in the abdominal fluid than in the peripheral blood. By 24 hours, the abdominal fluid urea begins to equilibrate with the blood urea. In our experience, the urea concentration in the abdominal fluid remains greater than the blood concentration for several days. Usually, a reagent strip ("azostick") determination can be used to differentiate urine from other types of abdominal fluid. If the results are equivocal, fluid and serum creatinine values are measured. When there is uroperitoneum, the concentration of the abdominal fluid creatinine should be greater than serum creatinine values.

The retrieved fluid is examined microscopically for the presence of bacteria. A sample is submitted for bacteriologic culture and sensitivity.

Radiographic Studies

Survey radiographs of the abdomen may reveal enlargement and increased density of the retroperitoneal space following disruption of kidneys or ureters. If a kidney is displaced, asymmetrical, or not seen on a plain radiograph, an excretory urogram is done before exploratory surgery to delineate the kidneys. An absent or nonfunctioning kidney may preclude removal of a damaged opposite kidney. Because radiographic contrast material can produce hypotension and bradycardia, the animal should be rehydrated and normotensive before excretory urography. The excretory urogram is also quite accurate in detecting ureteral injury. Bladder tears are best delineated by positive contrast cystography, but if urethral damage is suspected, a retrograde urethrogram is performed first. If the urethral injury is confirmed, an excretory urogram is done instead of a retrograde cystogram, to avoid catheterizing the injured urethra. A complete discussion of urologic radiography is presented in Chapter 6.

EMERGENCY MANAGEMENT

Shock, respiratory distress, and severe hemorrhage are managed before treatment of injuries to the urinary tract. Broad-spectrum antibiotic administration is initiated because of tissue trauma. Surgical treatment of specific organ injury is discussed in Chapter 22.

Hemoperitoneum

An animal with severe hemorrhage from any abdominal organ, including the kidney, is treated for shock. An exploratory laparotomy is performed, if bleeding continues, to diagnose and control the source of bleeding.

Uroperitoneum and Uremia

A uremic animal is a poor anesthetic and surgical candidate for repair of urinary tract injury. The urine in the abdomen is drained, and the animal is rehydrated. Diuresis is induced with additional fluid therapy. Diagnostic findings are reviewed to determine whether prerenal azotemia or primary renal failure is worsening the postrenal azotemia. See Chapter 8 for discussion of fluid therapy in renal failure.

The urine can be drained simultaneously from a peritoneal catheter placed into the abdomen and a urethral catheter terminating at the trigone. Both the peritoneal and the urethral catheters are connected to closed collection systems. Once diuresis is established, dilute urine produced by the kidneys dilutes the abdominal fluid, which is removed through the peritoneal catheter. Instillation of lavage fluid is not necessary.

Placement of a Peritoneal Catheter[4]

The bladder should be empty before the peritoneal catheter is inserted. The peritoneal catheter is placed using a local anesthetic in a depressed or quiet animal. In an active dog, a narcotic analgesic (oxymorphone, 0.1 to 0.2 mg/kg IV), which can be reversed (naloxone, 0.02 mg/kg IV) is used. Intravenous ketamine (2 to 4 mg/kg) can be used in cats. Aseptic technique is essential to prevent contamination of the abdominal cavity. A small incision is made through the skin approximately 2 cm caudal to the umbilicus (Fig. 21–1A). A sterile rubber feeding tube with multiple holes or a manufactured per-

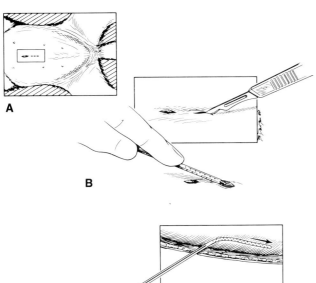

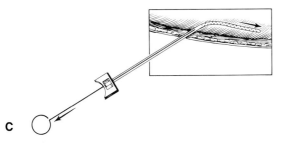

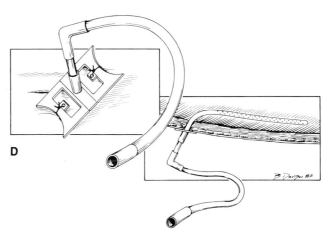

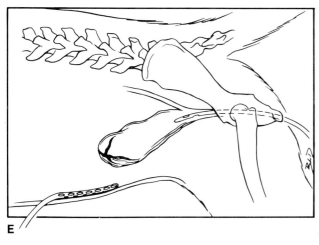

FIG. 21–1. Placement of a peritoneal catheter. (A) A small incision is made through the skin approximately 2 cm caudal to the umbilicus. (B) The manufactured peritoneal catheter and stylet is inserted directly through the linea alba. (C) The catheter is directed caudally, and the stylet is removed. (D) The catheter is secured to the skin and attached to an adapter, which is attached to a sterile collection set. (E) The peritoneal catheter should lie near the body wall with the tip near the bladder. A urethral catheter is placed with its tip within the urinary bladder trigone (From Stone, E.A.: Urologic surgery—an update. *In* Nephrology and Urology. Edited by E.B. Breitschwerdt. New York, Churchill Livingstone, 1986; with permission.)

itoneal catheter (Abbot Laboratories, Chicago, IL 60064) is used. For insertion of a rubber feeding tube, a small incision is made through the skin and into the linea alba. The manufactured peritoneal catheter comes with a stylet and can be inserted directly through the linea alba (Fig. 21–1B). The catheter is directed caudally, and the stylet is removed (Fig. 21–1C). The catheter is secured to the skin and attached to a sterile collection set (Fig. 21–1D). The catheter should lie near the body wall, close to the bladder (Fig. 21–1E).

MEDICAL VERSUS SURGICAL MANAGEMENT OF URINARY TRACT TRAUMA

Blunt Urinary Tract Trauma

The choice of medical or surgical management of blunt urinary tract trauma depends on the location and degree of injury. The great majority of renal parenchymal injuries are best treated by observation. Small urinary extravasations seal spontaneously.

Hematuria, without other problems, is not an indication for surgery. The animal should be kept quiet in a cage, and its vital signs, clinical status, and hematocrit should be serially monitored until the urine grossly clears of blood. If the hematuria persists, further diagnostic tests are needed. See Chapter 2 for evaluation of hematuria. Of course, deterioration of clinical status or hematocrit necessitates re-evaluation and possibly surgery.

Uroperitoneum is initially managed medically with urine drainage, using a peritoneal catheter and by fluid therapy as already described. Small bladder and urethral tears may heal spontaneously, if the bladder is kept decompressed with a urethral catheter. Surgical repair is often indicated, however, to assess the extent of damage accurately.

Penetrating Urinary Tract Trauma

All penetrating wounds to the abdomen should be surgically explored as soon as the animal is stable. The purpose of the exploratory surgery is not only to evaluate and treat urinary tract injury, but also to assess the integrity of surrounding abdominal viscera and vasculature.

REFERENCES

1. Burrows, C.F., and Bovee, K.C.: Metabolic changes due to experimentally induced rupture of the canine urinary bladder. Am. J. Vet. Res., 35:1083, 1974.
2. Crowe, D.T., Jr., and Crane, S.W.: Diagnostic paracentesis and lavage in the evaluation of abdominal injuries in dogs and cats: Clinical and experimental investigations. J. Am. Vet. Med. Assoc., 168:700, 1976.
3. Kolata, R.J.: Diagnostic abdominal paracentesis and lavage: Experimental and clinical evaluation in the dog. J. Am. Vet. Med. Assoc., 168:697, 1976.
4. Stone, E.A.: Urologic surgery—an update. In Nephrology and Urology. Edited by E.B. Breitschwerdt. New York, Churchill Livingstone, 1986, pp 75–88.

22

Surgical Therapy for Urinary Tract Trauma

RENAL INJURY

Following a midline abdominal incision, the abdomen is quickly explored, and bleeding from any major vessel is controlled with manual pressure or clamping. If major hemorrhage from a kidney or renal vessel is suspected, the aorta is located by using the duodenum and mesoduodenum as a natural retractor (see Fig. 10–2). The affected renal artery and vein are identified and occluded near the aorta and caudal vena cava with a vascular clamp. Once hemorrhage is controlled, the right kidney is inspected. The left kidney is examined using the colon and mesocolon for retraction (see Fig. 10–1). The peritoneal covering is not removed unless there is continuing bleeding from the renal parenchyma because disruption of the peritoneal covering may initiate renewed hemorrhage from the kidney.

Contusions and intracapsular fractures are not disturbed. Bleeding from a small hole can be tamponaded with a plug of fat or omentum. To treat laceration of the capsule and kidney, the parenchyma is minimally debrided, the edges are pressed together, and the capsule is sutured with 4–0 monofilament absorbable suture. If parenchyma is missing or fragmented, the wound is debrided, and omental or pararenal fat with attached blood supply is laid into the defect and sutured to the capsule at the edges of the wound to help hold it in place. Maceration of one renal pole necessitates partial nephrectomy to remove the damaged tissue, preserving as much parenchyma as possible. Nephroureterectomy is performed when the renal pedicle or one half or more of the kidney is damaged. Optimally, the function of the opposite kidney is determined before surgery by an excretory urogram. If one kidney has uncontrollable bleeding or severe renal pedicle injury, however, the surgeon has no option but to remove the damaged kidney. Prognosis is guarded if the function of the remaining kidney is unknown at the time of surgery.

PROCEDURES

Nephroureterectomy

The peritoneal attachments to the kidney are cut (Fig. 22–1A). The attachments are not torn because this disrupts the renal capsule and causes bleeding from the exposed surface of the kidney. Damage to the kidney is assessed, and a decision is made regarding complete or partial excision.

For nephroureterectomy, the kidney is elevated, and the renal pedicle is cleaned of fascial attachments, using a moistened sponge. The cranial pole of the kidney is rotated medially to reveal the renal vessels. (Fig. 21–1B). The renal artery is located on the cranial dorsal surface of the renal vein (Fig. 21–1C). The renal vessels are not clamped before ligation, unless it is necessary to control hemorrhage, because clamping increases the chance of accidental tearing. Nonabsorbable ligatures are placed proximally and distally on the renal artery (Fig. 22–1D). A transfixation ligature is placed distal to the proximal ligature for additional security. To make a transfixation ligature, a ligature is first placed around the vessel, using suture material swedged to a taper-point needle. The needle is passed through the vessel distal to the ligature. A knot is tied using the suture tag from the ligature and the suture attached to the needle, completing the transfixation ligature (Fig. 22–1D, insert). The renal vein is ligated. The left renal vein ligature is placed distal to the renal vein's confluence with the gonadal vein. The renal artery and then the renal vein are severed (Fig. 22–1E).

The ureter is dissected free, ligated, and severed at its junction with the bladder (Fig. 22–1F). The ureter is divided after the renal vessels are ligated to prevent congestion of urine in the kidney. Removing the entire ureter prevents reflux of urine and a possible nidus for infection in a residual ureteral stump.

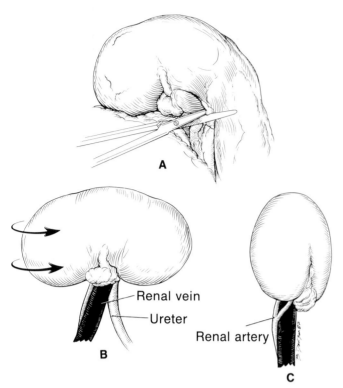

FIG. 22–1. Nephroureterectomy. (A) The peritoneal attachments to the left kidney are cut. (B) The cranial pole of the kidney is rotated medially to reveal the renal vessels. (C) The renal artery is located on the cranial dorsal surface of the renal vein.

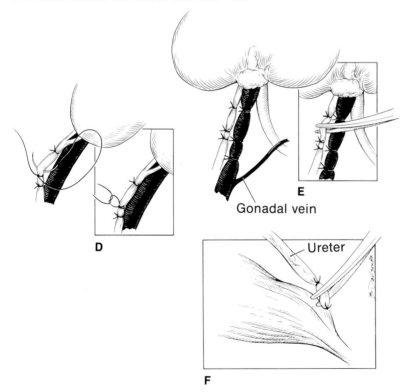

FIG. 22–1. (*Cont.*). (D) Nonabsorbable ligatures are placed proximally and distally on the renal artery. A transfixation ligature is placed just distal to the proximal ligature (insert). (E) The renal vein is ligated. The left renal vein ligature is placed distal to the renal vein's confluence with the left gonadal vein. The renal artery and then the renal vein are severed. (F) The ureter is dissected free, ligated, and severed at its junction with the bladder.

Partial Nephrectomy

After the kidney is elevated as described for nephroureterectomy, a vascular clamp or tourniquet is placed on the renal artery. Sutures are passed through the renal parenchyma, using a straight needle, dividing it into thirds at the site of resection (Fig. 22–2A,B). The sutures are grasped with hemostats. The first throw is made in one of the sutures, and it is slowly tightened to cut through the renal parenchyma and occlude the vascular supply (Fig. 22–2C). The ligature is tied. The other two sutures are tied similarly. The renal parenchyma is amputated distal to these ligatures (Fig. 22–2D,E). Small bleeding vessels within the parenchyma are ligated or cauterized. Because the capsule is friable and frequently damaged, it is not used to cover the cut surface. Instead, omentum is placed over the cut surface and tacked to the renal capsule (Fig. 22–2E). The kidney is repositioned, and a few sutures are placed between the kidney and body wall to prevent rotation and occlusion of the renal vessels.

URETERAL INJURY

The treatment for damaged ureters depends on the location of the injury. Preoperative excretory urographic studies often help localize the region involved. The precise area of ureteral injury can often be found at surgery by catheterizing the ureter following a ventral cystotomy. If the lesion is still not visible, 1 ml of methylene blue or indigo carmine is injected intravenously to disclose small areas of urine extravasation where bluish discoloration appears in tissue.

Damage to the distal ureter is managed by implanting healthy ureter into the bladder (*ureteroneocystostomy*) as close to the trigone as possible without tension. In cats, successful implantation of the ureter may require microsurgical techniques. If the middle portion of the ureter is damaged, ureteroneocystostomy is preferable to ureteral anastomosis because of the greater risk of leakage and stricture with anastomosis. Tension on the ureteroneocystostomy site can be reduced by anchoring the bladder cranially (*psoas cystopexy*) and moving the kidney caudally (*renal descensus*). By using a cystopexy, up to 6 cm of distal ureter in a 15-kg dog can be removed and a ureteroneocystostomy performed without tension.[1] A bladder-tube flap ureterostomy (Boari flap), in which bladder wall is fashioned into a tube for anastomosis to a shortened ureter, is not recommended because stricture is a common complication.[1]

If the ureter cannot be implanted, *ureteral anastomosis* can be accomplished successfully in medium-sized to large dogs. A *nephrostomy catheter* is used to drain urine away from the anastomotic site when the ureter is too small for stenting with available ureteral catheters. In a cat or small dog with a normal opposite kidney, nephroureterectomy is the treatment of choice, unless microsurgical capabilities are available for ureteral anastomosis.

Certain details are especially important in surgery involving the ureter. Whenever the ureter is mobilized,

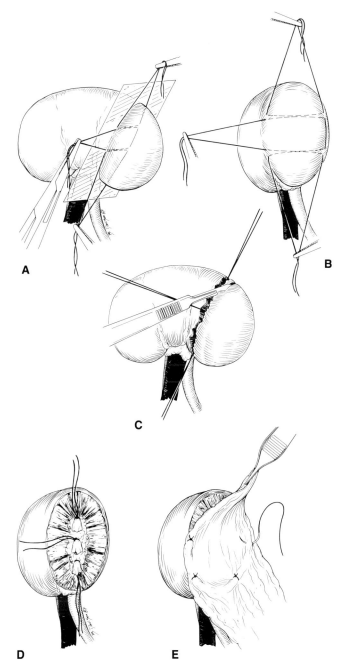

FIG. 22–2. Partial nephrectomy. (A, B) Sutures are passed through the renal parenchyma, using a straight needle, dividing it into thirds at the site of resection. (The renal artery clamp has been omitted for the sake of clarity.) (C) The first throw is made in one of the sutures, and it is slowly tightened to cut through the renal parenchyma and occlude the vascular supply. The ligature is tied. The other two sutures are tied similarly. The renal parenchyma is amputated distal to these ligatures. (D) The parenchyma is inspected, and small bleeding vessels are ligated or cauterized. (E) Omentum is placed over the cut surface and tacked to the renal capsule.

adventitial attachments should be divided as far from the ureter as possible, to avoid ureteral ischemia from disruption of ureteral blood supply within the adventitia. For the same reason, electrocoagulation of bleeding vessels should be carried out as far as possible from the ureter. The ureter is not handled with forceps. Instead, the adventitia is grasped and used to manipulate the ureter.

PROCEDURES

Ureteroneocystostomy

A ligature is placed on the most distal portion of healthy ureter. The ends of the ligature are left long to use in handling the ureter. The ureter is mobilized by cutting the peritoneum covering the ureter, taking care not to damage the adventitial sheath and blood supply. A ventral cystotomy incision is made (see Fig. 19–5). The original ureteral opening is identified and catheterized. The ureteral stump is ligated near its entrance into the bladder.

The site of the ureteroneocystostomy is as far distal as possible without tension. A small circular piece of mucosa is excised at the proposed site. A hemostat is used to punch through the bladder wall at an oblique angle (Fig. 22–3A). A long intramural tunnel (five times ureteral diameter) has been advocated to prevent urine reflux, but this is not feasible in a thin-walled dog or cat bladder. Also, a long tunnel in the mobile dome of the bladder could cause kinking of the ureter; thus, it is not recommended. A hemostat is used to grasp the ends of the ureteral ligature and draw the ureter into the bladder

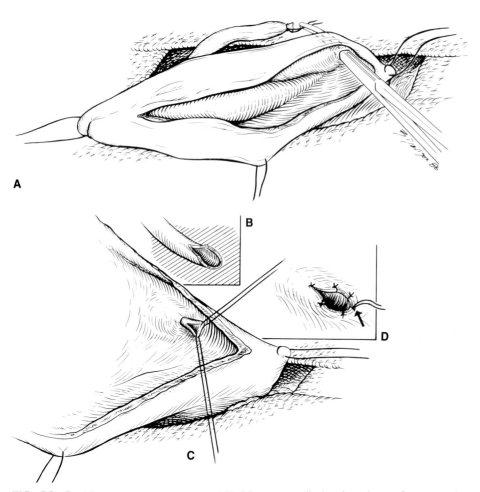

FIG. 22–3. Ureteroneocystostomy. (A) After a small circular piece of mucosa has been excised at the proposed site, a hemostat is used to punch through the bladder wall at an oblique angle. The hemostat is used to grasp the ends of the ureteral ligature and draw the ureter through the tunnel into the bladder lumen. (B) The end of the ureter is severed proximal to the ligature. A short longitudinal incision is made opposite the ureteral vessel to increase the circumference of the terminal ureter. (C) Two 5–0 to 6–0 absorbable retention sutures are placed through the ureter and are used to hold the ureter within the bladder. (D) A suture is passed through the tip of the ureter between the two retention sutures. It is then passed through the bladder muscle and mucosa and tied (arrow). This distal suture ensures firm fixation of the ureter within the bladder. The retention sutures are placed through bladder mucosa and tied. Three additional ureter to bladder mucosa sutures are placed as needed.

lumen. The end of the ureter is sharply severed proximal to the ligature. A short, longitudinal incision is made opposite the ureteral vessel (Fig. 22–3B). This incision, termed *spatulating*, increases the circumference of the terminal ureter. Two 5–0 to 6–0 absorbable retention sutures are placed through the ureter and are used to hold the ureter within the bladder (Fig. 22–3C). A distal suture is passed through the ureter, bladder muscle, and mucosa, between the two retention sutures, and tied. This distal suture ensures firm fixation of the ureter within the bladder. The retention sutures are placed through bladder mucosa and tied (Fig. 22–3D). Additional sutures are placed from the ureter through the bladder mucosa as needed. In small dogs in which postoperative edema could obstruct the ureteroneocystostomy, one end of a 3.5 Fr catheter is passed into the ureter through the ureteroneocystostomy, and the other end is passed into the urethra and exited through the distal urethral opening. Closure of the cystotomy and abdominal incisions is routine. The ureteral catheter is secured with suture to the vagina or prepuce, connected to a closed collection system, and removed in 2 days.

Psoas Cystopexy

Psoas cystopexy or fixation of the craniolateral bladder wall to the psoas fascia or psoas muscle (sometimes called a "psoas hitch") is used to compensate for inadequate ureteral length and to relieve tension on a ureteroneocystostomy.[2] Psoas cystopexy cannot be used on a contracted or scarred bladder or when the blood supply to the bladder is compromised.

After a ventral cystotomy, the end of the ureter to be implanted is brought through the bladder wall, as already described. The ureter is not sutured in place until the cystopexy is completed. The index finger is inserted into the bladder and used to move the bladder dome toward the proximal ureter. Two or three nonabsorbable sutures are placed from the craniolateral wall of the bladder, just lateral to the ureteral implantation site, and into the psoas fascia or psoas muscle. These sutures are tied securely to anchor the bladder wall to the psoas muscle (Fig. 22–4). The ureter to bladder anastomosis is performed as described (Fig. 22–3B,C,D).

If necessary, the same procedure is repeated on the opposite side, but the bladder must first be stretched to determine the best location for the second ureteral implantation. After bilateral ureteral implantation and cystopexy, the cranial bladder is closed transversely to relieve tension on the incision site.

Renal Descensus

The kidney is completely mobilized by incising peritoneal and fascial attachments. The kidney is gently pushed, caudally and medially. With the kidney held in this position, the capsule and a small amount of parenchyma of the caudal pole are anchored to the body wall with three nonabsorbable sutures (Fig. 22–5). This procedure moves the proximal ureter caudally.

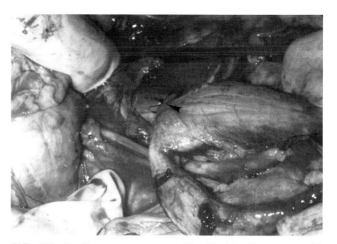

FIG. 22–4. Psoas cystopexy. The bladder is anchored in a more cranial position with sutures from the bladder wall to the psoas muscle (arrow). The ureter has been brought through the bladder wall in preparation for a ureteroneocystostomy.

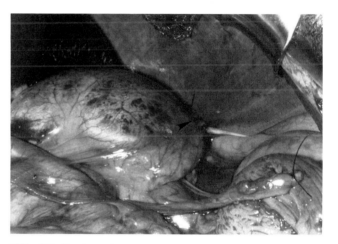

FIG. 22–5. Renal descensus. The kidney has been mobilized and moved caudally and medially. The capsule and a small amount of parenchyma are anchored to the body wall with three nonabsorbable sutures (arrow). The severed ureter is lying on the bladder.

Ureteral Anastomosis

The ureter is freed from the peritoneum with care to preserve as much periureteral tissue as possible, to decrease the possibility of vascular compromise. The ends of each ureteral segment are severed at an oblique angle, starting on the vascular side (Fig. 22–6A). The avascular side is then incised longitudinally to increase the diameter of the ureter. One ureteral segment is rotated 180°, and a suture is placed through the tip of one segment into the angle of the longitudinal incision on the opposing ureteral end (Fig. 22–6B). After the first suture is tied, the remaining sutures are placed 2 mm apart and tied (Fig. 22–6C). A cystotomy is performed, and a flexible catheter is passed from the bladder into the ureter and past the anastomosis site to help prevent leakage.

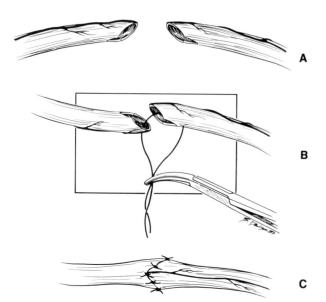

FIG. 22–6. Ureteral anastomosis. (A) The end of each ureteral segment is excised at an oblique angle starting on the vascular side of the ureter. A longitudinal incision is made on the avascular side. (B) One ureteral segment is rotated 180° and a suture is preplaced through the tip of one segment into the angle of the longitudinal incision of the other ureteral segment. (C) A second suture is preplaced from the tip of the other segment into the angle of the opposite segment. After these sutures are tied, the remaining sutures are placed 2 mm apart and tied.

The catheter should be small enough to insert easily without distending the ureter. If the catheter is long enough, it is exited through the urethra. Otherwise, the distal end is left in the bladder, and it is attached to a nylon suture, which is exited through the urethra and used to remove the catheter in 4 days.

If necessary, psoas cystopexy, renal descensus, or both can be done to reduce tension on the ureteral anastomosis.

Nephrostomy Catheter

With a small ureter, there may not be a ureteral catheter small enough to insert into the ureter and remain patent. In these instances, a nephrostomy catheter is placed to divert urine temporarily from the anastomotic site. An 8 Fr gauge Foley catheter, a straight rubber or Silastic catheter, or a specially designed nephrostomy catheter (C. R. Bard, Inc, Murray Hill, NJ 07974) can be used.

The nephrostomy catheter is placed during surgery before the ureter is anastomosed. A dilator, which can be an intravenous catheter, is passed into the ureter starting at the severed proximal end and exited through the renal cortex (Fig. 22–7A). A guidewire is passed through the dilator and exited through the end of the dilator. An 18-gauge needle is passed through the body wall and over the guidewire (Fig. 22–7B). The guidewire is exited through the needle and the body wall (Fig. 22–7C). After the needle is removed, the guidewire remains. A catheter is passed over the guidewire through the

body wall as the dilator is removed (Fig. 22–7D). The catheter is passed into the renal pelvis, and the guidewire is removed (Fig. 22–7E).

BLADDER INJURY

After a caudal midline or parapreputial abdominal incision, the bladder is examined and the tear located. The edges are debrided back to healthy tissue. The bladder is closed with a simple interrupted or inverting pattern through the serosa and muscularis without entering the lumen (see Fig. 19–5). The abdomen is lavaged with warm balanced electrolyte solution (10 ml/kg body weight) and suctioned dry.

URETHRAL INJURY

For sharp penetrating injuries, with at least one third of the urethral circumference still intact, surgical intervention may not be necessary. The urine is diverted by a cystostomy catheter (see Fig. 16–6) and a small urethral catheter. The position of the urethral catheter should be confirmed by radiography to ascertain that it is within the urethral lumen and not exiting through the damaged portion. If the catheter cannot be positioned from the external urethral orifice, a cystotomy is performed, and a catheter is passed from the bladder out the urethra. Once the tip of this catheter exits the urethral orifice, the tip is sutured to the tip of a second catheter. The first catheter is then pulled back into the bladder from the cystotomy incision, bringing the second catheter with it. The first catheter is removed from the bladder, and the cystotomy incision is closed. The second catheter remains in place, draining urine from the bladder out the urethral orifice.

Separation of the urethral ends following trauma necessitates surgical repair. A cystostomy catheter may be needed for several days to drain urine from the injured area and allow resolution of post-traumatic edema and tissue swelling. The approach to the urethra depends on the location of the injury. To access the pelvic urethra, a pubic or pubic and ischiatic osteotomy is required (see Fig. 10–4). If the urethra is avulsed from the bladder, a caudal midline incision is made, with preparation for pubic osteotomy if needed. Treatment of a traumatized prostatic urethra may entail partial or total prostatectomy (see Fig. 28–3). For perineal urethra injury, a midline incision over the urethra is used. Dissection continues to the retractor penile muscle, which is retracted laterally. The crura and bulbospongiosus muscles are separated at their raphe to expose the urethra.

Once the urethra is exposed, the damaged ends are debrided for 1 to 2 mm. If possible, an end to end anastomosis is performed using 4–0 absorbable suture in a simple interrupted pattern. Tension on the anastomotic site is minimized to prevent separation of the urethral ends and stricture.[3] Drains are placed near the urethra and exited through the skin. Urine is diverted by cys-

FIG. 22–7. Nephrostomy. (A) The nephrostomy catheter is placed during surgery before the ureteral anastomosis. A dilator, which can be an intravenous catheter, is passed up the ureter starting at the severed proximal end and out through the renal cortex. A guidewire is passed through the dilator. (B) The guidewire is exited through the end of the dilator. An 18-gauge needle is passed through the body wall and over the guidewire. (C) The guidewire is exited through the needle and the body wall.

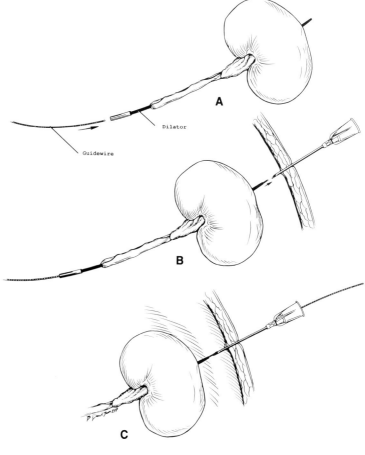

FIG. 22–7. (*Cont.*). (D) After the needle is removed, the guidewire remains. A catheter is passed over the guidewire through the body wall and into the renal parenchyma. As the catheter is advanced, the dilator is removed. (E) The catheter is passed into the renal pelvis, and the guidewire is removed.

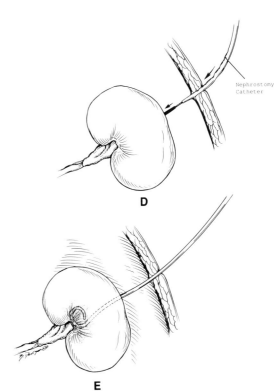

tostomy catheter, preferably, or a small urethral catheter for 5 days.

If the urethral ends cannot be apposed, a more proximal urethrostomy is done (e.g., scrotal urethrostomy, Fig. 16–7; perineal urethrostomy, Fig. 31–4). Severe damage to the pelvic urethra is difficult to manage. If 2 to 3 cm of undamaged urethra caudal to the prostate remain, prepubic urethrostomy is done. The procedure for dogs is similar to the procedure described for cats (see Fig. 13–2) except that the urethra caudal to the prostate is used to form the stoma. A subtotal prostatectomy may be necessary to mobilize the urethra and relieve tension on the urethra to skin suture line. Urinary incontinence is a potential complication of this procedure.

For a dog with a fractured os penis, an attempted is made to pass a small urethral catheter. If successful, the catheter is connected to a closed system while tissue edema decreases. If catheterization is unsuccessful, a prescrotal urethrotomy is performed. Alternatively, if the owners will permit castration of the dog, a scrotal urethrostomy can be done. If the fractured os penis is unstable, it is exposed, reduced, and immobilized with a fingerplate. Persistence of urethral obstruction necessitates a scrotal urethrostomy.

REFERENCES

1. Hamm, F.C., Peng, B., and Waterhouse, K.: Experimental studies on repair of injured ureter. Arch. Surg., *90:*298, 1965.
2. Middleton, R.G.: Routine use of the psoas hitch in ureteral reimplantation. J. Urol., *123:*352, 1980.
3. McRoberts J.W., and Ragde, H.: The severed canine posterior urethra: A study of two distinct methods of repair. J. Urol., *104:*724, 1962.

23

Postoperative Management and Surgical Complications of Urinary Tract Trauma

POSTOPERATIVE MANAGEMENT

If antibiotic administration was initiated before surgery, it is discontinued 24 hours after surgery, unless the culture results from the urine or ascitic fluid were positive. Continued monitoring of clinical status and vital signs for shock is indicated. Blood loss is evaluated with serial hematocrits. Azotemia should resolve rapidly after surgery. If it does not, renal function is reevaluated (see Chapter 3). An excretory urogram is performed 4 to 6 weeks after ureteral surgery to assess renal and ureteral size.

COMPLICATIONS

The types and incidence of complications after surgery for urinary tract trauma are not well documented. General postoperative complications are discussed in Chapter 11.

Abdominal Bleeding

Persistent postoperative bleeding suggests that a damaged vessel or organ was overlooked during the exploratory surgery. An activated clotting time and a platelet count are performed to assess coagulation status before considering operation. See Chapter 11 for evaluation of postoperative hemorrhage.

Hematuria

Hematuria following renal or bladder trauma should resolve within 1 week. If it continues, contrast-enhanced radiographic studies are indicated to look for anatomic abnormalities. Urine bacterial cultures are performed, and urinary tract infection is treated (see Chapter 18).

Urine Leakage

Leakage after repair of a damaged ureter or bladder is manifested by azotemia and ascites. Urine seeping from an operated ureter usually does not sequester in the retroperitoneal space because the peritoneum has been disrupted during the initial surgery. An excretory urogram should identify the location. Reoperation is indicated. Intravenous injection of methylene blue or indigo carmine (1 ml), which is excreted in the urine, may help locate the area of dehiscence during surgery.

A ureteroneocystostomy may leak urine when edema occludes the ureteral opening and increases urine pressure on the anastomosis. Occlusion is more likely to occur in cats and small dogs and can be avoided by maintaining a ureteral catheter for 2 days after surgery. At reoperation, the ureteroneocystostomy is examined to determine if placement of additional sutures will seal the leak. Usually it is necessary to detach the ureter from the bladder, close the opening, and make a new, more proximal ureteroneocystostomy. Before repairing a dehisced ureteral anastomosis, a nephrostomy catheter is placed to divert urine and increase the chances of an adequate fibrin seal.

Bladder dehiscence is corrected by removing all previously placed sutures, gently debriding the incision edges, and resuturing. Gentle tissue handling and precise placement of sutures are emphasized.

Azotemia/Uremia

Postoperative azotemia and subsequent uremia require careful evaluation to differentiate possible causes. Underlying renal dysfunction may have been present before the trauma (i.e., chronic renal failure) or induced by the trauma and the accompanying shock and hemorrhage. Following a nephrectomy, the remaining kidney may have inadequate function. Over several weeks, this kidney may hypertrophy and gain sufficient function. Surgical complications, such as urine leakage or urine outflow obstruction, can produce postrenal azotemia and uremia. The diagnostic procedures for azotemia and uremia are discussed in Chapter 3.

Ureteral Obstruction

Mild hydroureter and hydronephrosis are expected for several weeks after surgery. Progression should be monitored with repeat excretory urograms. If the partial obstruction worsens, reoperation is required to prevent irreversible kidney damage.

Following ureteroneocystostomy, extrinsic obstruction of the ureter can be caused by angulation of the ureter proximal to its entry into the bladder or failure to create a large enough opening into the bladder wall, which compresses the ureter as it enters the bladder. Stenosis of the implanted ureter is usually caused by ischemia from vascular compromise or tension on the anastomosis. To correct the obstructions, the narrowed terminal ureter is resected and reimplanted more proximally.

Stricture of an ureteral anastomosis is treated by resection and reanastomosis. If a tension-free anastomosis is not possible, even with psoas cystopexy and renal descensus, a nephroureterectomy is done.

Urethral Stricture

A urethral stricture can be either excised with anastomosis or bypassed by scrotal (see Fig. 16–7) or perineal urethrostomy (see Fig. 31–4) or prepubic urethrostomy (see Fig. 13–2). Management of urethral stricture is discussed in Chapter 16.

Urethral Fistula

A urethral fistula may develop when traumatic disruption damages not only the urethra but also the covering structures. It can also occur through a sutured area of urethra when the more distal urethra is obstructed. In this instance, an attempt to void through the strictured area produces excessive pressure proximally, forcing urine to leak through the weakened sutured area. No attempt should be made to close the defect with sutures even when the fistula is associated with wound dehiscence. The friable tissues will not hold sutures, and the defect will become larger. Instead, the skin edges should be loosely approximated with sutures. Urine diversion is continued with a cystostomy catheter and a small urethral catheter. If there is any question about the lumen size of the more distal urethra, a urethrogram is done. If the fistula is still present after 2 to 3 weeks of drainage, the area is explored and an attempt at debridement and primary closure is made. Often, a proximal diversion procedure (scrotal or perineal urethrostomy) is necessary.

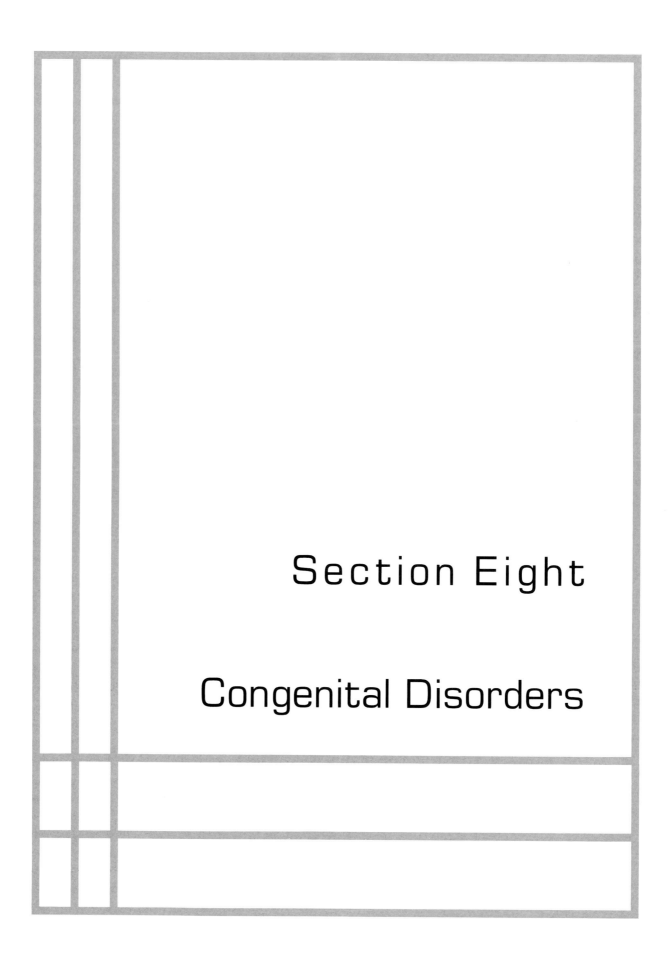

Section Eight

Congenital Disorders

24

Diagnosis and Medical Therapy of Congenital Disorders

ECTOPIC URETERS

Developmental Anomalies and Inheritance

Ureteral ectopia results from faulty differentiation or migration of the mesonephric and metanephric ducts, causing an abnormal routing of the ureter.[1] In female dogs, the ectopic ureter terminates most often in the urethra or vagina. Termination has also been reported in the cervix, uterus, and fallopian tubes.[2] In cats and male dogs, the ectopic ureter opens into the urethra.[3-5] Either or both ureters may be affected.

The condition occurs more frequently in Siberian huskies, Newfoundlands, English bulldogs, West Highland white terriers, fox terriers, golden retrievers, and miniature and toy poodles. Although breed predisposition is apparent, the mode of inheritance is unknown.[6] Bitches with ectopic ureters have had litters of puppies with no observed incontinence.[7] Ureteral ectopia is diagnosed infrequently in cats and male dogs. Concurrent urologic anomalies may include hydroureter (most common); absent, small, or misshapen kidneys; hydronephrosis; and tortuous or obstructed ureters.[8,9]

Morphologic types of ectopic ureter described in dogs include (1) intramural with a distal ureteral orifice, (2) intramural with no distal ureteral orifice, (3) ureteral troughs, (4) bilateral double ureteral openings, and (5) extramural.[7] Determination of the type of ectopic ureter is most accurately made during laparotomy and ventral cystotomy.

In our experience, intramural ectopic ureters are the most common type.[7] In this type, the ureter penetrates the serosa and detrusor musculature of the bladder in the usual or more distal location. In contrast to a normal ureter (Fig. 24–1), the submucosal segment continues through the urinary bladder trigone and opens distally in the urethra or vagina (Fig. 24–2). When a unilateral intramural ectopic ureter has no distal orifice, severe hydroureter and hydronephrosis develop.

With ureteral troughs, the ureter passes through the serosa and detrusor musculature of the bladder in the usual location. The opening through the bladder mucosa may be in a normal or more distal location. The ureter continues as a trough through the urethral sphincter (Fig. 24–3). Dogs with intramural ectopic ureters may have a better prognosis for surgical correction of incontinence than dogs with ureteral troughs.[7] A dog with double ureteral openings has a ureter that opens into the trigone in a typical fashion and then continues submucosally to a second more distal opening (Fig. 24–4).

An extramural ectopic ureter enters directly into the urethra or vagina without penetrating the bladder wall (Fig. 24–5). This is the only type reported in cats.[3,5]

Diagnosis

Animals with ectopic ureters are usually presented to the veterinarian because of continuous or intermittent urinary incontinence. Male dogs are more likely to have intermittent rather than continuous incontinence. Although ureteral ectopia is a congenital condition, adult dogs may be presented for the condition because of delayed diagnosis or owner reluctance to pursue therapy. Most dogs with ectopic ureters, even bilaterally, can void normally.[7]

All causes of incontinence are considered during the diagnostic workup (see Chapter 1). Excretory urography in conjunction with a pneumocystogram or double contrast cystogram is the best method for assessing the ectopic ureters and detecting other urologic anomalies[9] (see Chapter 6). Vaginourethrography is useful to assess the termination of the ectopic ureter. Radiography is not consistently useful in identifying the morphologic type of ectopic ureters.

The preoperative workup includes a urine specific gravity and a serum creatinine or urea nitrogen determination to identify renal compromise. Dogs with ec-

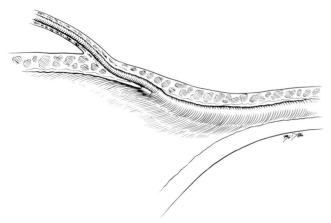

FIG. 24–1. Normal ureter. Ureter enters bladder wall, has a short submucosal segment, and opens into the trigone (schematic sagittal section).

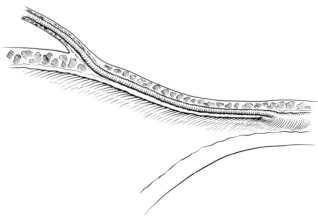

FIG. 24–2. Intramural ectopic ureter. Ureter passes through serosa and muscularis of bladder in usual location. Submucosal segment continues through the urinary bladder trigone to open distally (schematic sagittal section).

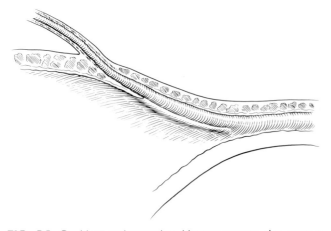

FIG. 24–3. Ureteral troughs. Ureter enters the serosa and muscularis of bladder in usual location. The opening through the bladder mucosa may be in a normal or more distal location. The ureter continues as a trough through the urethral sphincter (schematic sagittal section).

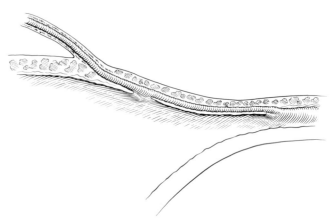

FIG. 24–4. Double ureteral openings. Ureter has one opening into the trigone in a typical location and continues submucosally to a second more distal opening (schematic sagittal section). (Figs. 24–1 to 24–4 from Stone, E.A., and Mason, K.L.: Surgery of ectopic ureters: Types, method of correction and postoperative results. J. Am. Anim. Hosp. Assoc., *26*:81, 1990; with permission.)

topic ureters frequently have urinary tract infection (UTI), so urine for complete urinalysis and bacteriologic culture is collected by cystocentesis before surgery, if possible, or during surgery. Urinary tract infection is treated with antibiotic therapy (see Chapter 18).

Some dogs with ectopic ureters have associated urethral sphincter mechanism incompetence, which causes persistent incontinence after surgery. The owners are warned about this possibility. Determining whether the dog's bladder is easy or difficult to express manually is warranted to help evaluate urethral competence. At referral centers, urethral pressure profilometry is used to assess urethra function before surgery. Abnormalities in urethral pressure, however, may be caused by the presence of an intramural ectopic ureter within the urethral wall. Thus, surgical correction is carried out even if the urethral pressure profile is abnormal, but the owner can be further advised of the possibility of continued postoperative incontinence.

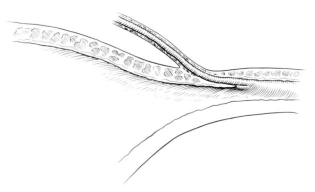

FIG. 24–5. Extramural ectopic ureter. Ureter enters directly into the urethra or vagina without penetrating the bladder wall.

PERSISTENT URACHUS

The fetal urachus lies within the umbilicus and joins the urinary bladder to the allantoic cavity. After birth, the urachus usually closes to become the middle ligament of the bladder. If the entire urachus remains open (persistent or patent urachus), urine dribbles from the umbilicus.

Diagnosis

The dog is usually presented for urinary incontinence. It may have urine scald on the ventral abdomen, a foul odor, and recurrent urinary tract infections. Definitive diagnosis is by contrast-enhanced cystography, demonstrating contrast material extending from bladder to umbilicus.

VESICOURACHAL DIVERTICULA

If the urachus closes except near the bladder, a blind pouch (congenital vesicourachal diverticulum) forms. Diverticula vary in size from a few millimeters to several centimeters. Positive contrast cystography diagnoses the diverticulum arising from the cranioventral surface of the bladder.

Vesicourachal diverticula may predispose dogs to recurrent urinary tract infection.[10] Retention of urine and bacteria within a diverticulum probably alters the ability of normal host defense mechanisms to remove bacteria from the bladder. Urinary tract infection may be controlled by antibiotic therapy, only to recur once the antibiotics are discontinued. Surgical excision in dogs with persistent UTI is recommended.

Congenital urachal diverticula in cats may spontaneously resolve or may remain. Many urachal diverticula in cats appear to be acquired and are associated with hematuria, dysuria, or urethral obstruction (see Fig. 12–6).[11] These acquired diverticula usually resolve with resolution of clinical signs. Urinary tract infection is uncommon in cats with signs of lower urinary tract disease. If persistent or recurrent UTI is documented, however, and the urachal diverticulum is still present, it is excised.

HYPOSPADIA

Hypospadia is a condition in male dogs in which the urethra opens on the ventral surface of the penis, at any place between the ischial arch and the normal urethral opening. Hypospadia occurs as a result of failure of the urogenital folds to fuse, with incomplete formation of the penis and penile urethra. The condition has not been reported in cats.

Diagnosis

The owners present the dog because of the anatomic abnormality or because of wet fur and foul odor. Diagnosis is made by visual examination (Fig. 24–6).

URETHRORECTAL FISTULA

Congenital urethrorectal fistulae are rare and develop because of incomplete formation of the cloacal urorectal septum between the urethrovesical and rectal segments.

Diagnosis

The primary symptom in dogs is leakage of urine through the anus. Some dogs simultaneously urinate from the urethra and the anus. Perineal urine scalding

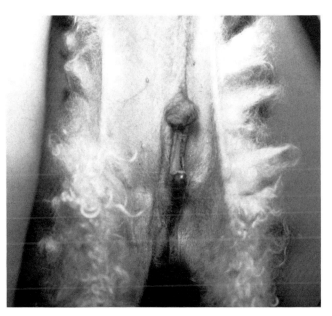

FIG. 24–6. Hypospadia in a 6-month-old miniature poodle.

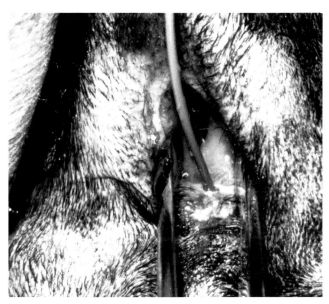

FIG. 24–7. Urethrorectal fistula in a 1-year-old miniature poodle. A catheter is positioned in the fistula. (From Osuna, D.J., Stone, E.A., and Metcalf, M.R.: A urethrorectal fistula with concurrent urolithiasis in a dog. J. Am. Anim. Hosp. Assoc., *25*:35, 1989; with permission.)

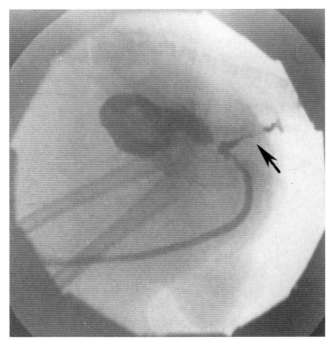

FIG. 24–8. Urethrorectal fistula (arrow) outlined with contrast material passing from urethra into the distal rectum. Mineralized opacity within bladder is a cystic calculus (fluoroscopical image of contrast cystogram and retrograde urethrogram). (From Osuna, D.J., Stone, E.A., and Metcalf, M.R.: A urethrorectal fistula with concurrent urolithiasis in a dog. J. Am. Anim. Hosp. Assoc., *25:*35, 1989; with permission.)

is often present. Chronic UTI may be a complicating factor because of fecal contamination of the bladder through the fistula. With the dog anesthetized, the bladder should be manually expressed and the anus and rectum examined for urine leakage and a possible opening (Fig. 24–7). Intravenous injection of indigo carmine (1

ml), which is excreted as a blue dye in the urine, may help identify the opening.

A combination of positive contrast cystography and retrograde urethrography is the best method of diagnosis if visual examination is unsuccessful.[12] On radiographs, contrast material is seen between the urethra and the distal rectum (Fig. 24–8).

REFERENCES

1. Owen, R.R.: Canine ureteral ectopia—a review 1. Embryology and etiology. J. Sm. Anim. Pract., *14:*407, 1973.
2. Owen, R.R.: Canine ureteral ectopia—a review 2. Incidence, diagnosis and treatment. J. Sm. Anim. Pract., *14:*419, 1973.
3. Filippich L.J., Read, R.A., Carlisle, C.H., et al.: Ectopic ureter in a cat—a case report. Aust. Vet. Pract., *15:*8, 1985.
4. Grauer, G.F., Freeman, L.F., and Nelson, A.W.: Urinary incontinence associated with an ectopic ureter in a female cat. J. Am. Vet. Med. Assoc., *182:*707, 1983.
5. Rutgers, C., Chew, D.J., and Burt, J.K.: Bilateral ectopic ureters in a female cat without urinary incontinence. J. Am. Vet. Med. Assoc., *11:*1394, 1984.
6. Hayes, H.H.: Breed associations of canine ectopic ureter: A study of 217 female cases. J. Sm. Anim. Pract., *25:*501, 1984.
7. Stone, E.A., and Mason, K.L.: Surgery of ectopic ureters: Types, method of correction and postoperative results. J. Am. Anim. Hosp. Assoc., *26:*81, 1990.
8. Dean, P.W., Bojrab, M.J., and Constantinescu, G.M.: Canine ectopic ureter. Compend. Contin. Educ. Pract. Vet., *10:*146, 1988.
9. Mason, K.L., Stone, E.A., Biery, D.N., et al.: Surgery of ectopic ureters: Pre- and postoperative radiographic morphology. J. Am. Anim. Hosp. Assoc., *26:*73, 1990.
10. Wilson, J.W., Klausner, J.S., Stevens, J.B., et al.: Canine vesicourachal diverticula. Vet. Surg., *8:*63, 1979.
11. Osborne, C.A., Kruger, J.M., and Johnston, G.R.: Feline vesicourachal diverticula. *In* Current Veterinary Therapy X. Edited by R.W. Kirk. Philadelphia, W.B. Saunders, 1989, p. 1153.
12. Osuna, D.J., Stone, E.A., and Metcalf, M.R.: A urethrorectal fistula with concurrent urolithiasis in a dog. J. Am. Anim. Hosp. Assoc., *25:*35, 1989.

25

Surgical Therapy for Congenital Disorders

ECTOPIC URETERS

General Concepts

A laparotomy is performed through a ventral midline approach. The kidneys and ureters are examined for abnormalities. The ventral cystotomy incision is extended through the trigone (see Fig. 19–5). The bladder interior is inspected for ureteral openings. In a normal bladder, both ureteral openings are visible within the trigone (Fig. 25–1).

The surgical technique for correction of an ectopic ureter depends on the degree of renal dysfunction and the morphologic type of the ectopic ureter.[1] When the kidney associated with the ectopic ureter is severely hydronephrotic or infected and the other kidney is functional, the involved kidney and ureter are excised (see Fig. 22–1).

Intramural Ectopic Ureter

With a unilateral ectopic ureter, visual inspection of the trigone via a ventral cystotomy reveals one ureteral opening in the typical location with no contralateral ureteral opening (Figs. 25–2, 25–3A). A submucosal ridge is usually seen over the pathway of the ectopic ureter. With bilateral ectopic ureters, no ureteral openings are seen within the trigone. If necessary, the proximal urethra can be occluded to make the ectopic ureters bulge beneath the submucosa.

To correct an intramural ectopic ureter, a 3- to 5-mm incision is made through the bladder mucosa and into the ureter at the typical location for a ureteral opening (Fig. 25–3B). If the ureter is very dilated, a small piece of ureter and bladder mucosa is excised to remove redundant tissue. The edges of the incised ureter are sutured to the edges of the incised bladder mucosa with 4–0 to 7–0 absorbable suture material (Fig. 25–3C). Selection of suture material size is based on the size of the

ureter. The distal portion of the ectopic ureter is incised longitudinally for 1 to 2 cm (Fig. 25–3D). The distal ectopic ureter is occluded by placing sutures through one side of the incised ureter, through the bladder wall, and through the other side of the incised ureter (Fig. 25–3E). Tying the sutures flattens the incised ureter and occludes the lumen. After ligation of the distal ureter, the surgeon attempts to pass a small catheter distally through the ureteral stoma. Inability to pass the catheter ensures that the distal ureter is occluded. (Previously we described a technique for occluding the distal ureter that kept the suture material out of the lumen.[1] Because we have had 3 dogs recanalize their ectopic ureters after that technique, we are now more concerned with permanent occlusion than with the risk of calculi formation from intraluminal sutures.)

Ureteral Troughs

The ureteral opening is identified, with the trough extending distally into the urethra (Fig. 25–4A). Surgical correction involves excising a strip of mucosa from each side of the trough and then closing the trough in a simple continuous pattern, using 4–0 absorbable suture material. Each suture bite includes both sides and the dorsal surface of the trough (Fig. 25–4B).

Double Ureteral Openings

Double ureteral openings are diagnosed by placing a catheter into a typically located ureteral opening and then passing it distally. To occlude the distal submucosal portion of the ureter, sutures are placed as described for intramural ureters.

Extramural Ectopic Ureters

An extramural ectopic ureter, in which the ureter opens into the urethra without coursing within the bladder

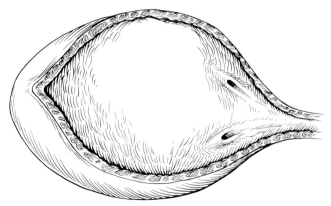

FIG. 25—1. Normal bladder trigone. Both ureteral openings are visible within the trigone.

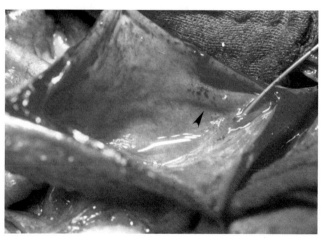

FIG. 25—2. Unilateral intramural ectopic ureter. Inspection of the trigone via a ventral cystotomy reveals one ureteral opening (catheterized) in the typical location with no contralateral ureteral opening. A large submucosal ridge is seen over the pathway of the ectopic ureter (arrow). (From Stone, E.A., and Mason, K.L.: Surgery of ectopic ureters: Types, method of correction, and postoperative results. J. Am. Anim. Hosp. Assoc., *26*:81, 1990, with permission.)

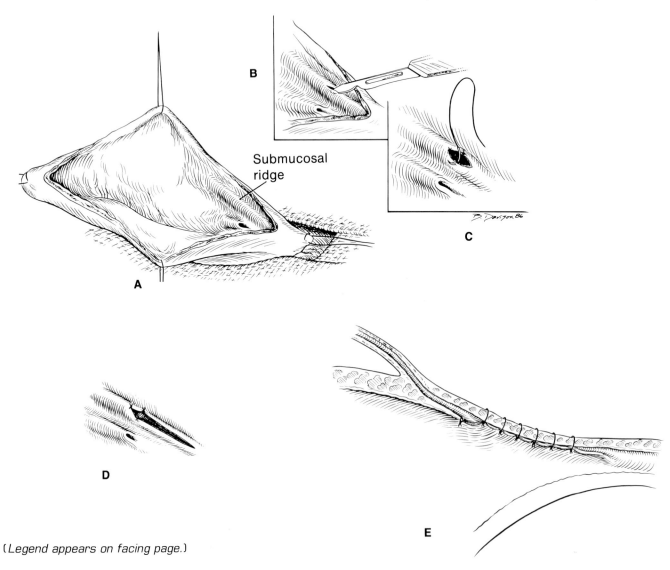

Submucosal ridge

(*Legend appears on facing page.*)

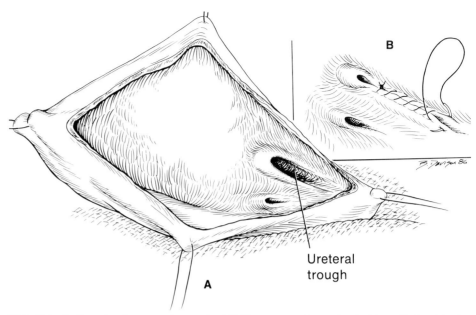

FIG. 25—4 Repair of ureteral trough. (A) The ureteral opening is identified, with the trough extending distally into the urethra. (B) After a strip of mucosa is excised from each side of the trough, the trough is closed in a simple continuous pattern, including both sides and the dorsal surface of the trough in each suture site. (From Stone, E.A., and Mason, K.L.: Surgery of ectopic ureters: Types, method of correction, and postoperative results. J. Am. Anim. Hosp. Assoc., *26*:81, 1990, with permission.)

wall, is suspected when no ureteral opening is seen within the trigone, and no submucosal bulge is elicited even with occlusion of the urethra (Fig. 25–5A). The ureter is identified external to the bladder and followed distally beyond the trigone. The ureter is severed as far distally as possible (Fig. 25–5B) and reimplanted into the trigone (ureteroneocystostomy), using the technique described in Chapter 22 (see Fig. 22–3). In a cat, microsurgical techniques may be necessary to implant the ureters successfully.

Ureteral catheters (3.5 Fr gauge) are placed for 2 days in cats and small dogs because postoperative edema may occlude small ureters. The catheters are exited through the urethra and attached to a closed collection device.

The trigone is closed with simple interrupted appositional sutures. The remaining incision in the urinary bladder is closed routinely (see Fig. 19–5).

PATENT URACHUS

Surgical correction of patent urachus requires excision of the entire urachus. A ventral midline skin incision is made from the umbilicus to the pubis. The urachus is identified, extending from the umbilicus to the bladder (Fig. 25–6). An elliptical incision is made around the umbilicus and its attached urachus. The urachus is traced back to the bladder, and a full-thickness circular

◄

FIG. 25—3 (A) Repair of intramural ectopic ureter. The submucosal ridge created by the ectopic ureter is identified. (B) A 3- to 5-mm incision is made through the bladder mucosa and into the ureter at the typical location for a ureteral opening. (C) The proximal and lateral edges of the incised ureter are sutured to the edges of the incised bladder mucosa with 4–0 to 7–0 absorbable suture material. (From Stone, E.A., and Mason, K.L.: Surgery of ectopic ureters: Types, method of correction, and postoperative results. J. Am. Anim. Hosp. Assoc., *26*:81, 1990, with permission.) (D) The distal portion of the ectopic ureter is incised longitudinally, starting at the new opening and continuing distally for 1-2 cm. (E) Sutures are placed through one side of the incised ureter, through the bladder wall, and through the other side of the incised ureter. Tying the sutures flattens the incised ureter and occludes the lumen.

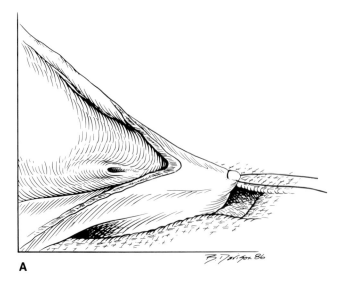

A

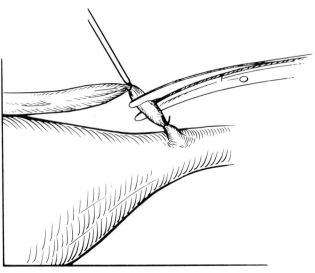

B

FIG. 25–5 Repair of extramural ureter. (A) No ureteral opening is seen within the trigone, and no submucosal ridge is apparent, even with occlusion of the urethra. (B) The ureter is ligated and severed as far distally as possible. (Creation of the ureteroneocystostomy is depicted in Fig. 22–3.)

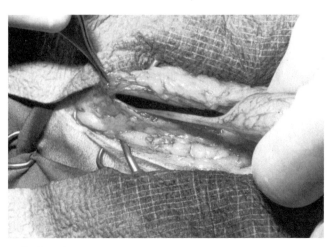

FIG. 25–6. Patent urachus (arrow) extends from umbilicus to bladder (held by fingers).

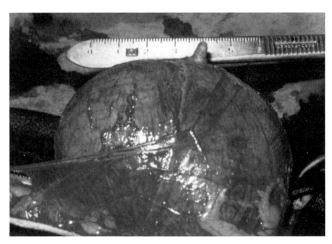

FIG. 25–7. Vesicourachal diverticulum protruding from the cranial dome of the bladder.

incision is made in the bladder wall around the urachus. The bladder is closed with simple interrupted sutures that do not penetrate the lumen. Abdominal wall closure is routine.

VESICOURACHAL DIVERTICULUM

Following a caudal abdominal incision, the vesicourachal diverticulum is identified (Fig. 25–7). The bladder wall is excised around the diverticulum, and the diverticulum is removed. The bladder is closed with simple interrupted sutures that do not penetrate the mucosa.

HYPOSPADIA

The type of surgical correction depends on the extent of the hypospadia. If the urethral opening is cranial to the scrotum, as depicted in Fig. 24–6, castration and scrotal urethrostomy (see Fig. 16–7) is the treatment of choice. If the urethral opening is in the perineal region, a perineal urethrostomy (see Fig. 31–4) is performed. The urethral groove and remnants of the prepuce and penis are excised.

URETHRORECTAL DIVERTICULUM

Warm water enemas are given the evening before and the morning of surgery. Antibiotic administration (metronidazole, 30 mg/kg once a day by mouth, and trimethoprim-sulfadiazine, 30 mg/kg bid (or q 12 hrs) by mouth) is initiated the day before surgery and continued for 24 hours after surgery. After the dog is anesthetized, catheters are placed in the urethra and in the rectum.

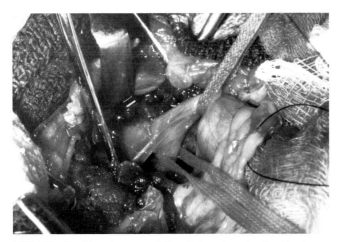

FIG. 25–8. Urethrorectal fistula is retracted by the lower umbilical tape. Upper umbilical tape is retracting the dilated proximal urethra. (From Osuna, D.J., Stone, E.A., and Metcalf, M.R.: A urethrorectal fistula with concurrent urolithiasis in a dog. J. Am. Anim. Hosp. Assoc., 25:35, 1989; with permission.)

A ventral abdominal incision is made from the umbilicus to the pubis. It may be necessary to do a pubic or pubic and ischiatic osteotomy (see Fig. 10–4) to gain exposure to the rectum and caudal urethra. After the fistula is identified, an umbilical tape is passed around it for retraction (Fig. 25–8). The fistula is severed near the urethra. The opening in the urethra is closed with 4–0 absorbable suture material in simple interrupted pattern. The fistula is traced to the rectum, where it is severed and the opening into the rectum closed in a similar pattern.[3]

REFERENCES

1. Stone, E.A., and Mason, K.L.: Surgery of ectopic ureters: Types, method of correction, and postoperative results. J. Am. Anim. Hosp. Assoc., 26:81, 1990.
2. Rawlings, C.A.: Correction of congenital defects of the urogenital system. Vet. Clin. North Am. Sm. Anim. Pract., 14:49, 1984.
3. Osuna, D.J., Stone, E.A., and Metcalf, M.R.: A urethrorectal fistula with concurrent urolithiasis in a dog. J. Am. Anim. Hosp. Assoc., 25:35, 1989.

26

Postoperative Management and Surgical Complications of Congenital Disorders

POSTOPERATIVE MANAGEMENT

Following ectopic ureter, patent urachus, or vesicourachal diverticulum surgery, routine management for cystotomy is done. Fluid therapy is continued until the dog is drinking on its own. The bladder is kept decompressed by allowing frequent voiding, preferably, or intermittent catheterization. Ureteral catheters, if used, are removed in 2 days. Urine scalding, secondary to chronic urine dribbling from ectopic ureters or a patent urachus, is treated with topical ointments and should resolve once the incontinence ceases. After a hypospadia repair, the urethrostomy site may bleed for several days. It may be necessary to hospitalize and tranquilize the dog to keep the dog calm and control hemorrhage. Any dog with urinary tract infection is treated and re-evaluated to ascertain effective therapy (see Chapter 18).

POSTOPERATIVE COMPLICATIONS

Ectopic Ureters

Urinary incontinence may persist after surgical correction of ectopic ureters in some dogs. The prevalence and causes of this complication are not fully understood, but ineffective surgical correction, abnormal vaginal anatomy, reduced bladder capacity, and primary urethral sphincter mechanism incompetence have all been implicated.[1-3] Dogs that remain incontinent following surgical repair require careful re-evaluation. Urethral pressure profilometry, available at referral centers, helps assess urethral sphincter function.

An excretory urogram, pneumocystogram, and vaginourethrogram are performed to diagnose a patent distal ureteral segment, following correction of an intramural ectopic ureter, and to assess the bladder and vagina. During an excretory urogram, contrast material is seen entering the bladder and continuing beyond the trigone, paralleling the urethra as it does in nonoperated intramural ectopic ureters. A vaginourethrogram may reveal reflux into the submucosal segment of an ectopic ureter. Inadequate occlusion may result from loosening of the ligatures around the distal segment or improper positioning of the ligatures during the initial surgery. For correction, a ventral cystotomy is performed, and the distal segment is ligated as in Fig. 25–3D, E.

A vaginourethrogram may also identify an abnormally shaped vagina, which may cause positional and sleep incontinence.[2] Abnormal sloping of the vagina in a cranioventral direction ("up and over" vagina) may allow urine to pool in the cranial vagina and to overflow intermittently as the dog changes position. Correction of this abnormality has been described.[4] Vestibulovaginal stenosis was initially thought to cause urine pooling cranial to the stenotic area.[5] A more recent study, however, found no significant association between the presence of vestibulovaginal stenosis and urinary incontinence.[6]

A bladder with decreased capacity can cause pollakiuria, which may be interpreted as incontinence. In our experience, a small bladder associated with ectopic ureters expands to normal size once urinary continence is established. If the dog is incontinent and a contrast cystogram reveals a small bladder, medical therapy should be initiated to try to restore continence and allow urine accumulation to expand the bladder.

Urinary tract infection can induce frequent voiding, which may be confused with incontinence and should be treated.

Medical therapy may be initiated to increase urethral sphincter function. Phenylpropanolamine (1.5 mg/kg tid by mouth) is an alpha adrenergic blocker that has been used successfully in some dogs with urethral sphincter mechanism incompetence after ectopic ureter surgery.[1,5] Alternatively, imipramine (0.5 to 1 mg/kg tid by mouth), a tricyclic antidepressant agent, can be tried.

Because this drug increases bladder capacity in addition to increasing urethral sphincter, it may be beneficial to dogs with small bladders and urethral incompetence.

Urinary incontinence secondary to incompetence of the urethral sphincter mechanism may be exacerbated by an intrapelvic, rather than intra-abdominal, bladder neck and proximal urethra.[6] A technique for moving the neck of the bladder to an intra-abdominal position by tacking the cranial vagina to the right and left prepubic tendons (colposuspension) has been described.[8] A study of the response to colposuspension in 150 bitches with incompetence of the urethral sphincter mechanism only (i.e., not ectopic ureters or other urinary tract abnormalities) indicated that 53% were completely cured, and the majority of the remainder became less incontinent.[9] The results in incontinent dogs with both incompetent sphincter mechanisms and previously operated ectopic ureters may not be as good. In the future, however, colposuspension should be considered for incontinent dogs that are unresponsive to medical therapy after successful repair of ectopic ureters.

PATENT URACHUS, VESICOURACHAL DIVERTICULUM

Complications following resection of a patent urachus or vesicourachal diverticulum are similar to those associated with cystotomy for any other reason (see Chapter 20).

HYPOSPADIA

Complications of scrotal and perineal urethrostomies are discussed in Chapter 17.

URETHRORECTAL DIVERTICULUM

If excessive urethral or rectal tissue is excised, stricture could develop. This problem is best avoided by severing the fistula level with the urethra and the rectum and closing the defects without inverting tissue.

REFERENCES

1. Stone, E.A., and Mason, K.L.: Surgery of ectopic ureters: Types, method of correction and postoperative results. J. Am. Anim. Hosp. Assoc., 26:81, 1990.
2. Holt, P.E.: Ectopic ureter in the bitch. Vet. Rec., 10:299, 1976.
3. Cotard, J.P., Collas, G., and Leclere, C.: L'ectopie ureterale chez le chien. A propos de onze cas. Rec. Med. Vet., 160:731, 1984.
4. Wykes, P.M., and Olson, P.N.: The vagina. In Textbook of Small Animal Surgery. Edited by D.H. Slatter. Philadelphia, W.B. Saunders, 1985, pp. 1672–1677.
5. Holt, P.E., and Sayle, B.: Congenital vestibulo-vaginal stenosis in the bitch. J. Sm. Anim. Pract., 22:67, 1981.
6. Holt, P.E.: Importance of urethral length, bladder neck position and vestibulovaginal stenosis in sphincter mechanism incompetence in the incontinent bitch. Res. Vet. Sci., 39:364, 1985.
7. Rigg, D.L., Zenoble, R.D., and Riedesel, E.A.: Neoureterostomy and phenylpropanolamine therapy for incontinence due to ectopic ureter in a dog. J. Am. Anim. Hosp., 19:237, 1983.
8. Holt, P.E.: Urinary incontinence in the bitch due to sphincter mechanism incompetence: Surgical treatment. J. Sm. Anim. Pract., 26:237, 1985.
9. Holt, P.E.: Long-term evaluation of colposuspension in the treatment of urinary incontinence due to incompetence of the urethral sphincter mechanism in the bitch. Vet. Res., 127:537, 1990.

Section Nine

Prostatic Disorders

27

Diagnosis and Medical Therapy of Prostatic Disorders

The normal anatomy and physiology of the prostate gland as well as the major causes for prostatomegaly are discussed in Chapter 4. Chapter 5 includes a description of the diagnostic techniques used to determine whether the prostate gland is normal or abnormal. The radiographic and ultrasonographic findings in prostatic diseases are discussed in Chapter 6. This chapter builds on these foundations by reviewing the clinical signs that are associated with various prostatic diseases and presenting a diagnostic plan to determine which disease is present. The medical therapy of each of the major diseases is discussed. Chapters 29 and 30 present the surgical therapy of prostatic diseases and the potential postoperative complications.

CLINICAL SIGNS

Clinical signs vary with the type and severity of prostatic disease (Table 27–1). Any prostatic disease except acute prostatitis can occur with no abnormal signs evident to the owner. Most prostatic diseases are associated with prostatomegaly. Early detection of these diseases may be possible by performing a yearly rectal examination on all mature male dogs. Probable avoidance of all prostatic diseases except neoplasia is one reason for advocating neutering young male dogs.

The major clinical problems for which dogs with prostatic disease are presented to veterinarians are discussed in this section. The types of prostatic disease that can produce each problem are listed, so that a list of reasonable differential diagnoses can be formulated based on the clinical problems. Problems with other organ systems that can produce these signs are not included.

Tenesmus

Fecal tenesmus may be caused by an enlarged prostate gland encroaching on the rectum in the pelvic canal.

Diseases that cause prostatomegaly are given in Table 4–1. Tenesmus may be the only abnormal sign associated with uncomplicated prostatic hyperplasia.

Dysuria/Urinary Incontinence

If prostatic enlargement is marked, dysuria from partial urethral obstruction may result. This is an uncommon sign in dogs in contrast to men because of differences in prostatic anatomy and physiology between the two species. With hyperplasia, the canine prostate gland tends to enlarge outward away from the urethra. Partial urethral obstruction is usually noted only in dogs with marked prostatomegaly associated with abscesses, cysts, or neoplasia. We have encountered only one dog in which partial urethral obstruction occurred from chronic prostatic inflammation and hyperplasia with minimal prostatic enlargement.

If a partial obstruction remains unresolved, the bladder detrusor muscle, urethra, or both may be damaged, resulting in urinary incontinence. Urodynamic (cystometric and urethral pressure profile) abnormalities are common in dogs with significant prostatic disease even if there is no history of incontinence.[1]

Urethral Discharge

A urethral discharge can result from abnormal prostatic fluid production as a result of cyst formation, from prostatic hemorrhage, or from exudation of pus. In each case, the fluid flows from the prostatic acini through the prostatic ducts into the urethra in sufficient quantities not only to reflux into the bladder, but also to drain out the urethral orifice. Other causes, besides prostatic disease, must also be considered for a urethral discharge (see Chapter 2). Any disease causing development of cysts, which communicate with the urethra or which result in prostatic inflammation or hemorrhage, can result in a urethral discharge. These include cystic hy-

TABLE 27–1. EXPECTED CLINICAL FINDINGS IN PROSTATIC DISEASES

Prostatic Disease	Possible Historical Problems	Physical Examination Findings	Complete Blood Count	Urinalysis/ Urine Culture	Biochemical Profile	Prostatic Fluid Evaluation	Radiography	Ultrasonography
Benign hyperplasia	Fecal tenesmus Urethral discharge No abnormal signs	Nonpainful, symmetrical prostatomegaly	Normal	Hematuria	Normal	Hemorrhagic Negative bacterial culture	Mild to moderate prostatomegaly	Diffusely hyperechoic with focal hypoechoic areas (cysts)
Paraprostatic cyst	Fecal tenesmus Dysuria/ incontinence Urethral discharge	Abdominal or perineal mass (fluctuant or firm)	Normal	Normal	Normal unless compression of ureters	Variable—normal or hemorrhagic	Asymmetrical prostateomegaly or "two bladders"	Large hypoechoic or anechoic mass
Squamous metaplasia	Fecal tenesmus Alopecia Hyperpigmentation Gynecomastia Pendulous prepuce (due to hyperestrogenism)	Mild to moderate prostatomegaly Abnormal testes Signs of hyperestrogenism	Normal	Normal	Normal	Mild inflammation Squamous cells	Mild to moderate prostatomegaly Accentuated colliculus seminalis	Diffusely hyperechoic
Acute prostatitis	Urethral discharge Depression/ anorexia Occasionally vomiting	Fever Caudal abdominal pain Occasionally a stiff, stilted gait	Leukocytosis	Hematuria Pyuria Bacteriuria	Normal unless septic	Usually not evaluated	Loss of detail in vicinity of prostate or normal	Diffusely or focally hyperechoic
Chronic prostatitis	Urethral discharge Recurrent urinary tract infection No abnormal signs	Normal Prostate may have variable consistency due to fibrosis	Normal	Hematuria Pyuria Bacteriuria	Normal	Purulent Positive bacterial culture	Normal or mild granular mineralization	Focally or diffusely hyperechoic
Abscessation	Fecal tenesmus Dysuria/ incontinence Urethral discharge Anorexia/ depression Recurrent urinary tract infection	Fever Occasionally peritonitis or sepsis Asymmetrical prostatomegaly	Leukocytosis	Hematuria Pyuria Bacteriuria	Possibly signs of sepsis— hypoalbuminemia, elevated serum alkaline phosphatase, hypoglycemia, hepatopathy, icterus	Purulent Positive bacterial culture	Asymmetrical prostatomegaly	Diffusely hyperechoic with focal anechoic area(s) Asymmetrical
Neoplasia	Fecal tenesmus Dysuria/ incontinence Urethral discharge Anorexia/ depression Weight loss	Fever Hind limb weakness or stiffness Asymmetrical prostatomegaly with focally firm areas	Normal (20% have leukocytosis)	Hematuria Pyuria	Normal unless azotemia from compression of ureters or increased serum alkaline phosphatase from bone metastasis	Hemorrhagic Purulent Negative bacterial culture	Asymmetrical prostatomegaly Granular mineralization Distortion of the prostatic urethra	Multifocally hyperechoic Asymmetrical

perplasia, bacterial infection, abscessation, and neoplasia.

Systemic Illness

Systemic signs of prostatic disease include fever, depression, pain in the caudal abdomen, a stiff gait in the rear limbs, vomiting, and leukocytosis (Fig. 27–1). These signs are usually associated with acute bacterial prostatitis, prostatic abscessation, or prostatic adenocarcinoma. Systemic signs associated with bacterial infection may be caused by severe local infection, secondary peritonitis, or secondary septicemia. With carcinoma, systemic signs may be caused by necrosis and inflammation associated with tumor growth exceeding blood supply or from metastasis, particularly to bone.[2,3]

Other systemic signs that may be seen with severe bacterial prostatitis or prostatic abscessation are evidence of liver disease (icterus, elevated liver enzymes) and liver dysfunction (abnormal liver function tests). Liver biopsies show minimal lesions.[4] Such a hepatopathy, referred to as reactive hepatopathy, is associated

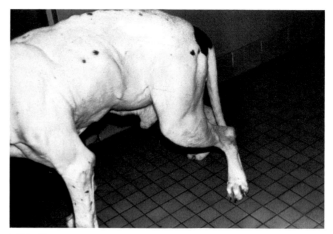

FIG. 27–1. A dog exhibiting pain in the rear limbs by standing up on its toes and slightly squatting. In this dog, the source of the pain was localized to the prostate gland by rectal palpation. The concurrent presence of fever, leukocytosis, and urinary tract infection with only mild prostatomegaly in this young adult supported a presumptive diagnosis of acute bacterial prostatitis.

with endotoxemia or septicemia caused by infection with *Escherichia coli*.[5] *E. coli* are the most common bacteria associated with prostatic infections. Another potential sign associated with *E. coli* endotoxemia is an obligatory polyuria/polydipsia suspected to be caused by inhibition of antidiuretic hormone (ADH) action by endotoxin (a form of nephrogenic diabetes insipidus).[4]

Abdominal Distention/Perineal Mass

Abdominal distention may be noted with very large paraprostatic cysts. Such large cysts may mineralize. If the cyst extends caudally, a firm mass may occur in the perineal area.

Urinary Tract Infection

Recurrent lower urinary tract infection (UTI) in male dogs is often caused by chronic bacterial prostatitis and may be the only abnormal sign associated with chronic prostatitis. If the underlying cause of the UTI is not suspected, routine antibiotic therapy may eliminate the bacteriuria. The prostatic infection will persist, however, and bacteria will reinfect the bladder when antibiotics are discontinued. Urinary tract infections are also common in dogs with acute bacterial prostatitis and with prostatic abscessation.

DIAGNOSTIC PLAN FOR SUSPECTED PROSTATIC DISEASE

The main diagnostic techniques for prostatic disease are history, prostatic palpation, cytologic examination of any urethral discharge, cytologic and microbiologic examination of prostatic fluid collected by ejaculation or after prostatic massage, complete blood count (CBC), urinalysis and urine culture, serum biochemical profile, radiography, ultrasonography, prostatic aspiration, and prostatic biopsy. The methods for most of these techniques are described in Chapters 5 and 6. This chapter focuses on interpreting the results.

Which tests to perform depends on the severity of the clinical signs. A history and physical examination, including rectal palpation, are indicated in all cases. If the dog is normal except for mild symmetrical prostatomegaly, prostatic hyperplasia is most likely and no further diagnostic testing or therapy is indicated. For dogs with clinical signs, the diagnostic plan includes a CBC, urinalysis, urine culture, and prostatic fluid cytology and culture. Depending on the severity of clinical signs, radiography, ultrasonography, and a serum biochemical profile may be indicated. On the basis of all these clinical findings, one should be able to determine in many cases what the likely diagnosis is and pursue therapy. If the diagnosis is still not evident or requires further confirmation (such as with suspected neoplasia or suspected infection with questionable culture results), prostatic aspiration, biopsy, or both can be performed.

History

A complete history is obtained including both the chief complaint and a review of the dog's overall health status. The nature, severity, duration, and progression of the abnormal presenting sign(s) are determined. Whether urination and defecation are normal is established. Any abnormality should be characterized. The occurrence of any systemic signs of illness (pain, depression, anorexia, vomiting), any lameness, or any changes in water intake or urine output may be important clues to the nature of the disease. Whether the dog is neutered, and, if neutered, why and when are important questions in relation to prostatic disease.

Prostatic Palpation

Prostatic palpation is essential to determine the presence and degree of prostatomegaly as well as the consistency of the gland (see Fig. 4–2). During the rectal examination, an attempt is made to palpate the iliac lymph nodes and to determine whether and to what degree the prostate gland encroaches on the rectal canal.

During the physical examination, the rest of the urinary and reproductive tracts is examined carefully. One should always note the reproductive status of the dog. If the dog is neutered, the prostate gland should be atrophied. If it is not small, it is abnormal, even if it is within normal size limits for an intact dog. Prostatomegaly in a dog neutered years previously is strongly suggestive of neoplasia (Fig. 27–2). Persistent prostatomegaly in a dog that was neutered because of prostatic disease indicates that the underlying disease is not uncomplicated benign hyperplasia. Prostatic cysts, abscesses, or neoplasia must be considered.

Diseases associated with the most severe prostatomegaly are cysts, abscessation, and neoplasia. With

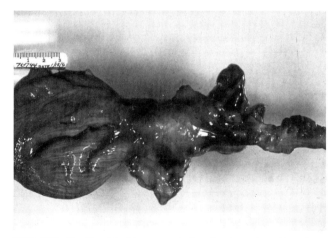

FIG. 27–2. The bladder, prostate gland, and urethra from a neutered dog presented for dysuria and inability to empty the bladder. Prostatic adenocarcinoma obstructing the prostatic urethra caused the clinical signs. Note that the prostate gland is not markedly enlarged but is markedly abnormal for a dog neutered when young. A much smaller, atrophied gland is expected after neutering.

these diseases, the gland is often asymmetrical and contains areas of varying consistency. Neoplastic areas are often of increased firmness. Palpation alone cannot be relied on for diagnosis, however, since areas of chronic inflammation also may be firm. Both inflammatory and neoplastic diseases can lead to enlargement of the iliac lymph nodes.

Mild prostatomegaly with maintenance of symmetry is most often associated with benign hyperplasia. The gland may develop a "cobblestone" type contour with cystic hyperplasia. Squamous metaplasia is also associated with mild prostatomegaly unless secondary abscessation develops.

The prostate gland may be normal in size and shape with either acute or chronic bacterial infection. With acute inflammation, there is usually discomfort on palpation and systemic signs of illness.

Urethral Discharge

If a urethral discharge is present, it should be examined microscopically. A light yellow discharge, somewhat similar to urine, may be seen with prostatic cysts that communicate with the urethra. Such a discharge must be compared to urine collected from the bladder at the same time to ensure that the problem is not urinary incontinence.

A hemorrhagic discharge may be found with cystic hyperplasia, acute or chronic infection, abscessation, or neoplasia. If the discharge also indicates inflammation, acute or chronic infection, abscessation, and neoplasia are much more likely than hyperplasia. Abnormal cells suggestive of neoplasia are rarely detected in urethral discharges, even when neoplasia is the cause of the discharge.

As noted in Chapter 5, urethral discharges are usually not cultured because of the normal distal urethral flora. If a quantitative culture, however, is performed as described in Chapter 5 and if a similar organism is cultured from urine collected by cystocentesis, the most likely diagnosis would be acute or chronic bacterial prostatitis or abscessation.

Semen Evaluation

The last fraction of an ejaculate is prostatic fluid (see Chapter 5). Both cytology and quantitative culture should be performed on the sample obtained.

Large numbers of white blood cells indicate inflammation, which is compatible either with infection or neoplasia but is not noted in hyperplasia. Hemorrhage can be found with hyperplasia, infection, or neoplasia. Abnormal epithelial cells suggestive of neoplasia are rarely seen in ejaculates, even in dogs whose prostatic disease is neoplastic.

The results of quantitative culture of the ejaculate are not easily interpreted because of possible and variable contamination by the normal urethral flora.[6,7] Because *E. coli* is the most common organism associated with prostatic infection, high numbers (> 100,000/ml) of it

with large numbers of white blood cells indicate infection. Likewise, high numbers of other gram-negative or gram-positive organisms with large numbers of white blood cells probably indicate infection if preputial contamination did not occur. Lower numbers of gram-negative or gram-positive organisms must be correlated with clinical signs, results of urinalysis and urine culture, and ejaculate cytology to determine significance.[6] Comparison with a urethral swab culture may be useful, as long as the dog does not have a urinary tract infection[7] (see Chapter 5). Remember that an abnormality in the ejaculate does not localize the problem to the prostate, since the testicles, epididymides, deferent ducts, and urethra also contribute to or transport the ejaculate.

Prostatic Massage

Because of the dog's pain, inexperience, or temperament, it is not possible to collect semen on all dogs with suspected prostatic disease. An alternative technique to collect prostatic fluid is prostatic massage (see Chapter 5). Remember that both the premassage and postmassage samples should be examined microscopically and by quantitative culture.

Cytologic evidence of purulent or mononuclear inflammation that is greater in the postmassage than premassage sample is strongly indicative of prostatic inflammation, caused by either infection or neoplasia. Cytologic evidence of hemorrhage, which is greater in the postmassage sample, is consistent with hyperplasia, infection, or neoplasia. Epithelial cells may also be evident in postmassage samples. Normal prostatic epithelial cells are cuboidal and uniform with central round to oval nuclei and moderate, lightly basophilic cytoplasm.[8] A few transitional cells are often seen that may be binucleate. In dogs with neoplasia, abnormal epithelial cells with characteristics of malignancy are often (but not always) seen in the postmassage samples.

To diagnose bacterial infection definitively by prostatic massage, numbers of bacteria must be greater in the postmassage than the premassage samples. As discussed in Chapter 5, the concurrent presence of bacterial UTI often interferes with interpretation of prostatic massage results. We usually perform cultures on prostatic massage samples only when UTI is absent or controlled.

Radiography

The radiographic characteristics of both the normal and abnormal prostate gland are presented in Chapter 6. Survey radiography is usually of limited benefit in diagnosis of specific prostatic diseases. In many dogs, the prostate can be palpated more accurately than it can be visualized on survey radiographs. Helpful findings for diagnosis, however, include the following. Poor contrast of caudal abdominal structures may exist with abscessation, carcinoma, and paraprostatic cysts. Asymmetrical shape is noted with abscess, neoplasia, and cysts.[9] Granular mineralization can be seen with inflammation or neoplasia; however, multifocal, irregularly distributed areas of mineralization are suggestive of prostatic carcinoma.[10] Marked prostatic enlargement is most often associated with abscessation, cysts, or neoplasia.[9,10] Enlargement of the iliac lymph nodes may be associated with either infection or neoplasia. All bones visible on the radiograph should be carefully examined for lytic lesions, suggestive of metastasis from prostatic adenocarcinoma (see Fig. 6–51).

Retrograde urethrography is often used to characterize further the prostate gland and its effects on the urethra (see Figs. 6–50, 6–52A). One must remember in interpreting the results that characteristics of the prostatic urethra vary with degree of bladder distention.[11] Narrowing of the prostatic urethra can be normal if the bladder is not distended.

To avoid variations in technique, distention retrograde urethrocystography has been recommended as the contrast study of choice.[12,13] With this method, the urinary bladder is palpably distended before retrograde infusion of the contrast media, using end-hole, balloon catheters. The normal diameter of the prostatic urethra is 1 to 2.7 times the diameter of the midpelvic membranous urethra (see Fig. 6–44). The prostate should be symmetrical around the urethra. The colliculus seminalis (urethral crest) may be visualized on distention urethrocystography in normal dogs but may be accentuated in dogs with squamous metaplasia of the prostate gland.[13,14] Mild urethroprostatic reflux is normal.[15] This normal reflux usually does not extend greater than one prostatic urethral diameter into the prostatic parenchyma. More extensive reflux can be seen with cysts, abscesses, and neoplasia. Massive, coalescent reflux is suggestive of abscessation or neoplasia (see Fig. 6–45). A narrowed prostatic urethra can be noted with neoplasia, abscessation, large parenchymal cysts, and rarely with hyperplasia.[10] If the prostatic urethra is markedly irregular, neoplasia is most likely (see Fig. 6–45). If the prostate is markedly asymmetrical in relation to the urethra, abscessation, parenchymal cyst, or neoplasia is most likely (see Figs. 6–49, 6–52A).[10] Although retrograde urethrography with bladder distention may allow better assessment of the prostatic urethra and prostate gland, the technique has potential complications. These include hematuria and induction of UTI in addition to the possibility of bladder rupture if significant bladder wall disease or injury is present.[16,17]

If the prostate is markedly enlarged, excretory urography is often necessary to determine whether ureteral obstruction is occurring. This is especially important in cases with clinical evidence of reduced renal function such as reduced concentrating ability or azotemia.

If prostatic neoplasia is a likely possibility, thoracic and abdominal radiographs should be examined for evidence of metastasis. The main metastatic route for prostatic adenocarcinoma is via pelvic lymphatics to the iliac lymph nodes, to the vertebral bodies, and to the lungs (see Fig. 6–51). Metastasis to other bones, however, most commonly ribs, long bones, and digits, is not uncommon.[2,3]

Ultrasonography

Prostatic consistency can be evaluated better with ultrasonography than with radiography (see Chapter 6; Fig. 6–48).[18,19]

A generalized increase in parenchymal echogenicity can be observed with any prostatic disease. Diseases such as inflammation and neoplasia have focal to multifocal areas of increased echogenicity, whereas cavitary diseases such as intraparenchymal cysts or abscesses appear focally hypoechoic to anechoic (see Fig. 6–54).[18] Ultrasonography can also differentiate paraprostatic cysts from other caudal abdominal masses (see Fig. 6–52).[18] Combining retrograde urethrocystography with ultrasonography may be of value because bladder distention can help in the ultrasonographic identification of the prostate gland. Ultrasonography can also provide guidance for aspiration and biopsy.[20]

Prostatic Aspiration

Diagnosis of prostatic disease can be aided by needle aspiration or biopsy (see Chapter 5). Ultrasonography can assist in directing the needle into abnormal areas. Aspirated material is examined cytologically. Any fluid obtained should be cultured for bacteria.

Aspiration can confirm a diagnosis of a prostatic cyst by finding a clear or serosanguineous fluid, which is neither inflammatory nor infected. Aspiration can also confirm a diagnosis of an abscess by the retrieval of pus, although this may be associated with dissemination of infection (see Chapter 5; Fig. 27–3). Aspiration of cells with characteristics of malignancy confirms neoplasia, whereas aspiration of squamous epithelial cells suggests squamous metaplasia.

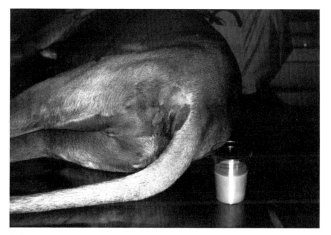

FIG. 27–3. Purulent fluid aspirated from the prostate gland, indicating abscessation. A portion of the fluid was collected aseptically for bacterial culture, and a portion was examined microscopically. After sample collection, as much fluid as possible was withdrawn through the same, single needle puncture.

Prostatic Biopsy

The techniques for both percutaneous and surgical prostatic biopsy are given in Chapter 5. An impression smear can be made from the biopsy for a rapid cytologic evaluation. Part of the biopsy specimen can also be placed in a sterile container and cultured for bacteria. The major portion of the biopsy specimen should be fixed and submitted for histologic examination.

The histologic results determine the tissue diagnosis as to hyperplasia, cystic hyperplasia, inflammation, or neoplasia. Bacterial organisms are usually not seen on histologic specimens. Positive cultures of prostatic fluid or tissue must be used to confirm a diagnosis of prostatic infection.

MEDICAL THERAPY

To institute appropriate therapy, one must make an accurate diagnosis. The diagnosis is based on the interpretation of results of appropriate diagnostic tests (see Table 27–1). In many cases, the results of these tests most strongly support one disease, and treatment can be based on a presumptive diagnosis without biopsy confirmation. In other dogs, a diagnosis may not be clear because of natural variation in the disease process as well as the common occurrence of more than one disease process within a prostate gland (e.g., hyperplasia plus infection). In this situation, prostatic tissue will need to be examined to make a definitive diagnosis. In any dog, if the response to therapy is not as would be expected for the suspected disease, further diagnostic evaluation should be performed. For example, you suspect a dog has prostatic hyperplasia and treat with castration. If there is no reduction in prostatic size after a few weeks, the disease is not uncomplicated hyperplasia but may be prostatic neoplasia or inflammation.

After establishing a presumptive or definitive diagnosis, therapy is instituted. This chapter reviews medical therapy for each major disease process. The pathophysiology of the diseases is also discussed briefly, but for a more complete review, other texts should be consulted.[21]

Benign Hyperplasia

Pathophysiology

Benign prostatic hyperplasia is an aging change that occurs in only two species, humans and dogs.[22] The development of hyperplasia is associated with an age-related change in the altered androgen to estrogen ratio and requires the presence of the testes.[23] Dihydrotestosterone within the gland probably serves as one hormonal mediator for hyperplasia.[24] Dihydrotestosterone may accumulate because of changes in catabolism and enhanced binding. Inhibitors of the final enzyme (5-alpha-reductase) in the synthetic pathway for dihydrotestosterone are promising for medical treatment of benign prostatic hyperplasia in the future.

Benign prostatic hyperplasia in the dog begins as glan-

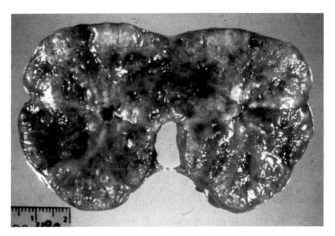

FIG. 27–4. A prostate gland with cystic hyperplasia; note the multifocal cystic areas, some of which appear hemorrhagic. Also note the mildly irregular, "cobblestone," contour of the gland. (Courtesy of Drs. W.A. Crowell and L.A. Cowan, College of Veterinary Medicine, University of Georgia.)

dular hyperplasia, as early as 2.5 years of age in some dogs.[25] After 4 years of age, the tendency to cystic hyperplasia begins,[25] appearing like a honeycomb on cross section (Fig. 27–4). Thus, intraprostatic cystic hyperplasia is an extension of glandular hyperplasia. Intraparenchymal cysts often communicate with the urethra and may be largest at the periphery of the gland.[26] The vascularity of the prostate is increased in hyperplasia, and the gland has a tendency to bleed.[26] Evidence of mild chronic mononuclear inflammation is also common[23,27] and seems to increase with age.[28] The cysts vary in size and contour and contain a thin, clear to amber fluid. In an individual dog, benign prostatic hyperplasia seems to develop rapidly (within 1 year after onset).[25]

Treatment

Treatment is required only if related abnormal signs are present (Fig. 27–5). The most effective treatment is castration, which results in a 70% decrease in prostate size.[26,29] The prostate gland begins to involute within days, and a palpable decrease in prostatic size is expected within 7 to 10 days. Prostatic secretion becomes minimal at 7 to 16 days after castration.[26,30] In both young and old dogs, prostatic weight declines most rapidly within the first month after castration.[31] In older dogs (> 6 years), prostatic weight continues to decline for 3 to 4 months.[26,31] With cystic hyperplasia, small irregular spaces may remain postcastration.[26]

If castration is not feasible, low doses of estrogens can be used. Estrogens depress gonadotropin secretion by the pituitary gland, which reduces the level of androgen secreted by the testes and results in prostatic atrophy. Diethylstilbestrol (DES) administered orally at 0.2 to 1 mg/day for 5 days has been recommended. In one study, 0.1 mg of injectable DES/day for 5 days markedly reduced prostatic secretory capability for 2 months.[32]

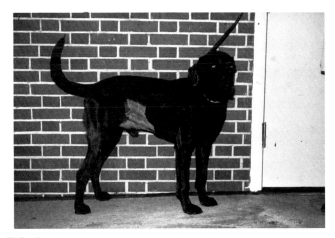

FIG. 27–5. A dog presented for a hemorrhagic urethral discharge and hematuria. The dog was normal otherwise, alert and active. Physical examination indicated mild prostatomegaly. On ultrasonographic examination, the prostate gland contained multifocal, small cystic spaces. Prostatic fluid was hemorrhagic but sterile. The presumptive diagnosis was cystic hyperplasia. Castration was effective in resolving the clinical signs.

The potential side effects of estrogen therapy must be compared with its clinical benefit in each dog. Toxicity is manifested by an initial leukocytosis with a left shift, followed by severe bone marrow depression with resultant anemia, thrombocytopenia, and leukopenia. These effects have been noticed with overdosage, with repeated administration, and at the recommended dose as an idiosyncratic reaction. In beagles, oral doses of 5 mg/day of DES resulted in death from estrogen toxicity within 2 months, whereas doses of 1 mg/day were tolerated for months without development of anemia.[33]

Although low doses of estrogens decrease prostatic size, repeated administration and overdosage can also cause growth of the fibromuscular stroma of the prostate, metaplasia of prostatic glandular epithelium, and secretory stasis.[26,34] These changes can result in further prostatic enlargement and a predisposition to cyst formation, bacterial infection, and abscessation.

The androgen receptor antagonist, flutamide, avoids the side effects of estrogens but is licensed only for use in men with prostatic neoplasia and is expensive. When this drug was administered to research dogs at 5 mg/kg/day orally, prostatic size decreased with no change in libido or sperm production.[35]

Megestrol acetate also has antiandrogenic properties. In men, megestrol reduces serum testosterone concentrations and competitively inhibits binding of dihydrotestosterone to intracellular receptors and inhibits 5-alpha-reductase.[36] The efficacy of megestrol for therapy of benign prostatic hyperplasia in dogs has not been studied. One group of authors, however, has recommended 0.55 mg/kg/day for 4 weeks.[37] Sperm numbers did not decrease, and one dog sired puppies while on therapy. The drug is not approved for this use, however, nor for any use longer than 1 month. Thus, the major use in dogs would be reserved for those animals whose owners desired further short-term use as a sire before castration.

Squamous Metaplasia

Pathophysiology

Squamous metaplasia of prostatic columnar epithelium is secondary to exogenous or endogenous hyperestrogenism.[26,32,34,38] The major endogenous cause is a functional Sertoli cell tumor. Estrogens also cause secretory stasis. The epithelial change and secretory stasis predispose to cyst formation, infection, and abscessation.

Treatment

Treatment requires removal of the source of estrogens, usually by castration in cases of endogenous hyperestrogenism and by discontinuation of medication in cases of exogenous hyperestrogenism. Squamous metaplasia of the epithelium is reversible.[26]

Paraprostatic Cysts

Pathophysiology

Occasionally a large cyst is found adjacent to the prostate and associated with it via a stalk or adhesions.[39] The cyst may also be closely associated with the dorsal wall of the bladder. These large cysts may be markedly enlarged prostatic cysts (prostatic retention cysts) or paraprostatic cysts of unknown origin.[39] They may be in the abdomen craniolateral to the prostate gland or in the pelvis caudal to the prostate, even extending to the perineum lateral to the anus. Some are in both sites. They can have a thin or thick wall with a smooth lining or masses of calcified material.[40,41]

Treatment

The recommended treatment for paraprostatic cysts is surgical excision or drainage (see Chapter 28). Castration is also recommended.

Bacterial Prostatitis

Pathophysiology

Bacterial prostatitis affects sexually mature male dogs. *E. coli* is the organism most frequently isolated, but infection with other gram-negative and gram-positive organisms is possible. Infection usually results from ascent of bacteria up the urethra, but it may also result from hematogenous infection, infection of bladder urine, and infection of semen.

Chronic prostatic infection may be a sequela to an acute infection or may develop insidiously without a prior bout of a clinically evident acute infection. It may be secondary to UTI, urolithiasis, or changes in prostatic architecture that interfere with prostatic fluid secretion, such as cysts, neoplasia, or squamous metaplasia. In dogs, lower UTI and prostatic infections are almost inseparable. Any male dog with a UTI should be considered to have a prostatic infection until proved otherwise, even if clinical signs are absent. The incidence of chronic prostatic infections in dogs is unknown. However, 6 to 10% of male dogs have UTI[42] and an accompanying prostatic infection would be expected.

Treatment of Acute Bacterial Prostatitis

An antibiotic is administered for 21 to 28 days. The choice of the antibiotic is based on results of urine culture and antibiotic sensitivity testing. The blood–prostatic fluid barrier is usually not intact in acute inflammation, allowing a wide initial antibiotic choice. If the presenting signs are severe, the antibiotic is initially administered intravenously with parenteral fluid support. Oral antimicrobials are used once the dog's condition improves. An oral antimicrobial with prostatic penetrance is preferred for the remainder of therapy (see next section on chronic bacterial prostatitis).

Because acute infections may become chronic, re-examination is performed 3 to 7 days after antibiotic therapy is completed. This examination includes a physical examination, urinalysis, urine culture, and examination of prostatic fluid by cytology and culture.

Treatment of Chronic Bacterial Prostatitis

Chronic bacterial prostatitis is difficult to treat effectively because the blood–prostatic fluid barrier is intact.[43] The blood–prostatic fluid barrier is based partly on the pH difference between the blood, prostatic interstitium, and prostatic fluid; partly on the characteristics of the prostatic acinar epithelium; and partly on the protein-binding characteristics of antibiotics.[44] The pH of blood and prostatic interstitium is 7.4. The pH of canine prostatic fluid is approximately 6.4.[6,45] The presence of a pH gradient of at least 1 pH unit between compartments allow the phenomenon of ion trapping to occur. The charged fraction of a drug will be greater on one side of the system depending on the pH. Since the uncharged fraction of a lipid-soluble drug equilibrates, there will be more total drug (charged plus uncharged) on the side of greater ionization. Most dogs with prostatic infection continue to have acidic prostatic fluid.[6,45,46] With acidic prostatic fluid, basic antibiotics with high pKa values, such as erythromycin, oleandomycin, clindamycin, and trimethoprim, ionize to a greater extent in prostatic fluid than plasma. In fact, prostatic fluid concentration of trimethoprim can exceed plasma concentrations by 2 to 10 times.[47,48] Distribution of nonionizable drugs such as chloramphenicol is not affected by pH differences.

Lipid solubility is also an important factor in determining drug movement across prostatic epithelium. Drugs with low lipid solubility cannot cross into the prostatic acini. Lipid-insoluble antibiotics include penicillin, ampicillin, cephalosporins, oxytetracycline, and the aminoglycosides. Chloramphenicol, macrolide antibiotics, trimethoprim, quinolones, and carbenicillin are examples of lipid-soluble drugs, which can potentially enter prostatic fluid.

Protein binding in plasma also determines the amount of drug available to enter prostatic fluid. Because protein binding prevents diffusion, only the fraction that is not bound to plasma proteins can diffuse across the membrane. With greater protein binding, less drug is available to cross the prostatic epithelium. This factor is probably less important than lipid solubility or pKa since biologic systems rarely reach equilibrium. Examples of drugs with significant protein binding are clindamycin and chloramphenicol.

Several quinolone antibiotics have been developed, some of which concentrate in human prostatic fluid and tissue and possibly in canine prostatic tissue. Most quinolones are amphoteric and lipid soluble between pH values of 6 and 8 with relatively low (10 to 40%) plasma protein binding.[49] Norfloxacin is a lipid-soluble, weak base with a high pKa and low protein binding that is concentrated in human prostate glands and has been reported to be effective in some cases of chronic prostatitis in men.[50] Enrofloxacin is marketed only as a veterinary product with claims of prostatic penetrance, at least in normal dogs. Enrofloxacin is partially metabolized to ciprofloxacin, a product marketed for humans, which is reported to penetrate the prostate gland and be effective in some men with chronic prostatitis.[50] Not all quinolones penetrate into the prostate. In dogs, rosoxacin and cinoxacin reached levels in prostatic fluid only 10% of plasma levels.[51]

Most of the penicillins and cephalosporins do not diffuse into prostatic fluid because they are lipid insoluble and weak acids.[52] An exception is carbenicillin indanyl sodium. In esterified form, carbenicillin is lipid soluble and uncharged and reaches prostatic fluid concentrations approximately 70% of plasma concentrations in men, but much lower concentrations were found in dogs.[53]

Current recommendations depend on whether a gram-positive or gram-negative organism is the infective agent. If the causative organism is gram-positive, erythromycin, clindamycin, chloramphenicol, or trimethoprim can be chosen based on bacterial sensitivity.[54] If the organism is gram-negative, chloramphenicol, trimethoprim, or enrofloxacin would be best (Table 27–2).

Antibiotics should be continued for at least 6 weeks.

TABLE 27–2. ANTIBIOTIC DOSAGES IN THE TREATMENT OF BACTERIAL PROSTATITIS

Drug	Dose (mg/kg)	Route
Chloramphenicol	50 q 8 hr	PO, IV, SQ
Clindamycin	5 q 8 hr	PO, IV, IM
Enrofloxacin	2.5–5 q 12 hr	PO, IM
Erythromycin	10 q 8 hr	PO
Trimethoprim/sulfa	15 q 12 hr	PO, SQ

Urine and prostatic fluid are recultured 3 to 7 days and 1 month after discontinuing antibiotics to ensure the infection has been eliminated, not merely suppressed. Prognosis for cure is only fair. Part of the difficulty in curing the infection is that there may be host abnormalities in defense against infection as well as the blood–prostatic fluid barrier. If initial therapy fails, a 3-month course of therapy should be instituted, bearing in mind any potential adverse effects of the drug chosen. For such long-term therapy, trimethoprim/sulfa is the best current choice. Trimethoprim/sulfa can result in keratoconjunctivitis sicca, however, or mild anemia as a result of folate deficiency. We administer folic acid (1 mg every 24 hours) when using trimethoprim at full dosage for longer than 6 weeks. The owner should be advised to return for re-evaluation should any abnormal ocular signs develop, especially, a mucous discharge.

Castration has been recommended as adjunctive therapy to reduce the quantity of prostatic tissue. In experimental chronic prostatitis in dogs, castration performed 2 weeks after induction of infection hastened spontaneous resolution of infection.[55] This research suggests that castration may be beneficial in resolving prostatic infection in clinical cases, but this remains to be proved, since time of castration after onset of infection may be important.

If oral antibiotics plus castration fail to cure the prostatic infection, only two options remain: low-dose antibiotic therapy or prostatectomy. Low-dose antibiotic therapy can be instituted to suppress any urinary tract infection so that the prostatic infection will be asymptomatic. Trimethoprim at 50% of the usual daily dose each night is useful for this purpose. Other drugs that have been used at one nightly dose include nitrofurantoin and cephalosporins.

Prostatectomy eliminates infected prostatic tissue and can be used in cases refractory to antibiotic therapy and castration. The surgical procedure is difficult, however, and urinary incontinence is a frequent sequela in advanced cases of prostatic disease (see Chapter 28). Urodynamic evaluation (cystometry and urethral pressure profilometry) should be done before prostatectomy to determine pre-existing abnormalities.[1] If significant pre-surgical abnormalities are present, incontinence is even more likely.

Prostatic Abscessation

Pathophysiology

Prostatic abscessation is a severe form of chronic bacterial prostatitis in which pockets of septic, purulent exudate develop within the parenchyma of the prostate gland (Fig. 27–6). Aerobic organisms similar to those causing bacterial prostatitis are most commonly isolated in dogs. Affected dogs are usually older (> 7 years), intact males.[56] Most present for depression and lethargy, dysuria, tenesmus, or hematuria. Approximately 10% appear to be in septic shock, and 18% were found to have generalized peritonitis.[56]

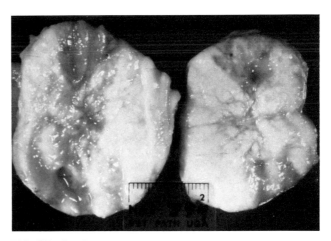

FIG. 27–6. A prostate gland with multifocal, abscessed areas. (Courtesy of Drs. W.A. Crowell and L.A. Cowan, College of Veterinary Medicine, University of Georgia.)

Diagnosis

Presumptive diagnosis is based on history, physical examination, hematology, urinalysis and urine culture, prostatic fluid cytology and culture, radiography, and ultrasonography. The diagnosis is confirmed by exploratory celiotomy. At surgery, the abscess contents are collected for cytology and for culture for aerobic bacteria, and a tissue section is obtained for microscopic examination.

Treatment

Surgical drainage or subtotal prostatectomy is currently the treatment of choice for large abscess pockets (see Chapter 28). The dog must be carefully evaluated and stabilized prior to surgery, however, if systemically ill. If not ill, delaying surgery until the causative organism can be identified by culture of urine or prostatic fluid allows administration of an appropriate antimicrobial intravenously during surgery to help prevent the development of sepsis during surgical manipulation.

If the dog appears septic (pale mucous membranes, tachycardia, delayed capillary refill, weak pulse), urine is collected for urinalysis and culture and antibiotic sensitivity testing, and blood is collected for CBC and a biochemical profile. An intravenous catheter is inserted and fluid support begun, initially with lactated Ringer's solution at a rapid rate (approximately 90 ml/kg/hr), with adjustment depending on response. If the dog is hypoglycemic in association with shock, intravenous dextrose is administered and response monitored. Electrolyte abnormalities should also be identified and corrected. Hypokalemia is the electrolyte abnormality occurring most commonly.[56]

In addition, intravenous antibiotic administration is begun, pending culture results. Based on prostatic penetration, chloramphenicol or trimethoprim are the drugs of choice. If the initial primary problem is bacteremia, however the main goal is to eliminate bacteremia. Because the usual infecting organism is *E. coli*, a bactericidal drug with a gram-negative spectrum should be selected. Aminoglycosides or cephalosporins are often used. Renal function should be carefully assessed, however, before and during use of aminoglycosides to avoid significant nephrotoxicity.

If the dog has signs of peritonitis (painful abdomen in addition to signs of sepsis), abdominocentesis or diagnostic peritoneal lavage is performed for confirmation and to obtain specimens for cytology and culture. In addition, peritoneal lavage can be used therapeutically in stabilizing the dog before surgery.

If prostatic enlargement has resulted in partial urethra obstruction, bladder and urethral function should be carefully assessed. Prolonged bladder distention may have resulted in bladder atony, leading to overflow incontinence, or the urethra or its innervation may have been adversely affected. Some assessment of bladder and urethral function is particularly important before prostatectomy, since abnormalities before surgery increase the likelihood of postoperative incontinence.[1] Even with drainage procedures, postoperative incontinence is common (approximately 50%).[56] An indwelling urinary catheter may allow the detrusor muscle to recover, but chronic distention and infection may irreversibly damage the bladder wall.

Castration is recommended in conjunction with prostatic drainage. In our experience, castration without abscess drainage leads to reduction of prostatic tissue but continuation of the abscess pocket(s).

After surgery, affected dogs must continue to receive antibiotic therapy, based on culture and sensitivity results. Intravenous antimicrobials should be continued until the dog's condition is stable. After improvement of clinical signs, the dog should be managed in the same way as a dog with chronic bacterial prostatitis.

If the dog's condition stabilizes on antibiotic therapy and the owner declines surgery, the dog can be managed with long-term antibiotic therapy as long as the owner realizes that the abscess will persist and potentially result in life-threatening infection.

Large prostatic abscesses are difficult and expensive to treat, with many potential complications.[4,56] In one survey, survival after surgical therapy was approximately 50% after 1 year.[4] In another survey, 25% of dogs died within 2 weeks of surgery, mainly as a result of septic shock.[56] These facts underscore the importance of aggressive treatment of chronic prostatitis to try to halt progression to abscessation.

Prostatic Neoplasia

Pathophysiology

The most common primary prostatic neoplasm in the dog is adenocarcinoma.[57,58] The second most common neoplasm affecting the prostate gland is transitional cell carcinoma.[57] Squamous cell carcinoma has been found in the prostate[59] as well as lymphoma[60] and other neoplasms that metastasized from another site. Note that all these neoplasms are considered malignant.

Prostatic adenocarcinoma tends to metastasize to the iliac lymph nodes and to vertebral bodies as well as to the lungs.[2,3] The tumor may grow into the neck of the bladder and obstruct the ureters. The colon and pelvic musculature may be invaded via direct extension through the prostatic capsule. The urethra may also become obstructed from neoplastic extension. Cysts, abscesses, and areas of hemorrhage can be found in association with neoplasia, making diagnosis difficult in some dogs.[57,58]

Prostatic adenocarcinoma arises in old dogs with a mean age of 9 to 10 years (Fig. 27–7).[2,58] Medium to large breed dogs seem to be more commonly affected. This neoplasm can develop in both intact and neutered males.[61] In fact, prostatic neoplasia should be highest on the list of differential diagnoses in an old dog that was neutered when young and presents for signs referable to prostatic disease or prostatic enlargement.

Diagnosis

A presumptive diagnosis is based on history, physical examination, hematology, urinalysis, cytology of prostatic fluid, radiography, and ultrasonography. Unless metastatic disease is evident radiographically, the diagnosis should always be confirmed by aspiration or biopsy since the prognosis is poor. If a surgical biopsy is obtained, a biopsy specimen should also be taken from the iliac lymph nodes.

Treatment

Once a diagnosis has been made, the owner should be advised that a cure is unlikely because this type of neoplasm is malignant and metastasis is likely to have occurred even if not clinically detectable.[62] Unfortunately, most prostatic adenocarcinomas are advanced at the time of diagnosis, and euthanasia may be the most humane course because effective therapy is unavailable at

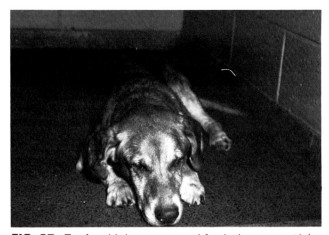

FIG. 27–7. An old dog presented for lethargy, partial anorexia, and dysuria. A markedly enlarged prostate gland was found on physical examination. Results of prostatic fluid evaluation, contrast-enhanced radiography, and ultrasonography all suggested neoplasia, which was confirmed by prostatic biopsy.

this time. If the owner elects therapy, the owner needs to understand that the goal is temporary control of the tumor and amelioration of clinical signs, rather than "cure." Earlier diagnosis may improve prognosis, emphasizing the importance of diagnostic pursuit of suspected prostatic disease in old dogs.

If the owner understands the poor prognosis but wishes to pursue therapy, a thorough search for metastasis is undertaken to allow a more accurate prognosis. Such a search includes thoracic radiographs (dorsoventral and both laterals). Contrast-enhanced radiographs of the lower urinary tract are necessary to evaluate the extent of neoplastic involvement. An excretory urogram is advisable if renal function is abnormal to determine if the ureters are occluded. A bone scan to detect metastasis to bone is also advisable where available.

Radiation therapy may be the treatment of choice if metastatic disease is not evident.[62] Intraoperative orthovoltage therapy has been recommended. Median and mean survival times for 10 dogs with radiotherapy were 114 and 196 days, respectively.[62] Three dogs with no evidence of metastatic disease appeared to be cured. The risk of postradiation fibrosis of the bladder must be considered because it can cause incontinence secondary to decreased bladder capacity.

Prostatectomy is alternative therapy, but the owner must be willing to accept the probable postsurgical development of urinary incontinence.[4] The longest reported postoperative survival has been 9 months, in a dog that had only small foci of neoplasia at the time of initial diagnosis.[4]

Palliative therapy that has been tried includes castration, estrogen therapy, and chemotherapeutic regimens designed for men. Veterinary experience with these treatments are limited, but hormonal therapy does not seem to be effective.[58,61,63] In fact, lack of decrease in prostatic size after castration or estrogen therapy may help differentiate neoplasia from other prostatic diseases.

REFERENCES

1. Basinger, R.R., Rawlings, C.A., Barsanti, J.A., et al.: Urodynamic alterations associated with clinical prostatic diseases and prostatic surgery in 23 dogs. J. Am. Anim. Hosp. Assoc., 25:385, 1989.
2. Leav, I., and Ling, G.V.: Adenocarcinoma of the canine prostate. Cancer, 22:1329, 1968.
3. Durham, S.K., and Dietze, A.E.: Prostatic adenocarcinoma with and without metastasis to bone in dogs. J. Am. Vet. Med. Assoc., 188:1432, 1986.
4. Hardie, E.M., Barsanti, J.A., and Rawlings, C.A.: Complications of prostatic surgery. J. Am. Anim. Hosp. Assoc., 20:50, 1984.
5. Fenster, L.F.: Reactive hepatopathy. Postgrad. Med., 76:62, 1984.
6. Barsanti, J.A., Prasse, K.W., Crowell, W.A., et al.: Evaluation of various techniques for diagnosis of chronic bacterial prostatitis in the dog. J. Am. Vet. Med. Assoc., 183:219, 1983.
7. Ling, G.V., Nyland, T.G., Kennedy, P.C., et al.: Comparison of two sample collection methods for quantitative bacteriologic culture of canine prostatic fluid. J. Am. Vet. Med. Assoc., 196:1479, 1990.
8. Thrall, M.A., Olson, P.N., and Freenmyer, F.G.: Cytologic diagnosis of canine prostatic disease. J. Am. Anim. Hosp. Assoc., 21:95, 1986.
9. Stone, E.A., Thrall, D.E., and Barber, D.L.: Radiographic interpretation of prostatic disease in the dog. J. Am. Anim. Hosp. Assoc., 14:115, 1978.
10. Feeney, D.A., Johnston, G.R., Klausner, J.S., et al.: Canine prostatic disease—comparison of radiographic appearance with morphologic and microbiologic findings: 30 cases (1981–1985). J. Am. Vet. Med. Assoc., 190:1019, 1987.
11. Johnston, G.R., Feeney, D.A., Osborne, C.A., et al.: Effect of intravesical hydrostatic pressure and volume on the distensibility of the canine prostatic portion of the urethra. Am. J. Vet. Res., 46:748, 1985.
12. Feeney, D.A., Johnston, G.R., Osborne, C.A., et al.: Dimensions of the prostatic and membranous urethra in normal male dogs during maximum distention retrograde urethrocystography. Vet. Radiol., 25:249, 1984.
13. Feeney, D.A., and Johnston, G.R.: Urogenital imaging: A practical update. Semin. Vet. Med. Surg., 1:144, 1986.
14. Jacobs, G., Barsanti, J.A., Prasse, K.W., et al.: Colliculus seminalis as a cause of a urethral filling defect in two dogs with Sertoli cell testicular neoplasms. J. Am. Vet. Med. Assoc., 192:1748, 1988.
15. Feeney, D.A., Johnston, G.R., Osborne, C.A., et al.: Maximum-distension retrograde urethrocystography in healthy male dogs: Occurrence and radiographic appearance of urethroprostatic reflux. Am. J. Vet. Res., 45:948, 1984.
16. Barsanti, J.A., Crowell, W.A., Losonsky, J., et al.: Complications of bladder distension during retrograde urethrography. Am. J. Vet. Res., 42:819, 1981.
17. Johnston, G.R., Stevens, J.B., Jessen, C.R., et al.: Complications of retrograde contrast urography in dogs and cats. Am. J. Vet. Res., 44:1248, 1983.
18. Feeney, D.A., Johnston, G.R., Klausner, J.S., et al.: Canine prostatic disease—comparison of ultrasonographic appearance with morphologic and microbiologic findings: 30 cases (1981–1985). J. Am. Vet. Med. Assoc., 190:1027, 1987.
19. Feeney, D.A., Johnston, G.R., Klausner, J.S., et al.: Canine prostatic ultrasonography—1989. Semin. Vet. Med. Surg. (Sm. Anim.), 4:44, 1989.
20. Smith, S.: Ultrasound-guided biopsy. Vet. Clin. North Am. [Sm. Anim. Pract.], 15:1249, 1985.
21. Barsanti, J.A., and Finco, D.R.: Canine prostatic diseases. In Textbook of Veterinary Internal Medicine. Edited by S.J. Ettinger. Philadelphia, W.B. Saunders, 1989, pp. 1859–1880.
22. Isaacs, J.T.: Common characteristics of human and canine benign prostatic hyperplasia. Prog. Clin. Biol. Res., 145:217, 1984.
23. Brendler, C.B., Berry, S.J., Ewing, L.L., et al.: Spontaneous benign prostatic hyperplasia in the Beagle. J. Clin. Invest., 71:1114, 1983.
24. Isaacs, J.T.: Changes in dihydrotestosterone metabolism and the development of benign prostatic hyperplasia in the aging beagle. J. Steroid. Biochem., 18:749, 1983.
25. Berry, S.J., Strandberg, J.D., Saunders, W.J., et al.: Development of canine benign prostatic hyperplasia with age. Prostate, 9:363, 1986.
26. Huggins, C., and Clark, P.G.: Quantitative studies of prostatic secretion II. The effect of castration and of estrogen injection on the normal and on the hyperplastic prostate glands of dogs. J. Exp. Med., 72:747, 1940.
27. James, R.W., and Heywood, R.: Age-related variations in the testes and prostate of Beagle dogs. Toxicology, 12:273, 1979.
28. Lowseth, L.A., Gerlach, R.F., Gillett, N.A., et al.: Age-related changes in the prostate and testes of the beagle dog. Vet. Pathol., 27:347, 1990.
29. Schlotthauer, C.F.: Observations on the prostate gland of the dog. J. Am. Vet. Med. Assoc., 81:645, 1932.

30. Huggins, C., Masina, M.H., Eichelberger, L.E., et al.: Quantitative studies of prostatic secretion. J. Exp. Med., *70:*543, 1939.
31. Berry, S.J., Coffey, D.S., Strandberg, J.D., et al.: Effect of age, castration and testosterone replacement on the development and restoration of canine benign hyperplasia. Prostate, *9:*295, 1986.
32. Mulligan, R.M.: Feminization in male dogs: A syndrome associated with carcinoma of the testes and mimicked by the administration of estrogen. Am. J. Pathol., *20:*865, 1944.
33. Tyslowitz, R., and Dingemanse, E.: Effect of large doses of estrogens on the blood picture of dogs. Endocrinology, *29:*817, 1941.
34. Berg, O.A.: Effect of stilbestrol on the prostate gland in normal puppies and adult dogs. Acta Endocrinol., *27:*155, 1958.
35. Neri, R.: Pharmacology and pharmacokinetics of flutamide. Urology, *34*(suppl):19, 1989.
36. Geller, J., Albert, J., Geller, S., et al.: Effect of megestrol acetate on steroid metabolism and steroid-protein binding in the human prostate. J. Clin. Endocrinol. Metab., *43:*1000, 1976.
37. Olson, P.N., Wrigley, R.H., Thrall, M.A., et al.: Disorders of the canine prostate gland: Pathogenesis, diagnosis and medical therapy. Compend. Contin. Educ. Pract. Vet., *9:*613, 1987.
38. Sherding, R.G., Wilson, G.P., and Kociba, G.J.: Bone marrow hypoplasia in 8 dogs with Sertoli cell tumor. J. Am. Vet. Med. Assoc., *178:*497, 1981.
39. Weaver, A.D.: Discrete prostatic (paraprostatitic) cysts in the dog. Vet. Rec., *102:*435, 1978.
40. Akpavie, S.O., and Sullivan, M.: Constipation associated with calcified cystic enlargement of the prostate in a dog. Vet. Rec., *118:*694, 1986.
41. Sisson, D.D., and Hoffer, R.E.: Osteocollagenous prostatic retention cyst: Report of a canine case. J. Am. Anim. Hosp. Assoc., *13:*61, 1977.
42. Kivisto, A.K., Vasenius, H., and Sandholm, M.: Canine bacteriuria. J. Sm. Anim. Pract., *18:*707, 1977.
43. Madsen, P.O., Jensen, K.M., and Iverson, P.: Chronic bacterial prostatitis: Theoretical and experimental. Urol. Res., *11:*1, 1983.
44. Stamey, T.A., Meares, E.M., and Winningham, D.G.: Chronic bacteria prostatitis and the diffusion of drugs into prostatic fluid. J. Urol., *103:*187, 1970.
45. Branam, J.E., Keen, C.L., Ling, G.V., et al.: Selected physical and chemical characteristics of prostatic fluid collected by ejaculation from healthy dogs and from dogs with bacterial prostatitis. Am. J. Vet. Res., *45:*825, 1984.
46. Baumueller, A., and Madsen, P.O.: Experimental bacterial prostatitis in dogs. Urol. Res., *5:*211, 1977.
47. Granato, J.J., Gross, D.M., and Stamey, T.A.: Trimethoprim diffusion into prostatic and salivary secretions of the dog. Invest. Urol., *11:*205, 1973.
48. Reeves, D.S., and Ghilchik, M.: Secretion of the antibacterial substance trimethoprim in the prostatic fluid of dogs. Br. J. Urol., *42:*66, 1980.
49. Vancutsem, P.M., Babish, J.G., Schwark, W.S.: The fluoroquinolone antimicrobials: Structure, antimicrobial activity, pharmacokinetics, clinical use in domestic animals and toxicity. Cornell Vet., *80:*173, 1990.
50. Schaeffer, A.J.: Diagnosis and treatment of prostatic infections. Urology, *36*(suppl):13, 1990.
51. Maigaard, S., Frimodt-Moeller, N., Hoyme, U., et al.: Rosoxacin and cinoxacin distribution in prostate, vagina, and female urethra in dogs. Invest. Urol., *17:*149, 1979.
52. Baumueller, A., and Madsen, P.O.: Secretion of various antimicrobial substances in dogs with experimental bacterial prostatitis. Urol. Res., *5:*215, 1977.
53. Nielsen, O.S., Frimodt-Moeller, N., Maigaard, S., et al.: Penicillamic acid derivatives in the canine prostate. Prostate, *1:*79, 1980.
54. Reeves, D.S., Rowe, R.G., Small, M.E., et al.: 23 further studies on the secretion of antibiotics in the prostatic fluid of the dog. *In* Proceedings, 2nd Int Symp Urinary Tract Infection, London, 1972, pp. 197–205.
55. Cowan, L.A., Barsanti, J.A., Crowell, W., et al.: Effects of castration on chronic bacterial prostatitis in dogs. J. Am. Vet. Med. Assoc., 199:346, 1991.
56. Mullen, H.S., Matthiesen, D.T., and Scavelli, T.D.: Results of surgery and postoperative complications in 92 dogs treated for prostatic abscessation by a multiple Penrose drain technique. J. Am. Anim. Hosp. Assoc., 26:369, 1990.
57. O'Shea, J.D.: Studies on the canine prostate gland. J. Comp. Path., *73:*244, 1963.
58. Weaver, A.D.: Fifteen cases of prostatic carcinoma in the dog. Vet. Rec., *109:*71, 1981.
59. Leib, M.S., Saunders, G.K., Dallman, M.J., et al.: Squamous cell carcinoma of the prostate gland in a dog. J. Am. Anim. Hosp. Assoc., 22:509, 1986.
60. Mainwaring, C.J.: Primary lymphoma of the prostate in a dog. J. Sm. Anim. Pract., *31:*517, 1990.
61. Obradovich, J., Walsh, R., and Goullaud, E.: The influence of castration on the development of prostatic carcinoma in the dog. J. Vet. Intern. Med., *1:*183, 1987.
62. Turrel, J.M.: Intraoperative radiotherapy of carcinoma of the prostate gland in 10 dogs. J. Am. Vet. Med. Assoc., *190:*48, 1987.
63. Dube, J.Y., Frenetta, G., Tremblay, Y., et al.: Single case report of prostate adenocarcinoma in a dog castrated 3 months previously: Morphological, biochemical and endocrine determinations. Prostate, *5:*495, 1984.

28

Surgical Therapy for Prostatic Disorders

SELECTION OF SURGICAL PROCEDURE

The selection of surgical procedure is dependent on the dog's condition, type of prostatic disease, owner's expectations, and surgeon's experience. Any dog with prostatomegaly should be evaluated to determine the cause (see Chapter 4). If benign prostatic hyperplasia is the most likely diagnosis, castration is recommended, unless the animal is used for breeding. Castration may also be recommended as adjunct therapy for chronic prostatitis. For medical treatment of benign prostatic hyperplasia and bacterial prostatitis, see Chapter 27. A prostate that is enlarged from benign prostatic hyperplasia should decrease in size within 1 month after castration. If it remains enlarged, further diagnostic tests are mandatory to detect other causes of prostatomegaly.

Prostatic Abscessation

Several options exist for surgical treatment of prostatic abscessation, which are used in conjunction with castration. Because abscessation can occur with prostatic neoplasia, biopsy specimens should be taken of any suspect tissue. *Prostatic drainage*, using drains placed through the prostatic parenchyma, is the easiest and least traumatic method. This treatment is often effective for transitory resolution of the current episode, but urinary tract infection (UTI) and recurrence of abscessation are major long-term complications.[1-4] Prostatic drainage is the procedure of choice if an animal is septic and a poor surgical candidate. Sepsis is monitored and treated as discussed in Chapter 27. Antibiotic therapy is started before surgery, preferably based on culture and sensitivity of prostatic fluid, and continued for at least 4 weeks after surgery. The dog is re-evaluated after surgery for recurrence of infection, using urine cultures and ultrasonography, if available. If abscessation or UTI recurs or persists after drainage, reoperation is indicated to repeat the drainage procedure or remove residual prostatic parenchyma by subtotal prostatectomy. The prostate should be smaller and easier to remove after drainage.

If the dog is not septic and is a reasonably good surgical candidate, *subtotal prostatectomy* ("fillet prostatectomy") is the preferred technique. With subtotal prostatectomy, the lateral and ventral prostatic parenchyma is removed except for a small amount surrounding the prostatic urethra. The dorsal region of the prostate is preserved unless it is involved in the disease process. Subtotal prostatectomy requires more operative time (2 to 4 hours) and produces greater tissue trauma than prostatic drainage. The incidence of reabscessation and persistent UTI is less than with drainage.[4] Because of the high incidence of postoperative urinary incontinence,[3,5] *excisional prostatectomy* is not recommended for prostatic abscessation, unless the prostatic urethra is necrotic or severely damaged.

Prostatic and Paraprostatic Cysts

After the cyst is located, its size and shape are evaluated. Dissection around the cyst must be meticulous to prevent damage to the innervation and blood supply of bladder and urethra. The ureters are protected and retracted early in the procedure. The urethra is identified by the preplaced urethral catheter. If the cyst narrows down to a stalk, the stalk can be ligated and severed and the entire cyst removed. When there is a broad attachment between the cyst and the prostate, the cyst wall is carefully excised. Remnants of the resection that are attached to the prostate are oversewn to prevent continued drainage from prostatic ducts and adhesion formation.[6] When cyst resection is impossible because of its large size and extensive adhesions, marsupialization is performed. The decision to marsupialize must be made before resection is initiated because partial excision precludes marsupialization.

Prostatic Neoplasia

Excisional prostatectomy is usually reserved for prostatic cancer confined to the prostate. Prostatectomy is difficult and should best be performed by an experienced surgeon. It may be prudent to obtain a biopsy specimen of the prostate and then refer it for definitive surgery and adjuvant therapy. If the probability of prostatic cancer is great, based on diagnostic evaluation, the dog can be referred without biopsy. This allows the primary surgeon to operate in an undisturbed field. Palliative procedures for urethral obstruction from prostatic cancer include placing a permanent cystostomy catheter (see Fig. 16–6) or making a permanent cystostomy (see Fig. 31–3).

SURGICAL PREPARATION AND APPROACH

If there is sufficient time before surgery, warm-water enemas are administered the day and evening before surgery, to decrease the volume of the distal colon and rectum and facilitate dissection. After the dog is anesthetized, a urinary catheter is placed and connected to a closed collection system to aid in identification of the urethra, to keep the bladder decompressed during surgery, and to measure urine output. A parapreputial abdominal incision is used to approach the prostate (see Fig. 10–3). Retention sutures are placed in the bladder to pull the bladder cranially and aid in exposure. The connective tissue band between the pubis and the ventral urethra is severed with scissors. If the prostate is intrapelvic or if an excisional prostatectomy is anticipated, a pubic or a pubic and ischiatic osteotomy is performed (see Fig. 10–4). Hypogastric, medial iliac, and lumbar lymph nodes are examined, and biopsy specimens are obtained if enlarged, in any dog with suspected prostatic neoplasia.

Suction should be always available during prostatic surgery to remove purulent material and lessen contamination of the abdomen. The prostate is isolated from the abdomen with moistened laparotomy pads.

PROSTATIC DRAINAGE

Dissection of periprostatic fat is minimized to prevent extension of the infection into periprostatic tissues. The abscess cavity is identified and some of the contents are suctioned, using a 22-gauge needle and syringe, and saved for aerobic and anaerobic bacterial culture. The remaining material can be removed with an 18-gauge needle and suction apparatus (see Fig. 7–3). A blunt opening is made in the abscess cavity ventral and lateral to the urethra. If the prostate contains multiple large abscesses, the surgeon's finger is used to break down loculations into one large cavity. The cavity is lavaged and suctioned. Representative biopsy specimens are taken of tissue with an abnormal appearance. A 5-mm Penrose drain is passed through the ventral opening into the cavity and exited lateral to the urethra and ventral to the prostatic vessels. Previously, a more dorsal exit

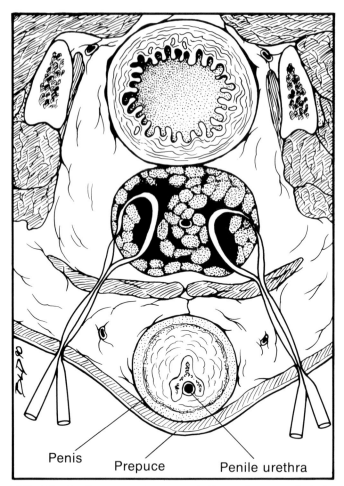

FIG. 28–1. Prostatic drainage. A 5-mm Penrose drain is passed through the ventral opening in the prostate, into the abscess cavity, and exited through the lateral wall of the prostate, ventral to the prostatic vessels.

Penis Prepuce Penile urethra

was recommended,[7] but it endangers the innervation to the urethra on the dorsal surface of the prostate and may be more likely to produce urinary incontinence.[1,2] The urinary catheter is used to locate and avoid damage to the urethra as the drain is passed. As the drain exits the prostate, it is passed along the lateral surface of the gland. Both ends of the drain are exteriorized through the same opening in the abdominal wall, lateral to the prepuce (Fig. 28–1). If the prostate has bilateral abscesses, the procedure is repeated on the opposite side of the prostate. The drains are secured to the skin and removed after 2 weeks.

SUBTOTAL PROSTATECTOMY[4]

The periprostatic fat is incised along the midline of the prostate and reflected from the ventral and lateral surfaces of the prostate, staying as close to the prostate as possible. Short prostatic vessels, directly entering the dorsolateral prostate, are ligated and severed or cauterized close to the prostate. Abscess cavities are suctioned as described for prostatic drainage. The cavities are opened, lavaged, and suctioned. Using electrocoagulation, the prostatic parenchyma is gradually excised from the lateral and ventral surfaces. The location of the urethra is identified by the urinary catheter. Vessels larger than 2 mm are ligated before transection. Adhesions to the rectum or other surrounding organs are cut, leaving a small amount of prostatic tissue attached. Approximately 5 mm of parenchyma around the urethra is preserved. If the dorsal region of the prostate is minimally involved in the disease process, it is left intact. Excised tissue is submitted for histologic examination.

Methylene blue (0.5 ml diluted in 10 ml saline) is slowly injected into the bladder, and the prostatic urethra is inspected for leaks. If no leakage of methylene blue is observed, the urethral catheter is removed the day after surgery. Leakage of methylene blue signifies urethral perforations, which are sutured with 4–0 absorbable suture material in a simple interrupted pattern. After repair of urethral defects, the urinary catheter is retained for 7 days to divert urine until the urethral perforations heal. When a large defect in the urethra cannot be repaired because of friable tissue or iatrogenic damage to the urethra, a cystostomy catheter (see Fig. 16–6), in addition to the urinary catheter, is placed to divert urine from the healing urethra. The catheters remain until a low pressure urethrogram reveals no leakage.

MARSUPIALIZATION

The prostatic or paraprostatic cyst is examined to ensure that it will reach the body wall (Fig. 28–2A). The cyst is aspirated, and fluid is saved for bacterial culture. The cyst is freed from any restricting adhesions. If necessary, the ductus deferens can be isolated, ligated, and severed. An oval stoma is made in the skin, subcutaneous fat, and ventral rectus muscle fascia, lateral to the prepuce. Muscle is separated by blunt dissection, and the peritoneum is incised. Retention sutures are placed in the cyst wall, and the cyst is suctioned dry. The retention sutures and then the cyst are passed through the stoma (Fig. 28–2B). The cyst wall is sutured to the ventral rectus muscle fascia with absorbable suture material in a continuous pattern. The cyst is incised (Fig. 28–2C) and flushed with 0.05% povidone-iodine solution. Excess cyst wall is excised, and the cut edges are sutured to the skin with simple interrupted nonabsorbable sutures (Fig. 28–2D).[8–10] If the cyst extends into the perineal region, a suction drain can be placed through the marsupialization stoma and into the caudal extent of the cyst. Marsupialization or drainage through the highly contaminated perineal area is not recommended.

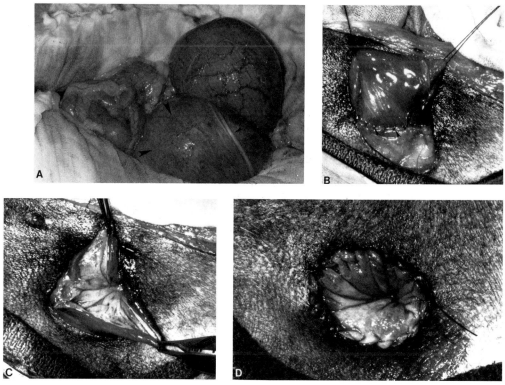

FIG. 28–2. Prostatic marsupialization. (A) A large prostatic cyst (large arrows) is lateral to the bladder and is crossed by the ductus deferens (small arrow). (B) After the stoma is made in the skin and the body wall, the aspirated cyst is passed through the stoma, using retention sutures for handling. The cyst is sutured to the external rectus sheath with absorbable suture material in a continuous pattern (arrows). (C) The cyst is incised. (D) After excess cyst wall is excised, the cut edges of the cyst are sutured to the skin with simple interrupted, nonabsorbable sutures.

EXCISIONAL PROSTATECTOMY

The exposure is similar to that described for subtotal prostatectomy except that the dissection extends to the dorsal surface of the prostate. The prostate is retracted laterally, and the ductus deferens are ligated and severed (Fig. 28–3A). The short branches of the prostatic vessels are individually ligated and cut. Care is taken to preserve the caudal vesical artery on each side (formerly known as urogenital artery), which is a branch of the prostatic artery (Fig. 28–3B). The dorsal fibrous band between the prostate and rectum is located and severed. For non-neoplastic conditions, the prostate is dissected from the neck of the bladder, leaving as much neck as possible. With an enlarged neoplastic prostate, it may be necessary to section part of the bladder neck to achieve acceptable tumor-free margins. In this instance, a ventral cystotomy is performed to identify ureteral openings.

Retention sutures are placed in the urethra distal to the prostate. The urethra is transected cranial and caudal to the prostate (Fig. 28–3C). It is helpful to leave the urinary catheter in place during the transection. A scalpel blade is used to cut through the urethra to the catheter. After removal of the prostate, the catheter is replaced in the bladder, and three polypropylene or nylon (4–0) sutures are preplaced from the proximal to the distal urethral edges (Fig. 28–3D). These sutures are tied, and simple interrupted sutures are placed to finish the urethral anastomosis (Fig. 28–3E). A cystostomy

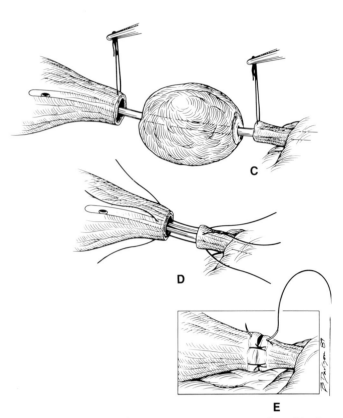

FIG. 28–3 (*Cont.*) (C) Retention sutures are placed in the urethra distal to the prostate. The urethra is transected as near as possible cranial and caudal to the prostate. A scalpel is used to cut circumferentially through the urethra down to the urethral catheter. (D) After removal of the prostate, the catheter is replaced into the bladder, and three sutures are preplaced from the proximal to the distal urethral edges. (E) Sutures are tied, and simple interrupted sutures are placed to finish the urethral anastomosis.

catheter is placed to divert urine (see Fig. 16–6) and to keep the bladder decompressed, thereby reducing tension on the anastomosis. The abdominal exit site for the cystostomy catheter is located so that the catheter does not pull the bladder and urethra cranially. Routine abdominal closure is performed. The urinary and cystostomy catheters are connected to closed collection systems. The urinary catheter is left in place for 2 to 3 days. The cystostomy catheter is removed in 7 days.

REFERENCES

1. Mullen, H.S., Matthiesen, D.T., and Scavelli, T.D.: Results of surgery and postoperative complications in 92 dogs treated for prostatic abscessation by a multiple Penrose drain technique. J. Am. Anim. Hosp. Assoc., 26:369, 1990.
2. Matthiesen, D.T., and Marretta, S.M.: Complications associated with the surgical treatment of prostatic abscessation. Prob. Vet. Med., 1:63, 1989.
3. Hardie, E.M., Barsanti, J.A., and Rawlings, C.A.: Complications of prostatic surgery. J. Am. Anim. Hosp. Assoc., 20:50, 1984.
4. Hardie, E.M., Stone, E.A., Spaulding, K.A., et al.: Subtotal prostatectomy using the neodymium:yttrium aluminum garnet laser in the dog. Vet. Surg., 19:348–355, 1990.

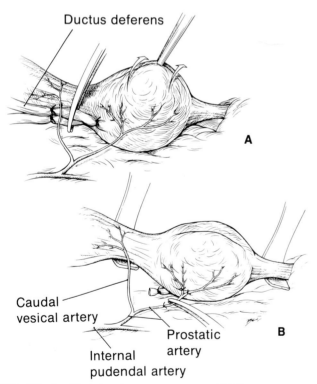

FIG. 28–3. Excisional prostatectomy. (A) The prostate is rotated laterally, and the ductus deferens are ligated and severed. (B) Short branches of the prostatic vessels are individually ligated and cut.

5. Basinger, R.R., Rawlings, C.A., and Barsanti, J.A.: Urodynamic alterations associated with clinical prostatic disease and prostatic surgery in 23 dogs. J. Am. Anim. Hosp. Assoc., 25:385, 1989.
6. White, R.A.S., Herrtage, M.E., and Dennis, R.: The diagnosis and management of paraprostatic and prostatic retention cysts in the dog. J. Sm. Anim. Pract., 28:551, 1987.
7. Basinger, R.R., and Rawlings, C.A.: Surgical management of prostatic diseases. Compend. Contin. Educ. Pract. Vet., 9:993, 1987.
8. Johnston, D.E.: Prostate. In Textbook of Small Animal Surgery. Edited by D.H. Slatter. Philadelphia, W.B. Saunders, 1985, p. 1635.
9. Hoffer, R.E., Dykes, N.L., and Greiner, T.P.: Marsupialization as a treatment for prostatic disease. J. Am. Anim. Hosp. Assoc., 13:98, 1977.
10. Lijour, L., and Lijour-Bac, B.: Kystes paraprostatiques chez le chien. Le Point Veterinaire, 20:787, 1988.

29

Postoperative Management and Surgical Complications of Prostatic Disorders

POSTOPERATIVE MANAGEMENT

The dog's clinical condition is closely monitored for signs of shock and disseminated intravascular coagulopathy for 24 to 48 hours (see Chapter 11). Long anesthesia and surgery times, release of endotoxins or bacteria from an infected prostate gland, and hemorrhage contribute to the development of shock. In one study, sepsis and shock developed in 33% of dogs surviving surgical drainage of prostatic abscesses.[1,2] Depending on the physiologic status of the dog before surgery, septicemia and shock may be more likely after subtotal or excisional prostatectomy because of greater tissue trauma and longer operations.[3] Blood pressure and urine output are measured for at least 24 hours after surgery and fluid therapy adjusted to establish a volume diuresis. Dogs with prostatic infection may be unable to concentrate urine and, thus, can rapidly become volume depleted, resulting in oliguria and acute renal failure. After fluid therapy is discontinued, free access to drinking water is essential.

A side brace (see Fig. 11–2) is placed on any dog with drains or a urinary or cystostomy catheter. The drains are cleansed with antiseptic soap. The drains are removed after 2 weeks. For dogs with prostatic drains, urinary tract infection (UTI), or both, antibiotics are continued for 4 weeks after surgery, and urine is recultured 1 week later.

Drainage from a marsupialization stoma usually ceases in 1 to 2 months, and the stoma contracts and closes. If the stoma begins to close prematurely, the stoma is carefully dilated with hemostats. If the stoma continues to drain after 2 months, the dog is re-explored and the shrunken cyst excised.

POSTOPERATIVE COMPLICATIONS

Peripheral Edema

Edema of the prepuce, ventral abdomen, scrotum, or hind legs can occur after prostate surgery.[1,2] Hypoproteinemia, fluid drainage into the subcutaneous space, and obstruction of vascular and lymphatic vessels contribute to edema formation. Once the inciting factors resolve, the edema usually subsides in 1 to 2 weeks.

Urine Leakage from the Urethra

Infrequently, urine may drip from prostatic drains, indicating a communication between the urethra and an abscess cavity.[1,2] Urine leakage is managed with the insertion of a urinary catheter connected to a closed collection system for 5 days. At the end of that time, a low-pressure, contrast urethrogram is performed. If any contrast material escapes from the urethra, the catheter is left in place for 10 more days, and the urethrogram is repeated. Persistent leakage after 15 days is rare and necessitates re-exploration. Necrotic areas are debrided, and urethral defects are closed, if possible. Urinary and cystostomy catheters are placed to divert urine from the site until a low pressure urethrogram reveals no leakage.

Urine leakage can also occur following subtotal prostatectomy, although the use of dilute methylene blue to identify urethral perforations at the time of the initial surgery greatly reduces the incidence of this complication. Dehiscence of a urethral anastomosis after prostatectomy usually occurs from 2 to 7 days after surgery. Urine accumulating in the abdomen causes decreased urine output, abdominal distention, and signs of uremia. An abdominocentesis reveals urine within the peritoneal cavity. A contrast urethrogram is used to detect anastomotic leakage. The contrast material must be injected at low pressure to prevent further disruption of the suture line. Small urethral leaks are treated with a urinary or cystostomy catheter and should seal within 3 to 4 days. With major dehiscence, urine is diverted by urinary and cystostomy catheter for 3 to 4 days to allow the periurethral tissue inflammation to regress, and then the urethra is explored and resutured.

Persistent Urinary Tract Infections

Urinary tract infection occurs commonly following prostatic drainage (> 60% of dogs).[1-4] Dogs should be monitored for UTI with urine culture and antibiotic sensitivity repeated every 2 months until two negative cultures are attained. If persistent or recurrent UTI remains a problem, subtotal prostatectomy should be considered, because bacterial antibiotic resistance increases with recurrent and persistent UTI. Following subtotal prostatectomy, UTI may be associated with the indwelling catheter, but it should resolve after the catheter is removed and appropriate antibiotics are administered. If a prostatectomized dog has recurrent UTI, the kidneys and lower urinary tract must be evaluated for pyelonephritis, anatomic abnormalities, such as bladder diverticulum, and urolithiasis.

Recurrence of Prostatic Abscessation

Reabscessation following prostatic drainage is caused by continuing prostatitis and UTI. Although concurrent castration shrinks the prostate, pockets of infection may remain. Of 89 dogs with multiple drain treatment for prostatic abscessation, 18% had reabscessation anywhere from 3 to 570 days after surgery (mean = 120 days).[1,2] Initial signs of reabscessation can be subtle, so it is important to monitor the dog routinely for UTI, as already discussed, and to repeat ultrasonographic examination, if available, every 2 months for a year after surgery. A prostate with reabscessation can either be redrained[1,2] or have subtotal prostatectomy. Severe injury to the urethra may necessitate excisional prostatectomy.

Urinary Incontinence

Some dogs with prostatic diseases are incontinent before surgery and may remain incontinent after surgery, regardless of treatment. Other dogs may become incontinent because of progression of the prostatic disease after surgery. A detailed history regarding the dog's voiding function is essential to identify these dogs and to forewarn the owners. In addition, polidypsia and poliuria, secondary to a urine concentrating defect in the kidneys, can contribute to the manifestation of incontinence.

Postsurgical urinary incontinence is very common fol-

lowing total excision of diseased prostates (93%; 13 of 14 dogs in one study[5]), particularly in dogs with neoplastic prostatic disease.[6] Subtotal prostatectomy for prostatic abscessation may also cause urinary incontinence, but the frequency and severity of the incontinence are less (e.g., nocturnal, responsive to drug therapy).[3] Prostatic drainage, using multiple drains exiting from the dorsal surface of the prostate, was associated with persistent incontinence in 25% (18 of 70) of dogs.[1,2] Urinary incontinence following the drain placement technique described in Chapter 28 should be less frequent because the two drains exit the prostate laterally and are less likely to disrupt urethral innervation.

Characterization of postoperative incontinence is important (see Chapter 1). Some incontinence may be transient, with restoration of control in 2 to 3 weeks. Once the type of incontinence is identified, pharmacologic treatment can be tried. In a practice situation without the benefit of urodynamic testing, the suggested drugs are administered for 2 weeks on a trial basis.

Normal Detrusor Muscle Function with Decreased Urethral Tone

This is the most common cause of urinary incontinence following prostatic surgery. An alpha adrenergic agonist, phenylpropanolamine, is tried (1.5 mg/kg tid by mouth).[7] Because the urinary incontinence may be caused by damage to urethral innervation from the surgery or the disease process, drug therapy may be ineffective.

Overflow Incontinence from an Atonic Bladder

Dogs with atonic bladders associated with prostatic disease have or have had functional or mechanical urethral obstruction. The tight junctions of the detrusor muscle have stretched, and the detrusor muscle is not functioning properly. Keeping the bladder decompressed by intermittent or indwelling catheterization may be sufficient therapy to allow reformation of tight junctions. If the bladder remains compromised, bethanecol, a cholinergic agonist, is administered (5 mg bid to tid by mouth).[7] The dose is slowly increased until the bladder responds or toxicity develops, as evidenced by diarrhea or gastrointestinal signs. The urethra must be patent during drug administration. If there is some question about urethral patency, a urinary catheter can be left in place until the efficacy of the drug is determined. If it is effective, the catheter is removed. Functional obstruction of the urethra is managed with concurrent administration of phenoxybenzamine (2.5 to 15 mg once a day by mouth), starting with the lower dose and increasing slowly.

Detrusor Instability

A dog with a spastic bladder may produce short bursts of urine that are mistaken for incontinence. Detrusor contractions may be controlled with oxybutynin, an anticholinergic drug (0.5 to 5 mg, bid or tid by mouth).[7]

REFERENCES

1. Mullen, H.S., Matthiesen, D.T., and Scavelli, T.D.: Results of surgery and postoperative complications in 92 dogs treated for prostatic abscessation by a multiple Penrose drain technique. J. Am. Anim. Hosp. Assoc., *26:*369, 1990.
2. Matthiesen, D.T., and Marretta, S.M.: Complications associated with the surgical treatment of prostatic abscessation. Prob. Vet. Med., *1:*63, 1989.
3. Hardie, E.M., Stone, E.A., Spaulding, K.A., et al.: Subtotal prostatectomy using the neodymium:yttrium aluminum garnet laser in the dog. Vet. Surg., *19:*348–355, 1990.
4. Hardie, E.M., Barsanti, J.A., and Rawlings, C.A.: Complications of prostatic surgery. J. Am. Anim. Hosp. Assoc., *20:*50, 1984.
5. Basinger, R.R., Rawlings, C.A., and Barsanti, J.A.: Urodynamic alterations associated with clinical prostatic disease and prostatic surgery in 23 dogs. J. Am. Anim. Hosp. Assoc., *25:*385, 1989.
6. Goldsmid, S.E., and Bellenger, C.R.: Urinary incontinence after prostatectomy in dogs. Vet. Surg., *20:*253, 1991.
7. Basinger, R.R., and Barsanti, J.A.: Urodynamic abnormalities associated with canine prostatic diseases and therapeutic intervention. *In* Current Veterinary Therapy X. Edited by R.W. Kirk. Philadelphia, W.B. Saunders, 1989, pp. 1151–1152.

Section Ten

Urinary Tract Neoplasia

30

Diagnosis and Medical Therapy of Urinary Tract Neoplasia

STEPHEN D. GILSON

Any urinary tract organ can be affected by neoplasia. Several authors have commented that tumors in the bladder are the most common, clinically recognized neoplasms of the urinary tract of dogs.[1,2] Epidemiologic studies do not support this clinical impression, finding a higher incidence of renal tumors, especially in cats.[3-7] Urinary tract neoplasms can be benign or malignant, primary or metastatic, and of epithelial or mesenchymal tissue origin. Older animals are most commonly affected, although a few types of neoplasia preferentially affect the young. Prostatic neoplasia is discussed in Chapters 27 through 29 and is not included in this chapter.

The causes of urinary tract neoplasms are largely unknown. Renal cell carcinoma is more common in male dogs, suggesting a hormonal link.[1,8-11] Data to support this theory are weak, however, and studies show conflicting results.[1,8-11] Metastatic neoplasms are most common in the kidney, probably because of the high renal blood flow and presence of extensive capillary beds. Environmental and metabolic carcinogens may also be associated with urologic neoplasms because the urinary tract is a major excretory pathway for many substances and their metabolites. Exposure to chemical carcinogens has been linked to increased incidence of renal and bladder cancer in humans.[12,13] A higher incidence of bladder cancer in dogs has been associated with exposure to organophosphates and other insecticides.[14] Bladder cancer may be more common in dogs than cats because of inherent metabolic differences, resulting in greater excretion of carcinogenic tryptophan metabolites in dogs.[15] As a storage organ, the bladder has prolonged contact with potential carcinogenic agents in the urine. In one study, a positive correlation was found between morbidity for canine bladder cancer and overall level of industrial activity in the host county of the veterinary hospitals.[16] Transitional cell carcinoma

was reported in three dogs following treatment with oral cyclophosphamide. A causal relationship was not established.[17]

DIAGNOSIS OF URINARY TRACT NEOPLASIA

Clinical Presentation

Most signs associated with urinary tract neoplasms are not specific for cancer, so a high degree of clinical suspicion is necessary. Signalment may offer helpful clues for diagnosis. Urologic tumors generally affect older animals (9 to 10 years)[3-9,18]; exceptions include renal lymphosarcoma (5 to 7 years),[19] nephroblastoma (< 4 years),[1,8] and botryoid or embryonal rhabdomyosarcoma (< 2 years).[20] Females are more commonly affected with ureteral, bladder, and urethral carcinomas[5,18,21] and males with renal cell carcinoma.[8-11] No breed predispositions are recognized; however, renal cell carcinoma and botryoid rhabdomyosarcoma occur more frequently in larger-breed dogs.[8,11,20] A syndrome of nodular dermatofibrosis and renal cystadenocarcinoma is uncommonly seen in German shepherd dogs.[22,23]

Clinical signs may help localize disease to the upper urinary tract, or lower urinary tract or may be nonspecific (Table 30–1). The source of clinical signs should be localized, whenever possible, to determine better an appropriate diagnostic plan. If hematuria is noted, the timing of blood within the urine stream may be a helpful localizing sign. Blood consistently at the end of urination suggests bladder origin, whereas blood at the beginning of urination suggests urethra or reproductive tract origin. Blood throughout urination can occur with hemorrhage from any urinary tract site. Thorough ab-

TABLE 30–1. CLINICAL FINDINGS OF URINARY TRACT NEOPLASIA*

Upper urinary tract
  Palpable renal mass
  Retroperitoneal pain
  Polyuria
Lower urinary tract
  Palpable bladder or urethral mass
  Pollakiuria
  Dysuria
  Urinary incontinence
  Bleeding from penis, vagina
Nonspecific
  Weight loss
  Anorexia
  Hematuria throughout urination

* None of these findings is pathognomonic for urinary tract neoplasia. Further diagnostic procedures are indicated.

TABLE 30–2. TNM CLASSIFICATION OF URINARY TRACT TUMORS

	Kidney	Bladder
T: Primary Tumor*		
T0	No evidence of tumor	
T1S		Carcinoma in situ
T1	Small tumor without deformation of kidney	Superficial papillary tumor
T2	Solitary tumor with deformation and/or renal enlargement	Tumor invading bladder wall with induration
T3	Tumor invading renal pelvis, ureter, or renal vessels	Tumor invading adjacent organs (prostate, uterus vagina, rectum)
N: Regional lymph node (RLN) involvement		
N0	No RLN involvement	
N1	RLN involved	
N2	Bilateral RLN	RLN and juxtaregional lymph nodes
N3	Other lymph nodes	
M: Distant metastasis		
M0	No evidence of metastasis	
M1a	Single metastasis in one organ, specify site	
M1b	Multiple metastases in one organ, specify site	
M1c	Multiple metastases in multiple organs, specify sites	

* The symbol "m" added to a T category indicates multiple tumors.

Data from Owen, L.N., ed.: TNM Classification of Tumors in Domestic Animals. Geneva, World Health Organization, 1980.

dominal and rectal palpation should be performed on all animals, and the external genitalia should be inspected. Urethral tumors may involve the entire urethral length extending into the bladder and vagina. Rectal palpation and vaginoscopy are very important in physical examination of older female dogs with hematuria and dysuria.

Hypertrophic osteopathy has been reported in dogs with atypical nephroblastoma, bladder carcinoma, and botryoid rhabdomyosarcoma with no apparent pulmonary lesions.[24,25] Affected dogs may present for limb swelling and no apparent urologic problem.

Diagnostic Procedures

General Diagnostic Procedures and Staging

Urinary tract tumors are staged using the TNM system developed for domestic animals by the World Health Organization (Table 30–2).[27] When urinary tract neoplasia is suspected, several general diagnostic procedures are routinely performed to assess the health of the animal and to stage the tumor, including evaluation of a complete blood count, serum biochemistry panel, and urinalysis. Survey radiographs are made of the abdomen and thorax, using three radiographic views of the thorax (i.e., ventrodorsal or dorsoventral view and *both* right and left lateral views).[28] Other diagnostic tests include contrast-enhanced radiography, ultrasound evaluation, and cytologic and histologic analysis. Special imaging studies, available at referral centers, include selective arteriography, caudal vena caval angiography, computed tomography, and nuclear scintigraphy. Specific applications of these techniques are discussed next.

Renal and Ureteral Neoplasia

Routine laboratory tests typically show only nonspecific abnormalities. Hemogram changes can include anemia from chronic renal failure or from neoplasia itself (chronic hemorrhage or anemia of chronic disease).[11] In a few animals with renal cell carcinoma, polycythemia can develop from excessive erythropoietin production.[11,29] On serum biochemistry, elevated liver enzyme concentrations may be associated with hepatic metastases. Azotemia may occur because of prerenal (hypovolemia), renal (tumor infiltration of both kidneys as occurs in feline lymphosarcoma), or postrenal (bilateral ureteral obstruction) causes. Urinalysis abnormalities include cylindruria, proteinuria, and gross or microscopic hematuria.[11] Neoplastic cells are rarely seen in urine sediment.

Imaging techniques useful for diagnosis of renal and ureteral tumors include survey abdominal radiographs, excretory urography, and ultrasonography (see Chapter 6). On abdominal radiographs, a primary renal neoplasm typically appears as a unilaterally enlarged or distorted kidney. Lymphosarcoma generally causes bilateral symmetrical renal enlargement, with minimal shape distortion (see Fig. 6-7). Survey abdominal radiographs are seldom diagnostic for ureteral tumors. Excretory urography is the most useful, widely available imaging technique for renal and ureteral tumors and was diagnostic in 97% of dogs with renal tumors.[11] Abnormalities seen with renal cancer include distortion of the shape or size of renal parenchyma or pelvic diverticula, nonuniform opacification, and retention of contrast medium (see Fig. 6-8A,B). Ureteral tumors appear as filling defects or irregularities of the ureteral wall; secondary hydronephrosis and hydroureter are common. Benign and malignant disease can seldom be differentiated by radiographic studies.

Ultrasonographic evaluation of renal neoplasms is more sensitive and specific than excretory urography but is not widely available in practice and is highly operator-dependent. Ultrasonography can detect earlier-stage tumors and more accurately differentiate cystic versus solid and benign versus malignant lesions than conventional radiographic techniques.[30-32] Neoplasms may appear hyperechoic or hypoechoic or have mixed echo patterns (see Fig. 6-8C). Renal lymphosarcoma is most characteristic, appearing as a diffuse hypoechoic lesion affecting both kidneys.[30-32] Ultrasound evaluation of the ureters is difficult. Hydroureter secondary to tumor obstruction can usually be identified, but detection of small tumors is often impossible.

Definitive diagnosis of renal and ureteral tumors is by cytologic or histologic evaluation. Cytologic samples are obtained by fine-needle aspirate in animals in which lymphosarcoma is highly suspected as a diagnosis (i.e., bilaterally enlarged kidneys that are not painful on palpation and have characteristic diffuse hypoechoic ultrasound pattern). A percutaneous cutting needle biopsy can also be used for suspected renal lymphosarcoma. Other renal tumors are often very vascularized, which increases the risk of hemorrhage and tumor spread after percutaneous aspiration or biopsy.[10,33]

With unilateral renal and ureteral tumors, excisional biopsy (i.e., complete removal of tumor with normal, healthy tissue margins) is best, as long as renal function in the remaining kidney is adequate. During laparotomy, biopsy specimens of regional lymph nodes (i.e., lumbar aortic nodes; Fig. 30–1) and any suspicious lesions in other organs are obtained.

If bilateral or widespread disease is present and lymphosarcoma has been excluded by cytology, incisional biopsies of the primary mass, regional lymph nodes, and abdominal metastatic lesions are obtained by laparotomy. Definitive diagnosis and determination of clinical tumor stage are necessary because therapy and prognosis vary with tumor type and extent of disease.

Bladder and Urethral Neoplasia

Routine laboratory tests generally show only nonspecific abnormalities. Hemogram changes are minimal (anemia of chronic disease may be present). Azotemia, if present, is generally secondary to bladder trigone or urethral obstruction. Urinalysis abnormalities may include hematuria, proteinuria, pyuria, bacteriuria, and presence of neoplastic cells.[6,7] Urine cytology should be carefully examined because hyperplastic and neoplastic transitional cells can have a similar appearance.

Of 70 dogs with bladder tumors, only 30% had abnormalities seen on plain abdominal radiographs.[6] Survey radiographs are helpful, however, to rule out other causes of chronic hematuria and dysuria such as urolithiasis. Contrast-enhanced radiographic techniques are diagnostic in 90 to 100% of animals.[6,7] Excretory urography is performed to determine if tumor invasion of the ureter and secondary hydroureter or hydronephrosis is present (see Fig. 6-13A,B). A double-contrast cystogram (see Chapter 6) is preferable to positive-contrast cystography for small tumors that may be obscured

FIG. 30–1. Regional lymph nodes.

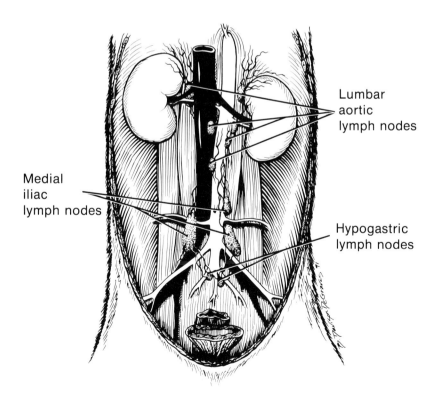

Lumbar aortic lymph nodes

Medial iliac lymph nodes

Hypogastric lymph nodes

by excessive radiopacity in the bladder. If urethral neoplasia or urethral invasion by a bladder tumor is suspected, positive-contrast vaginourethrography (female) or urethrography (male) should be performed (see Fig. 6-53). Radiographic changes seen with tumors of the bladder and urethra include mural thickenings or irregularities and luminal filling defects. Pyogranulomatous masses and polypoid cystitis, which have fair to good prognoses, may have the same radiographic appearance as a bladder neoplasm.

Other techniques for diagnosis of bladder and urethral tumors are ultrasonography, computed tomography, and cystoscopy. Percutaneous ultrasound examination may be used to evaluate the regional lymph nodes (hypogastric, medial iliac, lumbar aortic lymph nodes; see Fig. 30–1) but otherwise provide similar information to that gained from contrast-enhanced radiographic studies. Cystoscopy is the primary technique used for diagnosis of bladder tumors in humans, with a reported sensitivity and specificity of 100% following visual inspection of bladder and urethra and evaluation of cytologic and histologic samples.[34] The main shortcoming of cystoscopy is that it provides little information on depth of tumor penetration. The technique has been reported in dogs and cats.[35–37]

Pulmonary metastases of bladder and urethral tumors can appear as commonly recognized pulmonary nodules or consolidations or as a more subtle, diffuse interstitial increase in opacity.[38] Because this change can be confused with normal age-related increase in interstitial opacity, thoracic radiographs must be carefully reviewed.

Definitive diagnosis of bladder or urethral neoplasia is made cytologically or histologically. Histologic analysis may be more accurate because markedly hyperplastic transitional cells can be difficult to differentiate from neoplastic cells by cytology. Samples may be obtained without surgery from urine sediment, bladder or urethral washings, urinary catheterizations, and cystoscopic and vaginoscopic biopsies or brushings. Because the superficial inguinal nodes drain the vagina in the female and the distal urethra, penis, and prepuce in the male, they should be examined closely and aspiration or biopsy performed if suspicious.

An exploratory laparotomy solely for biopsy of a bladder or intrapelvic urethral tumor is usually not recommended because previous biopsy complicates excision during a second surgery. As described in Chapter 31, the surgeon should be prepared to obtain intraoperative cytology or analysis of frozen sections and then perform the primary excision and reconstruction. If this is not feasible, the animal can be referred, without a biopsy, for definitive diagnosis and therapy. In addition, great care should be taken when performing incisional biopsies of urinary tract tumors during laparotomy because of the risk of seeding tumor cells into normal tissues.[39]

Medical Therapy of Urinary Tract Neoplasia

Chemotherapy for urinary tract neoplasia is commonly available in practice, radiotherapy is frequently available on a referral basis, and research institutions are continuing to develop new treatment modalities such as immunotherapy, hyperthermia, and photodynamic therapy. The trend in treatment is toward multimodality therapies based on the expected biologic behavior of the specific tumor. This approach maximizes therapeutic benefit and minimizes treatment morbidity.

Surgery continues to be the mainstay of therapy for all benign and most malignant urinary tract neoplasms (see Chapter 31). This chapter discusses radiation and medical therapy of urinary tract tumors.

Renal and Ureteral Neoplasia

Renal cell carcinoma is often locally invasive, spreading by direct extension through the renal capsule and by invasion of the renal vein and vena cava.[8,10,11] Distant metastasis is also common,[8,10,11] and tumor cells move by hematogenous or lymphatic routes. Lungs, liver, lymph nodes, adrenal gland, brain, eyes, and bone are reported metastatic sites. A multimodality regimen that provides treatment for local tumor disease and distant metastases is indicated in most animals.

No detailed reports are available describing use of radiation or chemotherapy for treatment of renal cell carcinoma in animals. Surgical excision of renal cell carcinoma resulted in survival for more than 10 months for 20 to 30% of dogs.[10,11] Clinical conclusions cannot be made, however, because of poor correlation between tumor stage, type of treatment, and survival time. Treatment failures, when reported, were caused by distant metastases (up to 4 years later). Reports of treatment results for renal cell carcinoma are similar in humans.[12] Approximately 30% of humans with T1-stage and T2-stage tumors experience prolonged survival following surgery, with failure as a result of metastatic disease. Chemotherapy and radiotherapy have had little effect on survival (response rates < 10%).

Nephroblastoma usually affects young dogs and cats but can occur at any age. These tumors behave as low to moderate grade malignant neoplasms. They are frequently very large when diagnosed and most often grow by neoplastic invasion and benign compression of tissues. Lungs, liver, and lymph nodes are the most common sites of metastasis. Few reports are available describing treatment of nephroblastoma in dogs and cats. Increased survival time is reported following surgery.[8,11]

In dogs, renal lymphoma is one location of metastatic multicentric lymphoma.[40] Successful control of this disease has been described.[41,42] In cats, renal lymphoma is a distinct disease and constitutes approximately 15% of all feline lymphomas.[19] Affected cats range in age from 2 to 12 years (average 5 to 7 years), and approximately one half are FeLV-test-positive. Both kidneys are usually infiltrated by tumor, and central nervous system metastases are common.[19] Cats are usually presented in renal failure (a result of massive neoplastic infiltration) and require urgent supportive therapy and early initiation of chemotherapy. Renal lymphoma occurs bilaterally and is often widespread; thus, therapy must be systemic. Several chemotherapy protocols are available, and all appear to be equally effective.[19,43,44] Prognosis varies with tumor stage. Complete response rates occur in approximately 60% of cats and partial response rates in 30%, and average survival time is 6 months (range 1 week to > 5 years).[19] Cats that are FeLV-test-positive survive approximately half as long as FeLV-test-negative cats.[19] Morbidity associated with treatment is generally minimal. Patterns of treatment failure include local renal recurrence, metastasis to the central nervous system, and systemic recurrence.

Other uncommon tumors of the kidney and ureter include transitional cell and squamous cell carcinoma, renal cystadenocarcinoma, and various mesenchymal tumors. There are too few reports of these tumors to draw any conclusions about therapy. Most have been treated with surgery or not at all. Several animals have lived for more than a year following complete removal of a localized tumor, but distant metastases appear to be common, especially with epithelial tumors.[10,11] German shepherd dogs with renal cystadenocarcinomas can have prolonged survival with no treatment. Clinical morbidity is usually from associated fibrous nodules on the feet, skin, and subcutis.[22,23] Palliation is achieved by surgically removing painful or infected nodules. Ureteral tumors are rarely described, with surgical excision as the treatment.

Bladder and Urethral Neoplasia

Transitional cell carcinoma is the most common malignant tumor type of the bladder and urethra.[3,5–7,18,21,45] Squamous cell and adenocarcinoma occur infrequently and may arise from dedifferentiated transitional epithelium. In female dogs, urethral squamous cell carcinomas may be of primary origin because the distal two thirds of the urethra is lined with squamous epithelium.[45] Bladder tumors can occur as solitary, multiple, papillary, or diffusely infiltrative lesions. Depth of penetration varies from superficial (carcinoma in situ) to penetration of all muscular and epithelial layers. In humans (and probably animals), tumor invasiveness is highly prognostic and useful for determining appropriate adjuvant therapy.[13] Urethral tumors are usually diffuse and involve the entire urethral length by the time of diagnosis. Metastases occur in 30 to 60% of dogs with urethral tumors, and most frequently affect the regional lymph nodes and lungs.[18,45] Transitional cell carcinoma is more likely to metastasize than adenocarcinoma and squamous cell carcinoma.[45]

Effective treatment of most animals with transitional cell carcinoma requires both local and systemic therapy. For localized squamous cell and adenocarcinoma, surgery alone may be effective. Radiation therapy was combined with surgery to treat 18 dogs with transitional cell carcinoma of the bladder. Median survival was 15 months in dogs treated with intraoperative radiation[46] and 4 months in dogs treated with intraoperative radiation and fractionated radiation after surgery.[47] In both studies, complications were frequent, including incontinence, pollakiuria, cystitis, and stranguria. When a ureter was in the radiation field, hydroureter and hydronephrosis, secondary to ureteral fibrosis and stricture, occurred in almost all dogs. Treatment failures occurred at the primary site, regional lymph nodes, and distant metastatic sites, indicating that more effective local and systemic therapy is needed. Preoperative radiation therapy for bladder neoplasia in dogs has not been evaluated.

Two dogs with transitional cell carcinoma were treated with intra-arterial and intravenous cisplatin and radiotherapy.[48] Both dogs had partial responses to therapy (50 to 100% reduction in tumor volume) with minimal adverse effects from treatment. The dogs survived for 6 and 7 months.[48] Whether this would be an increase in survival time as compared with untreated dogs is unknown.

Few studies have evaluated chemotherapeutic agents for treatment of naturally occurring bladder and urethral tumors in dogs or cats. Several individual drugs have some activity against transitional cell carcinoma, but the numbers of animals treated were small.[49,50] In a comparative study of 31 dogs with transitional cell carcinoma, dogs treated with doxorubicin and cyclophosphamide survived significantly longer (259 days) than those treated with surgery alone (86 days) or intravesicular triethylenethiophosphoramide (57 days).[51] The extent of the disease, however, may not have been comparable.

Cisplatin was considered an effective drug for transitional cell carcinoma, but more recent reports are not encouraging. In 19 dogs, cisplatin administration at 50 mg/m^2 IV every 4 weeks resulted in no complete responses, three partial responses, and stable disease in nine dogs.[52,53] When administered at 60 mg/m^2 IV every 3 weeks, no complete or partial responses were seen; one of four dogs remained stable.[54] The poor efficacy seen with individual chemotherapy agents emphasizes the need for more effective multiple drug and adjuvant protocols.

Use of chemotherapy agents for treatment of bladder tumors has not been reported in cats. Survival time after surgical excision was 3 to 6 months, with tumor recurring locally.[7]

Immunotherapy has had limited use in dogs with bladder neoplasms. Partial surgical resection and intralesional bacillus Callamette-Guerin cell wall preparations in seven dogs resulted in two dogs "benefiting" from therapy and two dogs developing severe granulomatous reactions and urinary obstruction.[2]

Botryoid rhabdomyosarcoma and other sarcomas are seemingly best treated by wide surgical resection because metastases are uncommon. Intraoperative radiation therapy in conjunction with excision has been described,[46] but whether it improves survival is not known. Chemotherapy for mesenchymal tumors of the bladder has not been reported.

REFERENCES

1. Crow, S.E.: Urinary tract neoplasms in dogs and cats. Compend. Contin. Educ. Pract. Vet., 7:607, 1985.

2. Withrow, S.J.: Tumors of the urinary system. *In* Clinical Veterinary Oncology. Edited by S.J.Withrow and E.G. MacEwen. Philadelphia, J.B. Lippincott, 1989, pp. 312–324.

3. Osborne, C.A., Low, D.G., Perman, V., et al.: Neoplasms of the canine and feline urinary bladder: Incidence, etiologic factors, occurrence and pathologic features. Am. J. Vet. Res., *29:*2041, 1968.

4. Pamukcu, A.M.: Tumors of the urinary bladder. Bull. WHO, *50:*43, 1974.

5. Hayes, H.M.: Canine bladder cancer: Epidemiologic features. Am. J. Epidemiol., *104:*673, 1976.

6. Burnie, A.G., and Weaver, A.D.: Urinary bladder neoplasia in the dog: A review of seventy cases. J. Sm. Anim. Pract., *24:*129, 1983.

7. Schwarz, P.D., Greene, R.W., and Patnaik, A.K.: Urinary bladder tumors in the cat: A review of 27 cases. J. Am. Anim. Hosp. Assoc., *21:*237, 1985.

8. Baskin, G.B., and De Paoli, A.: Primary renal neoplasms of the dog. Vet. Pathol., *14:*591, 1977.

9. Hayes, H.M., and Fraumeni, J.F.: Epidemiologic features of canine renal neoplasms. Cancer Res., *37:*2553, 1977.

10. Lucke, V.M., and Kelly, D.F.: Renal carcinoma in the dog. Vet. Pathol., *13:*264, 1976.

11. Klein, M.K., Cockerell, G.L., Harris, C.K., et al.: Canine primary renal neoplasms: A retrospective review of 54 cases. J. Am. Anim. Hosp. Assoc., *24:*443, 1988.

12. Linehan, W.M., Shipley, W.U., and Longo, D.L.: Cancer of the kidney and ureter. *In* Cancer: Principles and Practice of Oncology. 3rd ed. Edited by V.T. DeVita Jr., S. Hellman, and S.A. Rosenberg. Philadelphia, J.B. Lippincott, 1989, pp. 979–1007.

13. Richie, J.P., Shipley, W.U., and Yagoda, A.: Cancer of the bladder. *In* Cancer: Principles and Practice of Oncology. 3rd ed. Edited by V.T. DeVita Jr., E. Hellman, and S.A. Rosenberg. Philadelphia, J.B. Lippincott, 1989, pp. 1008–1022.

14. Glickman, L.T., Schofer, F.S., and McKee, L.J.: Epidemiologic study of insecticide exposures, obesity and risks of bladder cancer in household dogs. J. Toxicol. Environ. Health, *28:*407, 1989.

15. Conzelman, G.M., and Moulton, J.E.: Dose-response relationships of the bladder tumorigen 2-naphthyline: A study in beagle dogs. J. Natl. Cancer Inst., *49:*193, 1972.

16. Hayes, H.M., Hoover, R., and Tarone, R.E.: Bladder cancer in pet dogs: a sentinel for environmental cancer? Am. J. Epidemiol., *114:*229, 1981.

17. Weller, R.E., Wolf, A.M., and Oyejide, A.: Transitional cell carcinoma of the bladder associated with cyclophosphamide therapy in 3 dogs. J. Am. Anim. Hosp. Assoc., *15:*733, 1979.

18. Wilson, G.P., Hayes, H.M., and Casey, H.W.: Canine urethral cancer. J. Am. Anim. Hosp. Assoc. *15:*741, 1979.

19. Mooney, S.C., Hayes, A.A., Matus, R.E., et al.: Renal lymphoma in cats: 28 cases (1977–1984). J. Am. Vet. Med. Assoc., *191:*1473, 1987.

20. Kelly, D.F.: Rhabdomyosarcoma of the urinary bladder in dogs. Vet. Pathol., *10:*375, 1973.

21. Strafuss, A.C., and Dean, M.J.: Neoplasms of the canine urinary bladder. J. Am. Vet. Med. Assoc., *166:*1161, 1975.

22. Lium, B., and Moe, L.: Hereditary multifocal renal cystadenocarcinomas and nodular dermatofibrosis in the German shepherd dog: Macroscopic and histopathologic changes. Vet. Pathol., *22:*447, 1985.

23. Cosenza, S.F., and Seely, J.C.: Generalized nodular dermatofibrosis and renal cystadenocarcinomas in a German shepherd dog. J. Am. Vet. Med. Assoc., *189:*1587, 1986.

24. Caywood, D.D., Osborne, C.A., Stevens, J.B., et al.: Hypertrophic osteoarthropathy associated with an atypical nephroblastoma in a dog. J. Am. Anim. Hosp. Assoc., *16:*855, 1980.

25. Brodey, R.S.: Hypertrophic osteoarthropathy in the dog: A clinicopathologic survey of 60 cases. J. Am. Vet. Med. Assoc., *159:*1242, 1971.

26. Halliwell, W.H., and Ackerman, N.: Botyroid rhabdomyosarcoma of the urinary bladder and hypertrophic osteoarthropathy in a young dog. J. Am. Vet. Med. Assoc., *165:*911, 1974.

27. Owen, L.N., ed.: TNM classification of tumours in domestic animals. Geneva, World Health Organization, 1980.

28. Spencer, C.P., Ackerman, N., and Burt, J.K.: The canine lateral thoracic radiograph. Vet. Radiol., *22:*262, 1981.

29. Gorse, M.J.: Polycythemia associated with renal fibrosarcoma in a dog. J. Am. Vet. Med. Assoc., *192:*793, 1988.

30. Walter, P.A., Feeney, D.A., Johnston, G.R., et al.: Ultrasonographic evaluation of renal parenchymal diseases in dogs: 32 cases (1981–1986). J. Am. Vet. Med. Assoc., *191:*999, 1987.

31. Walter, P.A., Johnston, G.R., Feeney, D.A., et al.: Applications of ultrasonography in the diagnosis of parenchymal kidney disease in cats: 24 cases (1981–1986). J. Am. Vet. Med. Assoc., *192:*92, 1988.

32. Konde, L.J., Park, R.D., Wrigley, R.H., et al.: Comparison of radiography and ultrasonography in the evaluation of renal lesions in the dog. J. Am. Vet. Med. Assoc., *188:*1420, 1986.

33. Wehle, M.J., and Grabstald, H.: Contraindications to needle aspiration of a solid renal mass: Tumor dissemination by renal needle aspiration. J. Urol., *136:*446–448, 1986.

34. Corwin, H.L., and Silverstein, M.D.: The diagnosis of neoplasia in patients with asymptomatic microscopic hematuria: a decision analysis. J. Urol., *139:*1002, 1988.

35. Cooper, J.E., Milroy, E.J.G., Turton, J.A., et al.: Cystoscopic examination of male and female dogs. Vet. Rec., *115:*571, 1984.

36. McCarthy, T.C., and McDermaoid, S.L.: Prepubic percutaneous cystoscopy in the dog and cat. J. Am. Anim. Hosp. Assoc., *22:*213, 1986.

37. Senior, D.F., and Sundstrom, D.A.: Cystoscopy in female dogs. Compend. Contin. Educ. Pract. Vet., *10:*890, 1988.

38. Walter, P.A., Haynes, J.S., Feeney, D.A., et al.: Radiographic appearance of pulmonary metastases from transitional cell carcinoma of the bladder and urethra of the dog. J. Am. Vet. Med. Assoc., *185:*411, 1984.

39. Gilson, S.D., and Stone, E.A.: Surgically induced tumor seeding in 8 dogs and 2 cats. J. Am. Vet. Med. Assoc., *196:*1811, 1990.

40. Rosenthal, R.C., and MacEwen, E.G.: Treatment of lymphoma in dogs. J. Am. Vet. Med. Assoc., *196:*774, 1990.

41. Postorino, N.C., Susaneck, S.J., Withrow, S.J., et al.: Single agent therapy with adriamycin for canine lymphosarcoma. J. Am. Anim. Hosp. Assoc., *25:*221, 1989.

42. Cotter, S.M.: Treatment of lymphoma and leukemia with cyclophosphamide, vincristine, and prednisone: I. Treatment of dogs. J. Am. Anim. Hosp. Assoc., *19:*159, 1983.

43. Cotter, S.M.: Treatment of lymphoma and leukemia with cyclophosphamide, vincristine, and prednisone: II. Treatment of cats. J. Am. Anim. Hosp. Assoc., *19:*166, 1983.

44. Jeglum, K.A., Whereat, A., and Young, K.: Chemotherapy of lymphoma in 75 cats. J. Am. Vet. Med. Assoc., *190:*174, 1987.

45. Tarvin, G.B., Patnaik, A., and Greene, R.: Primary urethral tumors in dogs. J. Am. Vet. Med. Assoc., *172:*931, 1978.

46. Walker, M., and Brieder, M.: Intraoperative radiotherapy of canine bladder cancer. Vet. Radiol., *28:*200, 1987.

47. Withrow, S.J., Gillette, E.L., Hoopes, P.J., et al.: Intraoperative irradiation of 16 spontaneously occurring canine neoplasms. Vet. Surg., *18:*7, 1989.

48. McCaw, D.L., and Lattimer, J.C.: Radiation and cisplatin for treatment of canine urinary bladder carcinoma. A report of 2 case histories. Vet. Radiol., *29:*264, 1988.

49. Ogilvie, G.K., Reynolds, H.A., Richardson, R.C., et al.: Phase II evaluation of doxorubicin for treatment of various canine neoplasms. J. Am. Vet. Med. Assoc., *195:*1580, 1989.

50. Crow, S.E., and Klausner, J.S.: Management of transitional cell carcinomas of the urinary bladder. *In* Current Veterinary Therapy VIII. Edited by R.W. Kirk. Philadelphia, W.B. Saunders, 1983, pp. 1119–1121.

51. Helfand, S.C., Hamilton, T.A., Jeglum, K.A., et al.: Comparison of three therapies for transitional cell carcinoma in the dog. *In* Proceedings for Veterinary Cancer Society 8th annual meeting, Estes Park, CO, 1988, p. 23.

52. Shapiro, W., Kitchell, B.E., Fossum, T.W., et al.: Cisplatin for treatment of transitional cell and squamous cell carcinomas in dogs. J. Am. Vet. Med. Assoc., *193*:1530, 1988.

53. Moore, A.S., Cardona, A., Shapiro, W., et al.: Cisplatin (cis-diammine dichloroplatinum) for treatment of transitional cell carcinoma of the urinary bladder or urethra. A retrospective study of 15 dogs. J. Vet. Intern. Med., *4*:148, 1990.

54. Knapp, D.W., Richardson, R.C., Bonney, P.L., et al.: Cisplatin therapy in 41 dogs with malignant tumors. J. Vet. Intern. Med., *2*:41, 1988.

31

Surgical Therapy for Urinary Tract Neoplasia

GENERAL PRINCIPLES OF ONCOLOGIC SURGERY

Surgical extirpation of contained urologic tumors, which requires early diagnosis, provides the best opportunity for cure. Although adjuvant therapies (e.g., radiation, chemotherapy) have augmented treatment opportunities, successful outcome often depends on the appropriate selection and performance of the operative procedure.

If there is a potential for surgical cure of a urologic tumor, an initial laparotomy for the sole purpose of biopsy is seldom desirable. Once a cystotomy has been performed for biopsy of a bladder tumor, for example, it is much more difficult to excise the tumor during a second surgery. The healing cystotomy wound incorporates normal tissue, which diminishes the amount of tissue suitable for bladder reconstruction. Thus, if the preoperative diagnosis of neoplasia is uncertain, the surgeon should be prepared to obtain intraoperative cytology or analysis of frozen sections and to perform the definitive surgical procedures. Alternatively, once there is a likely diagnosis of urologic cancer, the animal can be transferred, without a biopsy, to a referral center for definitive diagnosis and therapy. Access to cystoscopy may allow evaluation and biopsy before exploratory laparotomy.

The objectives of surgery for urologic cancer are to (1) obtain suitable biopsy specimens for accurate histologic diagnosis of primary tumor type and morphologic stage, (2) execute a precise extirpation without tumor spillage or contamination of normal tissues, and (3) perform a staging laparotomy to determine extent of intra-abdominal metastasis.

The surgeon carries major responsibility for accurate clinical staging and must obtain and record the following information: details of the operative procedure, location of the tumor, extent of local invasion and distant metastasis, location and magnitude of biopsies or excisions performed, and any tumor spillage or residual tumor. Intraoperative diagnosis, using cytologic or histologic analysis of frozen sections, can help determine if complete excision has been achieved. Marking the excision site with vascular clips may facilitate future radiographic mapping for radiotherapy.

Removal of lymph nodes (lymphadenectomy) may not improve surgical cure rates, but information gained from microscopic examination of excised nodes is essential for accurate prognostic staging. This information often cannot be obtained in any other way and is instrumental in determining adjuvant therapy.[1] The important lymph nodes to examine for *renal carcinoma* are the cranial lumbar aortic lymph nodes, which are variable in number and lie along the aorta and caudal vena cava from the diaphragmatic crus to the caudal mesenteric artery (see Fig. 30-1). For *bladder, prostate, and prostatic urethral cancer*, important nodes to examine are the hypogastric (formerly named internal iliac), the medial iliac (formerly named external iliac), and the lumbar aortic lymph nodes. The hypogastric lymph nodes lie between the internal iliac arteries, ventral to the seventh lumbar vertebra and the median sacral artery (usually paired, may have three on one side). The medial iliac lymph nodes are located between the deep circumflex iliac and the external iliac artery. The lumbar aortic lymph nodes of interest are caudal to the renal artery.

For *urethral cancer in the female*, the important nodes are the hypogastric and the lateral sacral lymph nodes. The lateral sacral nodes are not present in about 50% of normal dogs. They lie on each side of the median sacral artery and drain into the hypogastric lymph nodes. They usually cannot be seen during a routine exploratory laparotomy. If a pubic and ischiatic osteotomy is performed, however, these nodes should be examined. When urethral tumors invade the vagina and surrounding tissue, the superficial inguinal node should be aspirated and the cells examined. For *urethral cancer in the male*, the nodes to examine are the hypogastric and lateral sacral lymph nodes. The lymphatics of the distal urethra, penis, and prepuce drain into the superficial inguinal lymph node.[2]

Adherence to basic oncologic surgical principles is essential.[3] Urologic tumors are particularly susceptible to surgical implantation into normal tissues.[4] Drapes are used to protect the abdominal wall from tumor implantation. The tumor is isolated from the abdomen with laparotomy pads. Dissection is restricted to normal tissue with no disruption of tumorous tissue. Areas for resection are handled with retention sutures, rather than surgical instruments or fingers. After excision is completed, gloves and drapes are changed, and new instruments are used to close the wound. Contamination of the skin wound, particularly with urinary carcinoma cells, can seed tumor cells into the skin with resultant tumor growth.[4]

The tissue removed is submitted for histologic diagnosis, accompanied by a complete description of the clinical and surgical findings. The edges of the specimen can be marked with suture material or India ink to help the pathologist determine the completeness of the excision.

Coordination of surgical and adjuvant therapies requires cooperation and communication between surgeons, medical oncologists, and radiation therapists. To avoid interference with wound healing, surgery should be performed between 3 and 6 weeks after radiotherapy, and chemotherapeutics should not be administered for 7 days before and after surgery.[5]

SELECTION OF PROCEDURE

The choices of surgical procedures for urologic cancer are limited and involve partial or total excision of the affected organ, with urinary diversion, if necessary. The final decision of which procedure to perform may be made during surgery. If there is evidence of metastasis to regional lymph nodes or invasion of adjacent structures (e.g., body wall, adrenal gland, vessels, rectum), the decision may be to do nothing but obtain a biopsy specimen of the affected organ. Debulking (surgical cytoreduction) of urologic tumors may be indicated as a palliative procedure to relieve clinical signs (e.g., hematuria, stranguria). Debulking will probably not improve the efficacy of postoperative chemotherapy or radiation therapy, unless the tumor burden can be reduced to microscopic or milligram amounts.

Renal and Ureteral Cancer

Nephroureterectomy is performed for unilateral renal and ureteral cancer. Bilateral renal tumors are not treated surgically in dogs and cats. Bilateral multifocal renal cystadenocarcinoma affects German shepherd dogs and is associated with painful nodular dermatofibrosis of the foot pads. Excision of the lesions from the pads may give the dog pain relief.

Bladder Cancer

Solitary, Confined Lesion

Partial cystectomy is performed for tumors confined to a region of the bladder that allows removal of the tumor with a 2-cm margin of normal tissue. There should be no evidence of multifocal bladder cancer. Biopsies are taken to ensure that the remaining tissue margin is normal. Partial cystectomy with reimplantation of the ureter (ureteroneocystostomy) is used when one of the ureteral orifices is surrounded by tumor. Partial cystectomy may have a role in the palliation of hematuria and dysuria in animals with metastatic diseases.

The major advantage of partial cystectomy is the preservation of urinary tract continuity. We have found from clinical experience that after partial cystectomy with preservation of only enough bladder to ensure closure, animals initially urinate frequently. After a few months, however, they appear to regain normal voiding volume.

If the bladder cannot be closed, but the bladder neck, proximal urethra, and their neurovascular supply can be preserved, it might be possible to reconstruct a new bladder using a vascularized segment of ileum and jejunum.[6] When a tumor extends into the trigone region, however, complete cystectomy, as described subsequently, is necessary to remove all of the tumor.

Multiple Tumors; Trigone or Bladder Neck Tumors

When a tumor is obstructing urine flow and causing postrenal uremia, urine may be temporarily diverted by a cystostomy catheter (see Fig. 16–6) until therapeutic decisions are made. The catheter tract in the body wall and bladder can be excised during the definitive surgery. Temporary urinary diversion may also be used to bypass unresectable urinary tract tumors to allow time for response to other treatment modalities such as radiation therapy, hyperthermia, or chemotherapy.

Surgical excision of multiple bladder tumors or tumors that have extended into the bladder neck necessitates *total cystectomy and permanent urinary diversion. Ureterocolonic anastomosis* is the only urinary diversion procedure used in dogs that maintains continence after complete cystectomy, without an external collecting bag or catheterization.[7,8] Although trigone-colonic anastomosis has been described for dogs with bladder cancer,[9] it has limited usefulness because tumors that necessitate urinary diversion typically involve the trigone. Continent urinary diversion after cystectomy has not been described in cats.

A satisfactory surgical outcome following ureterocolonic anastomosis is most likely if dogs meet the following criteria: (1) serum creatinine level less than 1.5 mg/dl, (2) thoracic and abdominal radiographs negative for metastasis, (3) kidneys and ureters within normal limits on an excretory urogram, (4) fecal continence, (5) no hepatic or metabolic abnormalities. Whether complete cystectomy is curative depends on the stage of disease at the time of diagnosis and extirpation. Cystectomy should be curative for contained disease and may allow the use of adjuvant therapy to control metastatic disease.

Following ureterocolonic anastomosis, dogs void a watery mixture of feces and urine with a pungent odor. The owners must realize that after diversion, dogs should be allowed to defecate every 3 to 4 hours to prevent accumulation of urine and excessive absorption of urea and electrolytes from the colon. The dog needs careful monitoring for metabolic acidosis, hyperammonemia, and electrolyte abnormalities for the rest of its life. A complete discussion of postoperative management is presented in Chapter 32.

For some dogs or cats with bladder neck or urethral obstruction, a *permanent cystostomy* is a satisfactory palliative procedure for a few months. Ascending urinary tract infection may occur, but problems from pyelonephritis may not develop during the lifespan of the animal. The permanent cystostomy procedure is quick and has minimal surgical morbidity. Owners manage the animal with a diaper after surgery. Alternatively, a *permanent cystostomy catheter* (see Fig. 16–6) can be placed, using a de Pezzer mushroom catheter. After the catheter is inserted, it is clamped and the owners empty the bladder, using a syringe if necessary, three times a day.

Urethral Cancer

Tumors of the Pelvic Urethra

Resection of pelvic urethral tumors may necessitate ureterocolonic anastomosis for diversion. The pelvic urethra is accessed through a pubic and ischiatic osteotomy (see Fig. 10–4). When pelvic urethral tumors are adherent to surrounding pelvic structures such as the rectum, complete excision is difficult. In these instances, a more conservative procedure such as a permanent cystostomy or cystostomy catheter may be more appropriate than excision and urinary diversion.

If the tumor can be resected with preservation of proximal urethra and bladder-neck innervation, a *prepubic urethrostomy* (see Fig. 13–2), which preserves urinary continence, can be done in cats and female dogs. In male dogs, prepubic urethrostomy requires excisional or subtotal prostatectomy and may cause incontinence. Tumors of the prostate are discussed in Chapter 27. Prostatectomy is described in Chapter 28.

Focal urethral tumors are resected with as wide margins of normal urethra as possible. End to end anastomosis is performed using absorbable, synthetic suture material in a simple, interrupted pattern.[10] Excision of neoplasms of the distal urethra in the female dog necessitates destruction of the urethral orifice and resection of part of the vagina. The vaginal reconstruction creates a narrow tube that is anastomosed to the urethra. Satisfactory urinary continence was reported in three bitches after this "vagino-urethra" was passed through an incision in the clitoral fossa, spatulated, and sutured to the mucosa.[10] We have not done this procedure but would consider using it in dogs with resectable urethral tumors.

Tumors of the Extrapelvic Urethra in Male Dogs

Extrapelvic urethral tumors are usually excised and a new urethral opening made proximal to the excision. For tumors in the perineal and scrotal region, a *perineal urethrostomy* is performed. Excision of tumors in the preputial region necessitates a penile ablation followed by a *scrotal urethrostomy* (see Fig. 16–7).

PREPARATION FOR SURGERY

Possible sites of metastatic disease are thoroughly examined by palpation, radiography, and ultrasonography, if available. Arrangements are made for intraoperative cytology and frozen sections if their need is anticipated. Urologic tumors are often associated with urinary tract infection, so appropriate antibiotics, based on urine culture and sensitivity, are administered before surgery.

If ureterocolonic anastomosis is planned, the animal is started on a liquid diet 2 days before surgery. Enteral nutritional therapy, intravenous fluids, or both may be necessary. The day before surgery, administration of a broad-spectrum antibiotic (trimethoprim-sulfadiazine, 30 mg/kg once a day by mouth) and an antibiotic for anaerobic bacteria (metronidazole, 30 mg/kg once a day by mouth) is started. A warm-water enema is given the night before and the morning of surgery.

SURGICAL PROCEDURES

Nephroureterectomy

The nephroureterectomy procedure, as described in Fig. 22–1, requires modifications for the cancerous kidney and ureter.[11] When possible, the renal vessels are identified, ligated, and transected before mobilizing the kidney and tumor. To do this, the renal artery and renal vein are identified near the caudal vena cava. Using a right-angle clamp, a 2–0 nylon suture is passed around the renal vein. A second suture is placed distally at least 1 cm from the first. Neither is tied at this time. In a similar manner, a suture is passed around the renal artery near the vena cava. The suture is tied, but the artery is not transected. The sutures around the renal vein are tied, and the vein is divided. A second ligature is placed on the renal artery at least 1 cm distal to the first ligation. A transfixation ligature is placed near the proximal ligation (see Fig. 22–1D, insert). The artery is divided leaving a cuff of at least 0.5 cm, if possible. Isolation and ligation of the vessels in this manner allow early control of tumor vasculature, make isolation of the artery easier while the vein is patent and the kidney is not swollen, and permit venous ligation immediately after arterial ligation.

The ureter is divided between ligatures of 3–0 nylon at its entrance to the bladder. The kidney and peritoneal covering are dissected from the caudolateral abdominal musculature. If the tumor extends into the abdominal musculature, it may be necessary to excise the kidney and muscles en bloc.

Partial Cystectomy

A caudal midline or parapreputial abdominal incision is made. If the bladder is adhered to the body wall because of previous surgery for biopsy or partial cystectomy, the adhered region should be completely excised, i.e., full-thickness bladder and body wall removed en bloc. Laparotomy pads are placed to surround the bladder and to isolate it from adjacent structures. Retention sutures are placed near the proposed incision line (Fig. 31–1A). The initial cystotomy incision is made precisely to provide adequate tumor-free margins after the resection, while retaining maximal bladder volume. The retention sutures are used to maintain gentle lateral retraction on the cut edges of the bladder (Fig. 31–1B). The incision is extended to obtain adequate view of the bladder mucosal surface, and its length is dictated by the location and size of the tumor (Fig. 31–1C). If the ureteral orifices are near the planned excision, ureteral catheters are placed. If tumor obscures a ureteral orifice, intravenous indigo carmine (1 to 2.5 ml) will color the urine and aid in visualization.

Excision of the tumor is by sharp dissection, with at least a 2-cm margin of normal tissue removed. The specimen is carefully labeled as to its orientation. If the tumor is near the ureteral orifice, the orifice and distal ureter may be excised and the ureter reimplanted more proximally (ureteroneocystostomy; see Fig. 22–3). To prevent ureteral obstruction from edema after a ureteroneocystostomy or a major resection, ureteral catheters are placed and brought out through the urethra. The bladder remnant is closed with 4–0 absorbable suture material in a simple interrupted pattern. If closure is difficult, a Foley catheter can be inserted and the bulb expanded with sterile saline and used as a mold for reforming the bladder while suturing.

Total Cystectomy and Ureterocolonic Anastomosis[12]

A midline abdominal incision is made extending from umbilicus to pubis. Exposure of the pelvic urethra may require pubic or pubic and ischiatic osteotomy (see Fig. 10–4).

The ureters are inspected. If the ureter is greatly dilated, the ureterocolonic anastomosis is unlikely to have a successful outcome and the operative plan should be reconsidered. Otherwise, the ureters are divided between vascular clips or ligatures, 2 cm proximal to any neoplastic tissue. The ureter is freed from its retroperitoneal location, using care to preserve its adventitial covering and blood supply. The cranial and caudal vesical arteries and veins are ligated and severed. The ligaments of the bladder are cut. The urethra is ligated and severed at least 2 cm distal to tumor. In a male dog, a prostatectomy may be necessary (see Fig. 28–3). The bladder is removed.

Intestinal clamps are placed to isolate the descending

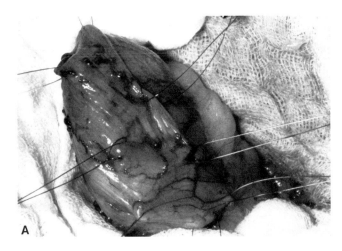

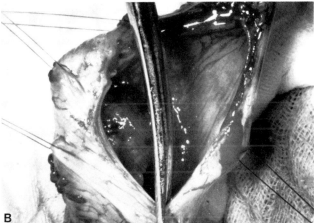

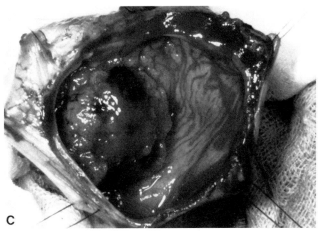

FIG. 31–1. Partial cystectomy. (A) Retention sutures are placed near the proposed incision line. (B) Retention sutures are used to maintain gentle lateral retraction on the cut edges of the bladder. (C) The incision is extended to obtain an adequate view of the bladder interior and to excise the tumor.

colon. The colon is positioned with clamps so that the antimesenteric side is uppermost. The ureters are laid along the colon without tension so that the surgeon can determine the location for the submuscular tunnels. It may be necessary to divide the duodenal-colonic ligament to prevent angulation of the right ureter. Retention sutures are placed in the colon, approximately 4 cm apart, to mark the proposed site of the submuscular flaps. The left ureterocolonic anastomosis should be approximately 0.5 cm distal to the right anastomosis to help preserve blood supply to the anastomotic site. The ureters are removed from the surface of the colon and isolated with sponges.

The left submuscular flap is prepared first. A 3.5-cm longitudinal incision is made on the antimesenteric surface through the colonic muscular fibers down to the mucosa. A 0.5-cm transverse incision is made at each end of the longitudinal incision (Fig. 31–2A). Retention sutures are placed at each end of the flap. Submuscular dissection, with fine scissors, is directed toward the mesenteric side of the colon to prevent devascularization of the flap (Fig. 31–2B). If the mucosa is inadvertently entered during creation of the flap, it should be closed with 6–0 synthetic absorbable sutures.

After the flap is prepared, the end of the left ureter is incised obliquely, starting on the side with vessels (Fig. 31–2C). The surface opposite the ureteral vessels is incised longitudinally for 2 to 3 mm to increase the diameter of the lumen. Two retention sutures of 6–0 synthetic absorbable material are placed through the ureter. A small circular opening is made in the colonic mucosa, approximately 0.5 cm proximal to the distal end

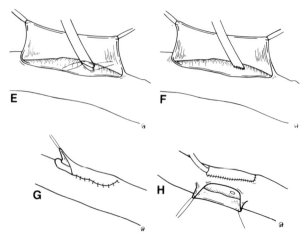

FIG. 31–2. (Cont.) (E) The ureteral retention sutures are passed through the proximal and distal edges of colonic mucosa surrounding the opening. (F) The ureter is sutured to the colonic mucosa, using precise mucosa to mucosa, simple interrupted pattern and 6–0 synthetic suture material. (G) The submucosal flap is closed over the ureter using simple interrupted 4–0 synthetic absorbable sutures. (H) The right ureterocolonic anastomosis is performed in a similar manner. The anastomotic site is approximately 0.5 cm proximal to the left anastomotic site. (Illustrations by Dr. J. Fujimoto, From Stone, E.A., Goldschmidt, M.H., and Walter, M.C.: Urinary diversion. Vet. Clin. North Am. [Sm. Anim. Pract.], 14:123, 1984; with permission.)

of the submucosal flap. This is done by picking up the mucosa with tissue forceps and excising a small piece with fine, curved scissors (Fig. 31–2D). The ureteral retention sutures are placed to anchor the ureter to the proximal and distal edge of the colonic opening (Fig. 31–2E).

The ureter is sutured to the colonic mucosa, using a precise mucosa to mucosa, simple interrupted pattern and 6–0 synthetic absorbable suture material (Fig. 31–2F). After the anastomosis is completed, the area is lavaged and suctioned to remove any contaminating material.

The submucosal flap is closed over the ureter using simple interrupted 4–0 synthetic absorbable sutures (Fig. 31–2G). Care is taken to avoid incorporating the ureter in the sutures and to avoid obstructing the ureter. A forceps should fit easily between the submuscular flap and the ureter. If it does not, the sutures are removed, the flap is repositioned more loosely, and the sutures are replaced. The right ureterocolonic anastomosis is performed in a similar manner. The right anastomotic site is approximately 0.5 cm proximal to the left anastomotic site (Fig. 31–2H).

Omentum is draped over the descending colon and tacked to the colonic serosa. Abdominal closure is routine. To ensure urinary outflow during recovery from anesthesia, a multiholed 8 Fr gauge tube is placed through the anus and into the colon, to serve as a rectal catheter, and sutured to the perineum. It is removed 24 hours after surgery. The dog is started on solid food 48 hours after surgery.

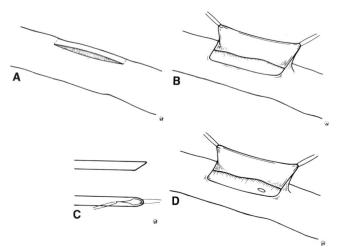

FIG. 31–2. Ureterocolonic anastomosis. (A) The left submuscular flap is prepared first. A 3.5-cm longitudinal incision is made through the colonic muscular fibers down to the mucosa. A 0.5-cm transverse incision is made at each end of the longitudinal incision. Retention sutures are placed at each end of the flap. (B) Submuscular dissection, with fine scissors, is directed toward the mesenteric side of the colon to prevent devascularization of the flap. (C) The end of the left ureter is incised obliquely, starting on the side with vessels. A 2- to 3-cm longitudinal incision is made opposite the vessels to increase the diameter of the lumen. Two retention sutures of 6–0 absorbable material are placed through the ureter. (D) A small circular opening is made in the colonic mucosa, approximately 0.5 cm proximal to the distal end of the submucosal flap. This is done by picking up the mucosa with tissue forceps and excising a small piece with fine, curved scissors.

Permanent Cystostomy

For a permanent cystostomy, a transverse incision is made one third the distance between the pubis and the umbilicus (Fig. 31–3A). In cats and female dogs, the incision is on the midline; in male dogs it is lateral to the prepuce. Because of skin tension in this region, a transverse incision makes a circular defect in the skin. A longitudinal incision is made through the linea alba after a midline skin incision (Fig. 31–3B) or through the rectus muscles and peritoneum after a parapreputial skin incision. The bladder is exteriorized and held with retention sutures (Fig. 31–3C). The bladder wall is sutured to the linea alba or ventral fascia of the body wall with absorbable sutures. The dome of the bladder is excised. The edges of the bladder are sutured to the skin, with nonabsorbable sutures, starting with the cranial and caudal sutures (Fig. 31–3D). The remaining sutures are placed (Fig. 31–3E).

Canine Perineal Urethrostomy

A urethral catheter is placed. A pursestring suture is placed around the anus. The dog is positioned in dorsal recumbency, with its front legs pulled caudally, its rear legs pulled cranially, and its tail hanging over the edge of the table (Fig. 31–4A). A midline skin incision is

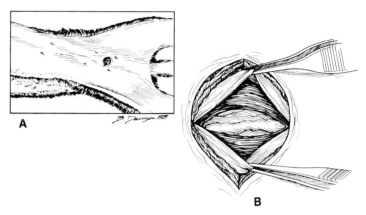

FIG. 31–3. Permanent cystostomy. (A) A transverse incision is made one third the distance between the pubis and umbilicus on midline in cats and female dogs, as illustrated here. (B) A longitudinal incision is made through the linea alba.

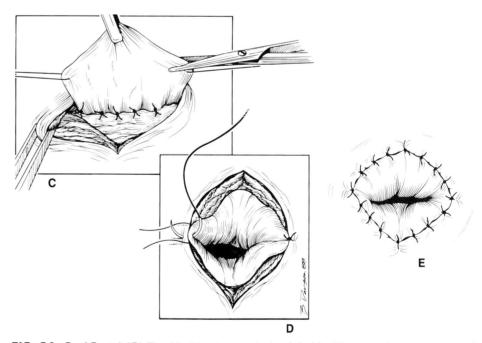

FIG. 31–3. (*Cont.*) (C) The bladder is exteriorized, held with retention sutures, and sutured to the linea alba. (D) The dome of the bladder is excised. The edges of the bladder are sutured to the skin, starting with the cranial and caudal sutures. (E) The remaining sutures are placed.

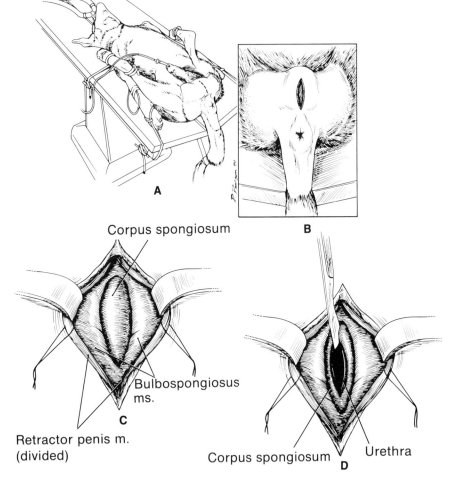

Corpus spongiosum

Bulbospongiosus ms.

C

Retractor penis m.
(divided)

Corpus spongiosum   Urethra

D

FIG. 31—4. Perineal urethrostomy. (A) After a catheter is placed in the urethra and a pursestring is placed around the anus, the dog is positioned in dorsal recumbency, with front legs extended caudally, rear legs extended cranially, and the tail draped over the edge of the table. (B) A midline skin incision is made, starting 2 cm from the anus and extending ventrally 3 cm. (C) The subcutaneous tissue is incised down to the retractor penile muscle, which is divided longitudinally on the midline. In a small dog, the retractor penile muscle can be retracted laterally. The bulbospongiosus muscles are separated along the median raphe, revealing the corpus spongiosum. (D) A 1- to 2-cm longitudinal incision is made through the corpus spongiosum and urethra.

made, starting 2 cm from the anus and extending ventrally 3 cm. The subcutaneous tissue is dissected down to the retractor penile muscle, which is retracted laterally (Fig. 31–4B). In a large dog, the retractor penile muscle can be divided longitudinally along its midline. A forceps is placed beneath the penis to elevate it from the incision. The bulbospongiosus muscles are separated along the median raphe, revealing the corpus spongiosum (Fig. 31–4C). The penis is grasped between thumb and forefinger for stabilization, and a 1 to 2 cm longitudinal incision is made through the corpus spongiosum and urethra (Fig. 31–4D). The incision is made directly on midline to avoid the very vascular bulb of the penis. The tunica albuginea is sutured to the subcutaneous fascia (3–0 absorbable suture, simple interrupted pattern), to reduce tension on the skin to urethra suture line (Fig. 31–4E). The urethra and attached corpus spongiosum are sutured to the skin with 4–0 nonabsorbable monofilament suture material. Two proximal sutures are placed at 10 o'clock and 2 o'clock (Fig. 31–4F). Sutures continue distally for 2 cm. At the distal end of the incision, the urethra is ligated with a nonabsorbable suture placed around the urethra and beneath the skin (Fig. 31–4G). The final urethra to skin sutures are placed at 5 o'clock and 7 o'clock. Any remaining skin is closed routinely (Fig. 31–4H).

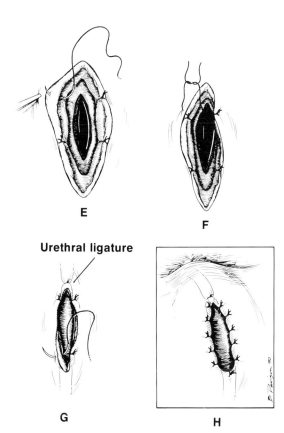

E

F

Urethral ligature

G

H

FIG. 31—4. Perineal urethrostomy. (A) After a catheter is placed in the urethra and a pursestring is placed around the anus, the dog is positioned in dorsal recumbency, with front legs extended caudally, rear legs extended cranially, and the tail draped over the edge of the table. (B) A midline skin incision is made, starting 2 cm from the anus and extending ventrally 3 cm. (C) The subcutaneous tissue is incised down to the retractor penile muscle, which is divided longitudinally on the midline. In a small dog, the retractor penile muscle can be retracted laterally. The bulbospongiosus muscles are separated along the median raphe, revealing the corpus spongiosum. (D) A 1- to 2-cm longitudinal incision is made through the corpus spongiosum and urethra.

REFERENCES

1. Herr, H.W.: Bladder cancer: Pelvic lymphadenectomy revisited. Surg. Oncol., *37*:242, 1988.
2. Evans, H.E., and Christensen, G.C.: The lymphatic system. *In* Miller's Anatomy of the Dog. Edited by H.E. Evans and G.C. Christiansen. Philadelphia, WB Saunders, 1979, pp. 802–841.
3. Gilson, S.D., and Stone, E.A.: Principles of oncologic surgery. Compend. Contin. Educ. Pract. Vet., *12*:827, 1990.
4. Gilson, S.D., and Stone, E.A.: Surgically induced tumor seeding in 10 animals. J. Am. Vet. Med. Assoc., *196*:1811, 1990.
5. Gilson, S.D., and Stone, E.A.: Management of the surgical oncology patient. Compend. Contin. Educ. Pract. Vet., *12*:1074, 1990.
6. Schwarz, P.D., Egger, E.L., and Klause, S.E.: Modified ''cup-patch'' ileocystoplasty for urinary bladder reconstruction in a dog. J. Am. Vet. Med. Assoc., *198*:273, 1991.
7. Stone, E.A., Walter, M.C., Goldschmidt, M.H., et al.: Ureterocolonic anastomosis in clinically normal dogs. Am. J. Vet. Res., *49*:1147, 1988.
8. Stone, E.A., Withrow, S.J., Page, R.L., et al.: Ureterocolonic anastomosis in 10 dogs with transitional cell carcinoma. Vet. Surg., *17*:147, 1988.
9. Bovee, K.C., Pass, M.A., Wardley, R., et al.: Trigonal-colonic anastomosis: A urinary diversion procedure in dogs. J. Am. Vet. Med. Assoc., *174*:184, 1979.
10. Davies, J.V., and Read, H.M.: Urethral tumors in dogs. J. Sm. Anim. Pract., *31*:131, 1990.
11. Das, S.: Radical nephrectomy: Thoracoabdominal extrapleural approach. *In* Genitourinary Cancer Surgery. Edited by E.D. Crawford and T.A. Borden. Philadelphia, Lea & Febiger, 1982, pp. 30–40.
12. Stone, E.A., Goldschmidt, M.H., and Walter, M.C.: Urinary diversion. Vet. Clin. North Am. [Sm. Anim. Pract.], *14*:123, 1984.

32

Postoperative Management and Surgical Complications of Urinary Tract Neoplasia

POSTOPERATIVE MANAGEMENT AND COMPLICATIONS ASSOCIATED WITH URINARY TRACT NEOPLASIA

The tumor histopathologic results are reviewed and correlated with the clinical and surgical findings. If there are discrepancies between the clinician's analysis and the pathologist's interpretation, the clinician should discuss the case with the pathologist. Depending on tumor type and stage, postoperative adjuvant therapy may be indicated.

Postoperative diagnostic techniques, as detailed here, are used to detect tumor recurrence or metastasis as early as possible. Any recurrence of signs (e.g., hematuria, dysuria) after surgery is immediately investigated. The asymptomatic animal is monitored for tumor recurrence and metastasis at 1, 2, 3, and 6 months after surgery and then every 6 months. A case history is obtained, and physical examination is performed, including careful palpation of the surgical site. Thoracic radiographs are used to detect distant metastasis. Contrast-enhanced radiographic studies and ultrasonographic evaluation, if available, of the urethra or bladder may be indicated. Biopsy specimens of any suspicious lesions are obtained for a definitive diagnosis.

POSTOPERATIVE MANAGEMENT AND COMPLICATIONS ASSOCIATED WITH THE SURGICAL PROCEDURE

Nephroureterectomy

Urine production is monitored after surgery by observation of voiding or by measurement of urine output with intermittent catheterization or an indwelling catheter. If urine output decreases, the catheter is aspirated and flushed to ensure patency. Hypotension, hypovolemia, and dehydration are assessed and corrected, if necessary. If urine production remains low, a diuretic is administered (see Chapter 8).

Partial Cystectomy

If ureteral catheters have been placed, they are connected to a closed urine collection system and removed after 2 days. Hematuria may persist for 3 to 4 days. After excision of greater than 50% of the bladder, the animal urinates frequently and may appear to be incontinent. In most animals, bladder volume increases after a few months, and the animal retains urine for normal intervals. Urinary tract infection is treated with appropriate antibiotics based on bacterial culture and sensitivity.

Urine leakage after partial cystectomy produces azotemia and ascites. An excretory urogram should identify the location. If a cystogram is performed, the amount of contrast material is decreased to correspond to the reduction in bladder volume. Once the leak is confirmed, surgical repair is indicated. Injection of indigo carmine or methylene blue (1 ml) into the bladder during surgery may help locate the area of dehiscence.

If the ureteroneocystostomy is leaking, it is examined to see if it is possible to place additional sutures to seal the leak. Usually, it is necessary to sever the ureter at its entrance to the bladder, close the opening, and make a more proximal ureteroneocystostomy. Placement of a ureteral catheter for 2 days after surgery should help the anastomotic site to seal and prevent ureteral occlusion from edema.

If the cystectomy incision line has partially opened, a few sutures on each side of the dehiscence are removed and the area resutured. Gentle tissue handling and precise placement of sutures are essential. Urine is drained for 4 days, through a cystostomy catheter or an indwelling urethral catheter.

Unilateral ureteral obstruction may not be apparent unless an excretory urogram reveals dilation of the ureters. Some degree of ureteral dilatation is expected after ureteral transplantation because of edema and altered peristalsis. Surgically induced dilation should resolve in 3 to 6 weeks and should not progress.[1] Excretory urography should be performed at the 1-month evaluation and then repeated within 2 weeks if the ureter is dilated. Progression or persistence of hydroureter suggests ureteral obstruction. Obstruction is caused by twisting the ureter before its entry into the bladder, constriction as it passes through the bladder wall, stenosis, ischemia, granulation tissue, or tumor at the reimplantation site. For correction, the terminal ureter is severed and reimplanted more proximally.

Total Cystectomy and Ureterocolonic Anastomosis[1,2]

Because operative time for total cystectomy and ureterocolonic anastomosis is 4 hours or greater, the immediate postoperative concern is recovery from anesthesia. Blood pressure, hematocrit, blood glucose concentration, and urine output are monitored closely. Intravenous lactated Ringer's solution (5 ml/kg/hr) is administered until the dog resumes drinking. The rectal catheter is retained for 2 days or until the dog voids on its own.

Long-term management of a dog after ureterocolonic anastomosis is aimed at preventing hyperammonemic encephalopathy, hyperchloremic acidosis, and uremia. The owner must understand that the dog has special needs and requires close attention (Table 32-1). The veterinarian must be cognizant of changes inherent in rerouting urine into the intestinal tract. For example, dosages of drugs eliminated by the kidneys may need to be adjusted because active drug or metabolites can be absorbed from the colon with resultant increased blood levels. This is particularly important for nephrotoxic drugs.

After ureterocolonic anastomosis, urine ammonia is absorbed from the colon and converted into urea by the liver. A low-protein diet may decrease the amount of

---

TABLE 32-1. MANAGEMENT OUTLINE FOR DOGS WITH URETEROCOLONIC ANASTOMOSIS

Educate owner about dog's unique requirements
Allow frequent voiding
Administer sodium bicarbonate
Treat with antibiotics for at least 1 month
Adjust dosages for drugs eliminated by kidney
Perform excretory urogram at 1, 3, and 6 months
Be prepared to treat electrolyte, acid-base, and ammonia
  abnormalities

---

ammonia produced. Allowing the dog the opportunity to evacuate the colon frequently (every 4 hours) should lessen the amount of ammonia that is absorbed. With colonic stasis, bacterial ureases hydrolyze urea into ammonia, which increases the ammonia available for absorption. Increased ammonia absorption also occurs whenever urine volume is reduced, and the urine is concentrated. Problems that decrease fluid intake or produce dehydration such as nausea, vomiting, depression, or disorientation increase urine concentration of ammonia and reduce the stimulus for the dog to void.

Metabolic acidosis is prevented by administration of oral bicarbonate, which is rapidly absorbed. The dose of oral bicarbonate should be sufficient to raise the TCO_2 to 15 mEq/L. The initial dose is 2 grains/kg/day divided bid or tid, which is then adjusted based on TCO_2 measurements. Sodium bicarbonate comes as a mint tablet (5 and 10 grains) and is palatable to most dogs. Alternatively, bicarbonate of soda powder can be placed on food (1 tsp = 60 grains = 4 g).

Some dogs with ureterocolonic anastomosis develop ulcerative colitis, which makes the colon more absorptive and may decrease the dog's ability to maintain continence. Early detection and management of colitis may improve clinical signs and lessen the metabolic consequences. Unfortunately, the treatment of colitis is not well delineated, particularly in dogs with ureterocolonic anastomosis. The use of a bulk fiber laxative may be beneficial because the fiber absorbs fluid and binds fecal material in the colon. The use of special diets and antimicrobial agents for colitis has been discussed.[4]

Metabolic acidosis following ureterocolonic anastomosis is probably related to colonic absorption of hydrogen or ammonium ions in conjunction with chloride ions. Uncontrolled acidosis results in anorexia, nausea, and vomiting and potentiates the colonic absorption of ammonia.

Owners should be warned that if the dog stops drinking or becomes depressed for any reason, it needs immediate attention. Hydration is maintained or re-established with subcutaneous or intravenous balanced electrolyte solution, while the reasons for the cessation in drinking are determined. Baseline electrolyte and acid-base status is determined, in addition to a complete blood count and blood chemistry panel. If the dog develops signs of hyperammonemic encephalopathy or metabolic acidosis, the colon is immediately evacuated and lavaged with warm-water enemas. A rectal catheter is placed to prevent urine accumulation until the dog has stabilized. Fluid therapy is continued based on laboratory results.

Dogs with ureterocolonic anastomosis are expected to be azotemic because of absorption of colonic urea and increased hepatic ureagenesis secondary to increased portal ammonia from the colon. Azotemia can be exacerbated by prerenal influences during gastrointestinal and neurologic disturbances and by primary renal dysfunction. Pyelonephritis may develop in some dogs, even though a functioning submuscular flap is designed to prevent ureteral reflux. To lessen the possibility of pyelonephritis, dogs are maintained on broad-spectrum antibiotics (e.g., trimethoprim-sulfadiazine) for 1 month after surgery. At that time an excretory urogram is performed. If the ureters or renal pelvis is dilated, antibiotics are continued. If the pyelogram is normal, the antibiotics are discontinued and an excretory urogram is repeated every 3 months. If collecting system dilation occurs, antibiotic administration is started again. Dogs with acute pyelonephritis may become febrile and have an inflammatory leukogram. Blood for cultures should be collected and the dog started on intravenous antibiotics.

REFERENCES

1. Barber, D.L.: Postoperative radiography of the urinary system. Vet. Clin. North Am. [Sm. Anim. Pract.], *14:*31, 1984.
2. Stone, E.A., Walter, M.C., Goldschmidt, M.H., et al.: Ureterocolonic anastomosis in clinically normal dogs. Am. J. Vet. Res., *49:*1147, 1988.
3. Stone, E.A., Withrow, S.J., Page, R.L., et al.: Ureterocolonic anastomosis in 10 dogs with transitional cell carcinoma. Vet. Surg., *17:*147, 1988.
4. Chiapella, A.: Diagnosis and management of chronic colitis in the dog and cat. *In* Current Veterinary Therapy X. Edited by R.W. Kirk. Philadelphia, W.B. Saunders, 1989, pp. 896–903.

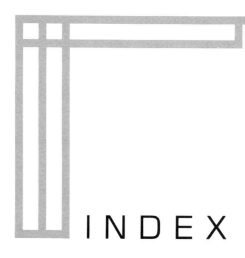

INDEX

Page numbers in italics indicate illustrations; numbers followed by "t" indicate tables.

Hypoadrenocorticism
  polyuria and, 7, 7t
Hypocalcemia
  in feline urethral obstruction, 125
  in renal failure, 94
Hypokalemia
  in urologic surgery, 109, 110t
  polyuria and, 7, 7t
Hypospadia
  diagnosis of, 203
  postoperative complications of, 211
  surgical therapy for, 208
Hypotension
  in urologic surgery, 109

I

Insulin
  in hyperkalemia, 94
Isoflurane
  in urologic surgery, 92, 94

K

Ketamine
  in feline urethral obstruction, 94
  in urologic surgery, 91–92, 94
Key-Gaskell syndrome
  in detrusor dysfunction, 13
Kidney
  abnormalities of, 57–60
  in urinary tract trauma
    surgical therapy for, 189, *190*, 191, *191*
  neoplasia of
    diagnosis of, 238–239
    medical therapy of, 240–241
  percutaneous biopsy of, 43–46, *44*, *45*
  radiographic examination of, 53–60, *54*, *55*, *56*, *57*, *58*, *59*, *60*, *61*
  surgical approach to, 100, *101*, *102*, 105
  surgical kidney biopsy of, *46*, 46–47
  ultrasonographic examination of, 53–60, *55*, *58*, *59*, *60*
  wound healing of, 107

M

Mannitol
  in renal disease, 93
Marsupialization
  as surgical therapy for prostatic disorders, 229, *229*
Meperidine
  in urologic surgery, 92
N-(2-mercaptopropionyl)-glycine
  in urolithiasis, 170, 171t
d,l-methionine
  in urolithiasis, 171, 171t
Methoxyflurane
  in urologic surgery, 92, 93
Micturition
  physiology of, 12, *12*
Mineral(s)
  in feline urethral obstruction, 121–122
Morphine
  in urologic surgery, 92
Myoglobinuria, 16–17

N

Naloxone
  in urethrotomy, 149
Natriuresis
  polyuria and, 7
Nausea
  control of, 97
Neoplasia
  of kidney
    diagnosis of, 238–239
    medical therapy of, 240–241
  of ureter
    diagnosis of, 238–239
    medical therapy of, 240–241
  of urethra
    diagnosis of, 239–240
    medical therapy of, 241

of urinary bladder
    diagnosis of, 239–240
    medical therapy of, 241
Nephrectomy
  definition of, 174
  partial
    in renal injury, 191, *191*
Nephrolith(s), 165, *165*
  bilateral, 175
Nephrostomy
  in ureteral injury, 194, *195*
Nephrotomy
  bisection
    in urolithiasis, 175, *175*, *176*, 177
  definition of, 174
  in urolithiasis, 174–175, *175*, *176*, 177, *178*, 180
Nephroureterectomy
  as surgical therapy in renal and ureteral cancer, 245, 246–247
  in renal injury, 189, *190*, 191
  postoperative management and complications with, 252
Nitrous oxide
  in urologic surgery, 92
Nocturia
  definition of, 5
Norketamine
  in urologic surgery, 92

O

Oliguria
  causes of, 9, 9t
  definition of, 5, 9
  diagnostic plan for, 9–10
Osteotomy
  cranial pubic, 101, *104*
  ischial, 101, *104*
  pubic, 101, *104*
Oxalate crystals. See also Urolith(s).
  in urinalysis, 41, *42*
Oxymorphone
  in renal disease, 94
  in urethrotomy, 149

P

Paraprostatic cysts, 31t, 32
D-penicillamine
  in urolithiasis, 170, *170*, 171t
Penis
  cross-section of, *152*
Perineal mass
  as sign of prostatic disorder, 217
Phenoxybenzamine
  as urethral relaxant, 132
Pollakiuria
  definition of, 5
Polydipsia. See also Polyuria.
  causes of, 8
  definition of, 6
  psychogenic, 8
Polyganglionopathy
  autonomic
    in detrusor dysfunction, 13
Polyuria
  causes of, 7, 7t
  definition of, 5
  differential diagnosis of, 7, 7t
  documentation of, 6
  in renal failure, 10t
  normal water balance and, 5–6, *6*
  obligatory, 7
  polydipsia and
    diagnostic plan for, 8–9
  primary, 7, 7t
  urine concentration tests for, 42–43
Potassium chloride
  in hypokalemia, 109, 110t
Potassium citrate
  in urolithiasis, 171, 171t
Prepuce
  surgical approach to, 100–101, *103*
Profilometry
  urethral, 50, *50*

Urinary tract (*Continued*)
    complications of, 197–198
    diagnostic tests for, 186
    emergency management of, 186–188, *187*
    medical versus surgical management of, 188
    surgical therapy for, 189, *190, 191,* 191–194, *192, 193, 194, 195,*
        196
Urination. See Micturition.
Urine
    abnormal color of, 16–17
    abnormal output and voiding of, 5–15
    abnormalities with, 16–23
    acidification of
        in feline urethral obstruction, 123
    bacterial culture of, 42
    collection of, *20,* 20–22, *21, 22*
    concentration tests of, 42–43
    dipstick tests of, 40
    extravasation of, 158
    leakage of
        as complication after prostate surgery, 232–233
        as complication of urinary tract trauma, 197
    pH of, 40
    protein in, 40, 42
    sediment examination of, 40–41, *41, 42*
    specific gravity of
        in azotemia, 26–27
        test for, 39–40
Urography
    excretory (intravenous), 54–60, *55, 56,* 56t, *57, 58, 59, 60, 61*
Urolithiasis
    clinical signs of, 165
    definition of, 161
    diagnosis of, 166t, 166–167, 168t
    dysuria and, 11, 11t
    medical therapy for, 168–172, 169t, 171t
    pathophysiology of, 161–165
    postoperative management of, 182
    prevention of, 170–172, 171t
    surgical complications of, 182
    surgical therapy for, 174–181, *175, 176, 178, 179, 180*
Urolith(s)
    analysis of, 167
    calcium oxalate
        diagnosis of, 162t, 162–164, *163,* 166t
        prevention of, 171, 171t
    calcium phosphate
        diagnosis of, 164, 166t
        prevention of, 171t, 172
    cystine
        diagnosis of, *164,* 164–165, 166t
        medical dissolution of, 170
        prevention of, 171t, 172
    feline urethral obstruction and, 119, *121*
    prevention of, 170–172, 171t
    silica

diagnosis of, 165, 166t
    prevention of, 171t, 172
struvite
    diagnosis of, 162, *162,* 162t, *163,* 166t
    medical dissolution of, 168–169, 169t
    prevention of, 170–171, 171t
urate
    diagnosis of, 162t, 164, *165,* 166t
    medical dissolution of, 169–170
    prevention of, 171t, 172
Urologic surgery, 83t, 83–90, *84, 85, 86, 88*
    anesthesia in, 91–96
    general approaches to, 100–101, *101, 102, 103, 104, 105,* 105–106,
        106
    hemorrhage in, 108–109
    hypokalemia in, 109, 110t
    postoperative management of, 107–113, *110,* 110t, *111, 112, 113*
    preoperative management of, 97–99
    restraint devices for, *110, 111,* 111–112
    shock in, 109
    surgical instruments for, 84, *85*
    suture material for, 83t, 83–84, *84*
    urinary catheters in, 85–88, *86, 87*
Uroperitoneum
    emergency management of, *187,* 187–188
    in urinary tract trauma, 185

V
Vesicourachal diverticulum(a)
    diagnosis of, 203, *203*
    in feline urethral obstruction, 123–124
    postoperative complications of, 211
    surgical therapy for, 208, *208*
Vomiting
    control of, 97

W
Water
    intake of
        in feline urethral obstruction, 122–123
Water balance
    antidiuretic hormone and, 6, *6*
    in polyuria, 5–6, *6*
Water deprivation test, 43
    in polyuria/polydipsia, 8–9
Wound(s)
    dehiscence of
        as complication of perineal urethrostomy, 141–142
        in urologic surgery, 112. *112*
    healing of
        in urologic surgery, 107–108
    infections of
        in urologic surgery, 112